Praise for Karen
Eat Well Live Well with Th...

Those of us who are sensitive or intoleran[t]... crease and dealing with these dietary require... Lee has carried out lengthy, in depth research and The Sensitive Foodie will come as a godsend. Not only is it an informative point of reference but, with its delicious recipes and tips, it will appeal to other members of the family who are not affected in the same way.

Bryony Hill, author of *Grow Happy, Cook Happy, Be Happy*

This book is a gem! I have been following Professor George Jelinek's Overcoming MS diet and lifestyle programme since 2018 and was recommended Karen Lee's Eat Well, Live Well course later that same year. I find her personally inspirational and am delighted she has written this book which I hope will not only help other people with MS, but many others who want to adopt a healthy whole-food, plant-based diet.

I thoroughly recommend this book to anyone who is looking to understand the theory behind why there is a health need for us all to move towards a more whole-food, plant-based diet and for anyone who is also looking for practical help with great recipes to make that fresh start.

Dr Cathryn Stokes MPhil MRCGP FRSM

Growth requires change, and disease reversal requires a shift in consciousness. By following Karen's passionate journey and personal stories through the insightful chapters, anyone can connect the dots to a higher consciousness and a healthier lifestyle. What I particularly love in Karen's work is the large number of recipes that are tried and tested. If we can marry health with taste, what more do we need? Karen has also loaded the book with tips to help you with your health journey, recognising that it's not easy to change habits but once the habits are changed, they become a way of life.

Dr Nandita Shah, Founder and Director of SHARAN-India

HEALING FROM THE INSIDE OUT

Managing autoimmune disease with a whole-food plant-based diet

KAREN LEE

WITH A FOREWORD BY DR SHIREEN KASSAM

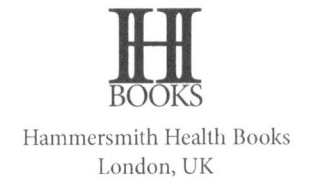

Hammersmith Health Books
London, UK

This first edition is published by Hammersmith Health Books – an imprint of Hammersmith Books Limited
82 Wandsworth Bridge Road, London SW6 2TF, UK
www.hammersmithbooks.co.uk

© 2026, Karen Lee

The right of Karen Lee has been asserted by her in accordance with the Copyright, Designs and Patents Act 1988.

All rights reserved. No part of this publication may be reproduced, stored in any retrieval system or transmitted in any form or by any means, electronic, mechanical, photocopying, recording or otherwise, without the prior permission of the publishers and copyright holder.

The information contained in this book is for educational purposes only. It is the result of the study and the experience of the author. Whilst the information and advice offered are believed to be true and accurate at the time of going to press, neither the author nor the publisher can accept any legal responsibility or liability for any errors or omissions that may have been made or for any adverse effects which may occur as a result of following the recommendations given herein. Always consult a qualified medical practitioner if you have any concerns regarding your health.

British Library Cataloguing in Publication Data: A CIP record of this book is available from the British Library.

Print ISBN 978-1-78161-258-3
Ebook ISBN 978-1-78161-259-0

Commissioning editor: Georgina Bentliff
Designed and typeset by: Julie Bennett, Bespoke Publishing Ltd
Cover design by: Madeline Meckiffe
Cover photograph: nadianb/shutterstock
Proof reading: Suzanne Elliott
Index: Dr Laurence Errington
Production: Anke Ueberberg
Printed and bound by: TJ Books, UK

Contents

Foreword by Dr Shireen Kassam	ix
Acknowledgements	xii
About the Author	xiv
Introduction	**1**
Chapter 1: What exactly is autoimmune disease?	
And why do I have it?	**13**
Introduction	13
Definition	13
Types of autoimmune disease	15
A snapshot of the immune system	17
What happens when the immune system goes rogue?	20
What causes autoimmune disease?	22
Don't despair – there is hope!	26
Chapter 2: Why gut health is so important	**29**
Introduction	29
Gut 101	29
The magical microbiome	32
So, what has the microbiome ever done for us…..?	33
What influences the make-up of a person's microbiome?	34
What is dysbiosis?	38
Summary	48

Chapter 3: Inflammatory foods — 49
   Introduction — 49
   Fat and saturated fat — 52
   Fats and gut health — 54
   Sugar — 57
   Salt — 60
   Dairy — 61
   Meat — 64
   Summary — 68

Chapter 4: What is a whole-food plant-based diet and why does it help? — 69
   Introduction — 69
   Why we need whole foods — 70
   A brief exploration of nutrient groups — 72
   Levels of processing and ultra-processed foods — 75
   Essential fibre — 78
   Healing nutrients — 84
   Polyphenols — 85
   Healthy fats — 87
   Summary — 90

Chapter 5: Starting your healing journey – Seven steps to healing from the inside out — 91
   Introduction — 91
   Step 1 – Eat more fresh vegetables and fruit — 92
   Step 2 – Eat healthy fats — 94
   Step 3 – Eat the rainbow — 96
   Step 4 – Variety — 99
   Step 5 – Minimally processed — 100
   Step 6 – Fill up with fibre — 102
   Step 7 – Feel empowered — 105

Chapter 6: But what about…? Myth busting — 107
   Introduction — 107
   Lectins — 110
   Oxalates — 112
   Nightshades — 113

Contents

Phytates	116
Gluten	117
But protein ... ?	119
'You must take lots of supplements'	122
Summary	123

Chapter 7: What am I actually going to eat? — **125**

Fruit	126
Berries	127
Other fruit	128
Vegetables	130
Cruciferous	130
Leafy greens	132
Roots and tubers	133
Bulbs and stems	135
'Fruit' vegetables	136
Fungi, algae and sea vegetables	137
Beans and lentils (legumes)	138
Grains	142
Nuts and seeds	144
Herbs and spices	145
Fermented foods	148
What about drinks?	150
Summary	151

Chapter 8: Final things to consider — **153**

Introduction	153
Go at your own pace	154
Learn new ways of cooking	155
Give your gut a break	157
Understand medications	161
Find your tribe (carefully)	163
Make a start – today!	165
Summary	167

The plant-based whole-food recipes   **169**
    Introduction to the recipes   173
    Three-day sample menu   175
    Breakfast   176
    Soups   188
    Salads   202
    Lunch or light meals   215
    Easy recipes   228
    Magnificent mains   243
    Baking   262
    Desserts   278
    Sauces and dressings   295
    Spreads and breads   304

Appendices   **317**
Appendix 1 – types of fibre   **318**
Appendix 2 – different groups of phytonutrients   **320**
Resources   **321**
References   **325**

Index   **339**

Foreword

By Dr Shireen Kassam

I am honoured to contribute the Foreword to this book by my friend and colleague, Karen Lee. Her work represents exactly the kind of practical, evidence-based guidance that is so urgently needed in today's healthcare service. Through her own lived experience of multiple sclerosis and her background as an intensive care nurse, Karen has combined personal insight with scientific understanding to create a resource that empowers others to take an active role in their health.

As a doctor, my professional life has been dedicated to improving the lives of people living with and beyond a diagnosis of cancer. I discovered the power of diet and lifestyle through my desire to better support my patients. Time and again, the evidence has shown that the choices we make in how we live, and particularly how we eat, are central to both preventing and managing diseases. Yet I am acutely aware of how difficult it can be for people to access information that is both scientifically robust and practically applicable. This is why Karen's book resonates so deeply with me.

Stories like Karen's are also the reason I was motivated to found Plant-Based Health Professionals UK, a non-profit dedicated to providing education on plant-based nutrition and lifestyle medicine. When I discovered the power of a whole-food plant-based diet, there was very little recognition of 'food as medicine' within medical education or the UK's National Health Service. This is slowly changing, but still not embedded into mainstream healthcare. As a result, we are missing out on one of the most powerful tools available to us for improving quality of life and our healthspan. Karen's story, and the evidence she brings together here, illustrate so clearly why this needs to change.

What is important to stress is that the knowledge in this book extends far beyond autoimmune disease. We do not need a different diet for each condition. A whole-food, plant-based diet supports all aspects of our physical and mental health. It reduces the risk of heart disease, type 2 diabetes, cancer, and dementia, while also helping to manage existing conditions more effectively. At the same time, it supports emotional wellbeing and resilience. This is because most chronic conditions share similar and overlapping mechanisms of disease development, such as chronic inflammation and an unhealthy gut microbiome. This unified, holistic approach to nutrition is one of the most empowering messages we can offer patients and the public alike.

Healing from the Inside Out succeeds in bringing together the latest evidence with lived experience, and presenting it in a way that is accessible, engaging, and profoundly hopeful. It offers readers not just theory, but concrete steps to take in their daily lives – steps that can make a tangible difference to health and wellbeing. At the same time, Karen never loses sight of the joy of food. The recipes are familiar yet imaginative, diverse and importantly nutritious and health promoting, proving that eating for health is not a sacrifice but a joy.

What I find particularly powerful about this book is its wider relevance. The adoption of a whole-food, plant-based diet not only promotes our personal health but also protects the health of our planet and our animal kin. As we face the twin crises of climate change and biodiversity loss, dietary change is one of the most impactful actions we can take as individuals. Karen's work aligns with my own ethical commitment to promoting human and planetary health in equal measure.

For me, this book is also a reminder that medicine is about more than prescriptions and procedures. It is about education, empowerment, and compassion. Karen embodies these qualities, offering readers a path that is grounded in science but illuminated by empathy and care.

Whether you are living with an autoimmune condition, supporting a loved one, or simply seeking to improve your health, *Healing from the Inside*

Out will guide, encourage and inspire you. It is a book to keep close at hand, to return to for advice, reassurance and, of course, delicious meals.

I wholeheartedly commend this book to you and am proud to stand beside Karen in championing this vital message: that healing is possible, that food is medicine, and that our choices can create a healthier, more compassionate world for us all.

Dr Shireen Kassam, Consultant Haematologist and Lifestyle Medicine Physician, Founder and Director of Plant-Based Health Professionals UK

Acknowledgements

It takes many people to create a published book – and time! I am blessed to have patient, supportive and sometimes long-suffering people in my life that have enabled my vision to come to fruition. Like the second album for musicians, the second book for an author can be a challenging task, especially when both managing a chronic health condition and life get in the way.

It's with this in mind that my upmost gratitude goes to my lovely husband Steve whose continued support, encouragement and sage advice have enabled me to complete this book. Listening to my moans, groans and episodes of self-doubt requires resilience, gracious love and episodes of selective deafness! And a big shout out to the rest of my wonderful little family, particularly my children Vicky and Ben who have grown into amazing young adults who make me proud every day.

I also have much gratitude for my lovely mum, Betty, who was so proud of my first book and most excited about this second one. Sadly, she passed away whilst I was in the process of writing it, so she'll not have the chance to tell everyone about her daughter, the writer. I feel she would have enjoyed reading it, though – she certainly enjoyed the cake recipes I made her.

A huge thank you goes out to my wonderful co-stars Rosa, Kate and Tricia, who allowed me to grill them about how their whole-food plant-based diet had made a difference to their symptoms (and life), then allowing me to share their nuggets of wisdom in this book. Each of their

Acknowledgements

stories is so inspiring and I'm so happy they allowed me to share this with a wider audience.

More thanks go to my lovely friend Maureen Gooding who took on the much needed role of first reader/sense checker. As a retired English teacher who found my grammar most annoying at times, and someone without health training or autoimmune disease, her encouragement and helpful feedback on readability and engagement were gratefully received.

I can't miss out a mention for Professor George Jelinek and everyone at Overcoming MS. The programme was a light in dark times, and I will be forever grateful to my colleague and friend Louise Seymour who unknowingly introduced me to it before I knew I needed it. The universe always provides, and in Overcoming MS it's not only provided incredible, accessible resources and community, but an opportunity to give back and support others.

A big thank you goes to Dr Shireen Kassam, not only for writing a lovely Foreword, but for also introducing me to Georgina Bentliff of Hammersmith Health Books. And my final thanks go to Georgina, for taking me on as a writer in the first place and believing that I could create something worth publishing! I hope it does you proud.

About the Author

Karen Lee (aka 'the Sensitive Foodie') is a qualified nutritionist and former intensive care nurse who has a passion for amazingly tasty food that's also great for health. Since receiving a diagnosis of multiple sclerosis in 2016, she has used diet and lifestyle to manage her condition and shares this knowledge with others through her website – The Sensitive Foodie Kitchen – as well as workshops, talks and online classes. She published her first book, *Eat Well Live Well with The Sensitive Foodie*, in 2019. She is a facilitator for the charity Overcoming MS which provides an accessible lifestyle medicine programme that supports people with MS. She also teaches medical students how to cook plant-based meals as part of the Cooking for the Climate module offered by Plant-Based Health Professionals UK and additionally works as their Events Manager, organising their nutrition and lifestyle medicine conferences. Karen lives in rural Devon with her husband and has two adult children.

Introduction

There's no getting away from it; having a life-long condition is pants. Being diagnosed with an autoimmune condition means your life has changed for good. That moment the doctor delivers the words 'you have…' (fill in the gap with your condition of non-choice) is never forgotten.

I was fortunate. My diagnosis was delivered in a clear, professional and kind way (as opposed to other horror stories I've heard) but it's a traumatic memory that stays with me still. It turns out, I'm great at denial. I so wanted there to be nothing wrong that reality crashed into my life as a most unwanted guest. Instead of listening to my consultant's explanation, my mind flipped into panic mode whilst an express train of emotion thundered through my head. All I could do was say the f-word repeatedly. Eventually my lovely husband told me to stop; he couldn't hear what the doctor was saying. One of us needed to listen. Or at least he did, because at that point I thought I knew what my new future was going to be.

It's often said that nurses are the worst patients. And from experience, I'd say that's true. Exposed to our patients' challenges, fears and individual peculiarities day in, day out, helps form a unique perspective on health, disease and what it is to be 'a patient'. We're used to telling others what to do and hate being told. Having seen all possibilities on the spectrum of 'sick', nurses tend to dismiss their own issues as not that bad because we've always seen worse. Especially when your work is in intensive care, looking after the sickest of the sick, dealing with potentially life-changing decisions every day, sometimes every moment. Even more so when you have worked in the speciality your diagnosis now comes under – neuroscience. This is why I was in so much denial. I couldn't be a patient, surely?

I have multiple sclerosis (MS), a long-term condition that affects the central nervous system and one of over 100 identified autoimmune conditions. In MS, the immune system attacks myelin, a fatty sheath covering nerves in the brain and spinal cord. Myelin protects nerves from heat, cold and damage but also enables impulses to travel super-fast to enable messages to reach their destination. Things like 'lift your hand from the flame' or 'this what you see' or 'you need a wee right now'. Once myelin is damaged and broken down, it can't be repaired, or not yet anyway. After the inflammatory episode passes, the damage left behind shows as scarring or white patches on MRI scans. These are 'sclerosis'. The 'multiple' part is when this scarring shows up in more than one place.

MS is considered an organ-specific autoimmune condition – the attacks happen in the central nervous system (CNS). The effects, however, can show up anywhere, as the CNS controls how the body functions. For me, it showed up as optic neuritis, acute inflammation of the optic nerve, a common first symptom of MS. It started as acute pain in my right eye that increased over a week. Then blurred vision, but in patches, followed by a strange white mesh effect. The day after this appeared, I lost all vision in that eye. It was most discombobulating.

After attending A&E at the eye hospital, I saw a lovely ophthalmic neurologist who undertook various tests to explore what was going on. Fortunately, the pain eased, and my sight returned over a few months. I was fine, right? But then pain started in my left eye, followed by blurring, but fortunately no sight loss. Then numbness in my left arm, next my left leg. When I started to drop things at work (not patients!) I acknowledged something was wrong but put it down to doing too much. I was working in ITU, running my business, The Sensitive Foodie, and had teenagers at home. I could not consider the possibility that something functional and potentially serious was going on.

Fortunately, my neurologist did and referred me to a specialist. I reluctantly endured a lumbar puncture (as horrendous as I thought it would be) and a selection of other tests. By the time we were sitting in

Introduction

the consultant's office for the results, all my symptoms had passed which supported my internal narrative that everything was fine. But of course, that's the nature of many autoimmune conditions – they flare up then calm down again, which is called 'remission'.

In the immediate days following my diagnosis, I went through an acute grieving process. There were many tears. I was so angry – with myself and my stupid body. I was full of fear and found myself in the lowest place I've been. I could no longer deny what was going on, even though I desperately wanted to. My anger turned to belligerence – I was not going to be beaten by this; I was not going to be a 'patient' but my own person. And to do that I needed additional knowledge. I already knew what MS was and how it could progress. What I needed was information on how to manage it and hopefully stop it getting worse. Fortunately, a colleague had told me about Overcoming MS (see Resources, page 321), an evidence-based diet and lifestyle programme that helped people with MS live well.

Being a patient
We all get ill. It's a fact. There's no shame in it. At times, you need to hand your power over to the medical professionals; they save lives. At some point, though, that power needs to be taken back, or at least to have shared custody. I've met too many people with long-term conditions who had no understanding about their health or medications. You don't need to be a medical professional, or even well educated, to have a basic grasp of how the body works or what happens when it goes wrong, as long as you have someone willing to explain it in an accessible way. Patients may feel disempowered, and reluctant to ask questions that might help them understand their condition, because they feel either that the doctor is too busy or that they've been dismissed or intimidated. They want to be a 'good patient' and not make a fuss. And maybe that's why nurses make such difficult patients – we know what to ask and are not afraid to do so! Information is power. Or rather, sound, practical and evidence-based information is empowering. It enables you to become an equal partner in your health, maybe even the boss. It also gives you hope. And optimism. Which is key to healing and living well.

As an ITU nurse, one of the things I appreciated about the highly regarded book *Overcoming Multiple Sclerosis* was the amount of research behind it. Authored by Professor George Jelinek, a now retired Professor of Emergency Medicine who has MS himself, it contains hundreds of references about diet, exercise, stress management and vitamin D, and their impact on MS.[1] Medications have a role, but Professor Jelinek realised that lifestyle changes were just as effective and gave control back to patients.

The main themes of the book run along the same lines as the pillars of lifestyle medicine that are becoming more mainstream in modern medicine. Here's a quick summary of the programme:

- An anti-inflammatory diet packed with nutrient-dense whole foods
- Supplementation of omega-3 fatty acids (cold-pressed flaxseed oil)
- Vitamin D supplementation as well as getting outdoors
- Exercise for overall health as well as brain health
- Using meditation and mindfulness techniques to reduce stress, improve sleep and promote brain plasticity
- Taking medications if needed
- Encouraging family members to live healthy lifestyles
- Making changes that work for life.

You may look at this and think 'well, that's not rocket science!' And you'd be right. But it is science-backed and implementable, if we choose to do so. It's a recipe for healthy life for everyone.

It's coming up to 10 years since my diagnosis of MS, an 'interesting' period of my life. Things have changed a lot. I am fortunate to have a supportive family and a husband who is willing to come on this wild journey with me. I have met some amazing people and learnt even more about just how amazing our bodies are – how, given the right tools and environment, we're programmed to heal, to live well in spite of all the things we throw at ourselves . We are a marvel.

Our innate ability to heal makes autoimmune disease an odd one. Why does a system designed to protect (the immune system) go into overdrive and become so confused it starts to attack 'self'? The answer to that is complicated and, in some ways, still unclear. As we will explore in Chapter

Introduction

1, there is no one single cause of autoimmunity. Rather there are multiple factors that build up over time until the body becomes overwhelmed and starts to fight against itself.

After my diagnosis with MS, I had a powerful sense of failure. What had I done so wrong it resulted in this? I should know better. I was at fault.

These feelings are completely normal, part of waking up to a life you didn't plan for, but essentially a waste of energy. Autoimmune disease is unbelievably exhausting enough (ask anyone with fatigue). You don't have any spare energy to waste! Playing the blame game doesn't help.

Instead, let your diagnosis be the spur to seeking solutions. What can be done to deal with this issue? If you are in an acute phase of the disease, your immediate options are limited, especially if you're hospitalised. The best thing you can 'do' at this time is become well enough to get home. Mindset is super-important during this time. Belief that you can and will get well, that you can and will be able to start on a holistic healing journey; that you can and will have a great life despite setbacks, is itself strong medicine. During my nursing career I have seen patients achieve the most incredible outcomes. With a burning desire and dogged determination, anything is possible.

Whilst there are many lifestyle changes to make, this book focuses on just one - food. I believe that eating 'well' is the cornerstone of health. Food is an established part of everyday life, an activity that's familiar and practical to adjust without too much upheaval. We eat, on average, three times a day, each an opportunity to support our bodies – or not.

Whilst food is essential for life, it can also harm. This is becoming increasingly apparent in the Western world with chronic health conditions, not just autoimmune disease, burgeoning alongside a food industry promoting cheap products with low quality nutrition and practically devoid of fibre. This will be explored in Chapters 2 and 3. Western medicine is still focused on trauma and infection, the major causes of death for thousands of years. Chronic health problems are approached in the same way – identify a single issue and deal with it rather than look at the person as a whole. Medical breakthroughs like antibiotics and vaccines alongside changes in lifestyle and relatively safer societies have reduced acute dangers to human health. However, our internal survival systems, developed over thousands of years, are being hacked by modern day behaviours like smoking, excess alcohol, nutrient-deficient food, sedentary jobs, ongoing stress and poor sleep. Long-term, chronic health conditions now account for 75% of all deaths worldwide,[2] higher in developed countries like the UK, US and the EU. Autoimmune conditions affect 10% of the Western population.[3] Long-term diseases are expensive and not just financially. They cost quality of life, society and lost potential.

That all sounds rather depressing. But it doesn't have to be as the cause of these issues can also be the solution. If the way we live is making us sick, why not change it so we can heal and live well again? If lifestyle is the underlying cause, why not make it the solution instead? Modern medicine can still play a part, just not the only one. When I started nursing back in the 1980s, there were no treatments for MS; you were just told to get on with it as best you could. Now there are multiple options that can slow the rate of disability and progression. Which is great news, but not the ultimate solution. That's when we come back to lifestyle, to finding out what you – what I – can do to live well with a chronic health condition. Or, even better, to prevent it from developing in the first place.

Lifestyle medicine must be the way forward in healthcare, a holistic approach instead of symptom management. This 'new' way of caring for patients in a holistic manner isn't rocket science though. Medicine has dived down into the microcosm of the human body and now we need to zoom back out and look at the macrocosm – the body as a whole, as well as its environment. The food we eat is a key part of that process, which for most people eating a Western diet pattern (low fibre, low veg and fruit; high meat, dairy and processed food) means a radical shift. But how do you make that dietary choice?

Unless you're single, have no family or friends and never go out, your food choices are always going to be influenced by the people around you. Making changes that are good for you have a ripple effect on the people closest to you as well as your social circle. This can be positive, but

Introduction

problematic. Making changes is hard. We like the easy options so, *how* do you know you are making the right choices for you? Especially when you're bombarded with multiple conflicting opinions.

The seven-step decision-making tool below may help. I believe all of the questions listed are important when you're making changes for health. Come back to these as you read the rest of this book to see if my suggestions fit these criteria.

We have a choice how to live our lives. I choose to live in a way that supports my health as well as the health of animals and Mother Earth. It's a win-win in my (admittedly rather dodgy) eyes. I choose to eat healthful plant foods that my body loves as much as my tastebuds. Being diagnosed with MS was a dark time, but I choose to see the light, to live as well as I can. And that's what I aim to share with you so you too can gain health for yourself, and the world around you.

I'm not alone in this journey to health with food, which is why you'll find three other voices dotted throughout the book, sharing their own inspiring stories of using a whole-food plant-based diet to manage autoimmune disease. Here's a quick introduction to these wonderful women, Rosa, Kate and Tricia.

Meet Rosa: Swollen, painful wrists sent Rosa to the doctor in 2018. Expecting to find out she had a joint problem, she was surprised, and devastated, to discover she had granulomas on her lungs and a diagnosis of sarcoidosis at the age of just 29. With the support of her family, Rosa changed from a meat-heavy diet to a vegan diet, then to a whole-food plant-based diet. Six months later, scans showed all the granulomas had gone – she was in remission. What amazing news! Heeding the warning she could relapse, Rosa continued with her whole-food plant-based diet, finding she had more energy and less cog-fog. In 2024, her consultant gave her the best news: her sarcoidosis was unlikely to return. With a physical job as a gardener, Rosa's fibromyalgia, cog-fog and energy have all improved over time. Now the whole family eat a whole-food plant-based diet and feel they are thriving.

SEVEN STEPS IN ASSESSING NUTRITIONAL ADVICE

1

IS IT EVIDENCE-BASED?

Whilst many influencers or gurus like to dismiss the experts, it's so important to look at the science. Particularly independent research that is not overtly, or covertly, influenced by the food industry. If you're not sure, look it up. Be curious. It's easy to find yourself in an echo chamber so independent verification is important.

2

IS IT ADAPTABLE?

Can you make it work for your everyday life? How much will it interfere with your family choices or social life? Can you eat like this at work? What about your favourite dishes – are there similar alternatives? Is it accessible for you – can you easily get your hands on fresh produce, for example?

3

IS IT AFFORDABLE?

If your budget is limited, what impact will changes have on your finances? Some health protocols include expensive ingredients or a range of pricey supplements. Can you afford it?

4

IS IT SUSTAINABLE?

A diagnosis of an autoimmune condition stays with you for life. Any beneficial changes need to be for the long, not short, term. Does the dietary pattern fit with that? Weight loss diets, for example, particularly extreme ones, that are followed for short-term benefit, see people piling on the pounds again when they return to their 'normal' way of eating. A restrictive programme like drinking only raw smoothies may work in the short term, but can you see yourself doing this forever? Long-term health requires long-term action.

Introduction

5

IS IT ENJOYABLE?

We eat three times a day. Will you enjoy eating this way all the time? If you hate all vegetables, fruit and beans, then a whole-food plant-based diet may not be the right choice for you. Or at least not at the start. Change doesn't have to be all or nothing from Day 1. If you allow yourself time and an open mind, you might be surprised by what you enjoy. I have worked with many people who couldn't imagine never eating meat or cheese again who are now repulsed by the thought of it.

6

DOES IT FIT WITH YOUR PERSONAL ETHICS?

Our choices affect the world around us and we all have a role to play in caring for it. The continual increase in demand for meat, for example, is having a detrimental effect on our climate, creating huge amounts of greenhouse gases and resource use, not to mention the exploitation of farmed animals and the loss of wild animals and ecosystems.

7

DOES IT WORK?

For you as an individual, this is the most important question of all. Does it improve your symptoms like pain and swelling? Can you get into remission – and stay there? Do you feel well? Or less fatigued? It's possible you may not feel brilliant for the first few days as your body adapts to your new way of eating. Maybe weeks. It takes time to adapt your tastebuds and reduce cravings. Give it time to work – after all, it's taken you years to get to this point of disease! You may need support from a nutritionist for a while if it's too challenging. If, after all this, you don't feel any benefits, then of course feel free to move on. Everyone is different. Do give it a good go, though, as you may well be surprised by what you find.

Meet Kate: Aged 40, Kate found herself bed-bound in constant pain wondering, if this was her life for the next 20 years, was it worth it? Recently diagnosed with psoriatic arthritis (even though psoriasis was not an issue then), Kate's body was swollen and painful and her days were spent sleeping in bed, unable to care for her young children. With steroids and medication, things slowly started to improve but she noticed the pain and swelling became worse after eating certain foods. Her rheumatologist suggested an elimination diet; this is when Kate discovered she reacted to red meat, bacon, cheese and eggs. After swapping to a vegan diet for ethical reasons 19 years ago, she felt her body improving so she could live her life once more. Although she managed to halve her medication, any lower triggered a flare up. Processed vegan foods and saturated fats still featured in her diet but a chance meeting in 2017 with a fellow runner led to another transformation – to a whole-food plant-based diet. Her body really started to heal and slowly she could reduce her medication without any side effects. Today, aged 62, she is medication- and pain-free and full of energy, able to run ultra-marathons!

Meet Tricia: Tricia's GP acted swiftly after she went to see her with severe abdominal pain and altered bowel habits in 2018. An urgent colonoscopy revealed a lower colon covered in multiple ulcers – well established Crohn's disease. Having suffered from intermittent bloating and pain for many years, it was still a shock. Tricia had changed to a vegan diet the year before so thought she was eating well. A delay in seeing a consultant gastroenterologist gave her time to explore dietary changes she could make, including a low-fibre diet, and she started to feel improvements. She was told medications would be necessary for the rest of her life, but these made her symptoms flare, so she decided to focus on diet and lifestyle. Over time, she slowly improved, gradually increasing the amount and range of plant foods that were increasingly whole. Seven years post-diagnosis, Tricia feels like her diagnosis of Crohn's disease wasn't real, even though she saw the ulcers on her colon lining. Now aged 74, she feels her gut health has transformed and she's truly living well.

So, now you know you can change the world as well as your health, it's time to assume the superman/woman pose and get going. Anyone fancy a spot of lunch first, though?

Notes on how to use this book

The first half of this book explores important issues around autoimmune disease, including what it is, what happens and the importance of gut health. Next we look at different types of food that promote or reduce inflammation before busting some myths about specific foods and autoimmune disease. Finally, we dive into the best whole plant foods to eat and address certain issues regarding making changes. The second half contains 100 tasty recipes for you to try, along with some guidance on how to use them and a suggested three-day meal plan.

Feel free to use this information however you want. Read through the whole first half or dip in and out – it's up to you. Or dive straight into the recipes and just start eating great food. The most important thing is to use it in a way that works for you, whether it's an overnight change or a slow transformation. Listen to your body, note the changes and let your tastebuds and microbiome enjoy the ride.

If you take certain medications, please do check the section on this in Chapter 8. In addition, if you have any food intolerances (common in most people with an inflamed, leaky gut), you may wish to continue to avoid these foods in the short term. As your gut heals, you should be able to start introducing them once more. Food intolerances and sensitivities are complicated and sometimes hard to identify using an elimination diet (the official recommendation). If this is an area you would like to explore, there is a whole section about this on my website (see Resources, page 321).

Chapter 1

What exactly is autoimmune disease? And why do I have it?

Introduction

If you're reading this, I'm assuming you have been diagnosed with an autoimmune disease or have been unwell and are waiting for a diagnosis. Alternatively, you may have a family member with one or two autoimmune conditions and know you are at risk of developing one. It's better to know what you are dealing with, because then, you can start doing something about it.

In this chapter, I am going to look at the official definition of autoimmune disease, explore the different types of autoimmune conditions, the risk factors and potential causes and what is going on inside that triggers a flare. This requires a certain amount of low-level physiology. I'll keep the medical jargon to a minimum though, as well as offer the option for more information if you're up for it. For now, let's have a quick look at what autoimmune disease is.

Definition

As far as we know today, autoimmune disease develops when the immune system (our internal defence) becomes confused, mistakenly identifying healthy cells and tissues for foreign, attacking them as they would any invader. If this continues, the sustained attack causes damage and results in an autoimmune disease.[1]

Currently, there are around 100 officially identified autoimmune conditions.[2] Some are familiar names like lupus, rheumatoid arthritis, coeliac disease and multiple sclerosis. Others are less well known, such as Evan's syndrome, Goodpasture's syndrome and linear IgA disease. Individually, these life-altering conditions affect fewer people than heart disease or cancer. Grouped together, however, autoimmune disease is huge and affects people of all ages. Some treatments are available but often come with nasty side effects and impact normal life.

A study from 2023 revealed that 10% of the UK population has one or more autoimmune conditions.[3] That's approximately 6.7 million people. In the US, it's around 50 million people. To put that in perspective, in the UK there are 7.6 million people with heart disease and 4.6 million with diabetes. There are major preventative and treatment programmes in place for those conditions. But not for autoimmune disease. Maybe that's because the root causes are not well understood. Or that it's not recognised as a collective. But as 75% of people with autoimmune conditions are women, it could also be it's just been overlooked. It's just as important and serious as the better known conditions; it's a leading cause of death in women under 75 in both the UK[4] and the US.[5]

Autoimmune disease affects all ages, but many are diagnosed when people are in their 20s, 30s and 40s. This can have a huge impact on careers, income and family responsibilities and dynamics, as well as the potential for years of medical intervention. These all come with a huge cost – financial, emotional, social and psychological. People with autoimmune disease are at increased risk of other chronic health conditions too.[6] Many chronic health conditions, like type 2 diabetes, heart disease and cancer, have the same key feature as autoimmune disease – chronic low-level inflammation. If you have one or more autoimmune diseases, you also have an increased risk of mental health conditions like depression and anxiety.[7]

A well-functioning immune system will identify a harmful substance (an antigen) like a virus, bacterium, cancer cell or toxin, forming proteins called antibodies that protect the body if the antigen appears again. With autoimmune disease, this goes awry, and some antibodies fail to tell the difference between healthy and dangerous cells. Instead, these antibodies start to attack normal cells, which causes damage, sometimes permanently.

So now we have a definition of autoimmunity, let's have a look at the different types of autoimmune condition before diving into a bit more detail about what's going on in the immune system.

Types of autoimmune disease

I've already mentioned there are over 100 different autoimmune diseases – but don't worry, I'm not going to list them all here! If you're interested, I've added a link to a comprehensive list in the Resources section. Whilst each one is different, they tend to fall into two groups – organ specific and systemic (or non-organ specific).

In organ-specific conditions, only one organ is attacked, but the effects may be experienced throughout the body. For example, in multiple sclerosis, the direct damage is in the brain and central nervous system but the effects manifest throughout the body as the signalling for organ function is impacted.

In systemic or non-organ-specific conditions, multiple organs or tissues can be attacked at the same time. Conditions like rheumatoid arthritis affect one or more joints. Systemic lupus erythematosus (SLE or 'lupus') can affect different organs at the same time like the skin, joints, kidneys, brain and even blood cells.

Some conditions are tricky and fall between the two categories, and you can have more than one autoimmune disease affecting different parts of the body.

The effect on organs and tissues from autoimmunity varies with each condition, ranging from destruction of specific cells or tissues, promotion of excess organ growth or interfering with normal function and operation. Many conditions affect parts of the body involved with sending signals that control and maintain essential functions, like the thyroid gland, pancreas or adrenal glands. Other conditions have a major impact on connective tissues, muscles and joints. It's all very inconvenient!

Each condition has its own set of signs and symptoms. However, many are common between all and can include crippling fatigue, chronic pain, flu-like symptoms or low-grade fever, changes in skin or mucous membranes and generally feeling pretty rough but without knowing why.

Unfortunately, autoimmune conditions are renowned for being difficult to diagnose. The symptoms can often be a ragbag collection ranging from odd sensations to rashes to complete loss of function. Unless you present with a classic symptom of a specific condition, like sight loss (optic neuritis), specific skin lesions (in psoriasis) or even an acute crisis resulting in an emergency admission, it can be hard to pin down a diagnosis or even to get a doctor to take you seriously. In my experience, medical staff are reluctant to start with a life-changing diagnosis. A good thing really, otherwise anyone with pins and needles or a random rash could undergo stress, and even treatments, they don't need. However, when you are the person struggling to get someone to take you seriously, it can be supremely frustrating and stressful.

Interestingly, receiving a diagnosis is a huge relief for many people. The imagination can take you to some dark places; the actual problem is not always as bad as they thought it might be. A diagnosis can be the start of moving towards some form of recovery. For others though, it can be devastating. Many people need to go through the grieving process to come to terms with the news. I certainly did. In just a moment, your future changes; the unknown is frightening. I believe the first two years after diagnosis are the most stressful for most people, which is unfortunate as stress aggravates autoimmune disease. However, taking positive action and regaining some control are key steps in turning things around. In many cases, all is not lost, just different.

> **Rosa's story:** Finding her diagnosis overwhelming, Rosa had a difficult time after being diagnosed with sarcoidosis at such a young age (29), and had dark thoughts and anxiety about what her future might hold. Getting the right support was crucial, and today both her mental and physical health have improved.

Chapter 1

A snapshot of the immune system

Human beings are so complex. We have evolved into intelligent, resilient and adaptable beings over millions of years. To survive the dangers and challenges we all face every day, our bodies developed intricate processes and systems for protection that enable us to survive and thrive.

To protect us from the dangers of the outside world, our skin and gastrointestinal tract (GIT) provide secure barriers that, when intact, keep our internal 'world' safe. If an unwanted 'invader' breaks through either of these, the immune system, a complex, multifaceted network of cells, tissues and organs, is on hand to rapidly identify, secure and destroy it. This network is split into two parts – innate immunity and learned (or adaptive) immunity. Both work in partnership but have different functions.

The innate immune system

We are born with innate immunity. It's our first line of defence against any micro-organisms or foreign substances that enter the body. It's response is rapid, and we wouldn't survive without it. If an invader gets past the protective skin or GIT, the innate immune system kicks off by releasing a cascade of different types of white blood cells, all with a specialised role. Chemicals are released to dilate tiny portals in blood vessels so larger killer cells can enter and deal with the problem. Scavenger cells (phagocytes) are also released – these surround the foreign body and start to break them down. This increased leakiness and influx of immune cells causes the area to become red and inflamed. There may be pain too. You will have seen the localised effect of this process on a cut hand or grazed knee. It's become red hot and swollen and often leaks gross yellowy/green pus which eventually dries up and heals. That's your innate immune system doing its job rather marvellously.

If a bacterium or virus gets into the body's system, this process kicks in on a much larger scale. This is what makes you feel poorly with a fever, aches and pains and maybe a headache. Your energy drops and all you want to do is sleep. These are the signs of acute inflammation. On the inside, your body is working hard to deal with the issue. Blood vessels become leaky all over the body to enable scavenger cells to reach the bacterium or virus that's attempting to make a home where it's not welcome. Your body temperature rises to create a hostile environment the invader can't thrive in. Next come the natural killer (NK) cells. These guys identify cells or tissues that have been invaded by a virus or other pathogen and secrete toxins to destroy them before too much damage is done.

Specialist compounds activate each phase of this immune cascade to enable such a swift response to danger. Once the job is complete and the area is safe and secure, messages are released to tell these guards to stand down. Turning the immune response and associated inflammation off is as important as switching it on – it's an energy- and resource-heavy process.

Is the innate immune system involved in autoimmune disease? It certainly is. But not alone. The learned (adaptive) system is just as involved, if not more.

The learned (adaptive) immune system

So, what is the learned immune system? As we are surrounded by potential threats to survival, humans (and many other animals) evolved a secondary immune system which develops after birth. After an invader, or antigen, enters the body, this part of the immune system learns to identify it as friend or foe so it can recognise it again in the future. Specialised proteins called antibodies are formed for each antigen – we'll come back to these shortly. This system allows the compounds we need, like nutrients, into the body without too much drama but responds appropriately to danger. It enables us to adapt to our environment; hence it's also called the adaptive immune system.

The learned immune system takes a little longer to work than the innate as it needs to identify the target and create the right 'tag' to destroy or tolerate it. Antibodies should only attach to an antigen if it's a precise match, like a lock and key. This enables the immune system to target specific cells on subsequent attacks instead of triggering a full-body response. You may just feel a little under the weather or may not know there's even been a problem.

This is the basis of immunisation; giving the body a low or inactive dose of a bacterium or virus that enables your body to recognise and learn how to overcome it. It's clever stuff.

The learned immune system includes specific types of white blood cell (or lymphocytes) secreted from the thymus gland, called T cells and B cells, made in the bone marrow. B cells produce antibodies, also known as immunoglobulins (because having one name is just too simple!). All three elements – T cells, B cells and antibodies – have their own specialist roles but also work together as a team alongside the innate immune system. This creates a strong and resilient defence squad. They communicate by direct activation or via tiny messenger proteins called cytokines. You may be familiar with the term 'cytokine cascade' from the Covid-19 pandemic, referring to critically ill patients overwhelmed by the virus and subsequent immune response. Fortunately, this extreme reaction is rare; most of the time, cytokines are carrying their messages in a calm and controlled manner, to keep everything ticking along just as it's needed.

How does the immune system separate 'us' from 'them'?

You may be wondering how the immune system differentiates between your own cells and an antigen. Molecules on the surface of the cell is the answer. Antigens have different molecules on their surface compared to those found naturally in the body. Hence, when the invader enters the body, the immune system is immediately alerted and gets to work. Antibodies are made in huge amounts and are located throughout the body, including in the skin, lungs, tear ducts and saliva. They're also found in breast milk; these help kick-start the immune system from birth.

Antibodies are key to keeping us safe from a multitude of antigens that might do us harm. However, they can turn rogue and start attacking host cells instead, becoming 'autoantibodies'. This is not always a bad thing, though. Autoantibodies clean up oxidised (damaged) proteins and fats as well as dead cells and general waste that needs clearing out. Unfortunately, the immune system sometimes gets confused and starts to produce excess amounts of autoantibodies that attack a specific organ or system. That's when autoimmune disease occurs.

There are too many elements of the incredible immune system to explore here so I'm going to leave it at this very low-level explanation. If you are curious and want to know more about the immune cascade, cell roles and what immunoglobulins do, you'll find plenty more information on the website for this book.

For now, though, let's have a look what is going on in the immune system to create enough havoc for the body to turn on itself.

What happens when the immune system goes rogue?

My low-level description of the immune system may make it look simple, but it's not! Multiple processes are constantly in action, working to keep our bodies safe. All systems in the body have evolved to work best within an often narrowly defined equilibrium. This is how we stay 'well'. However, sometimes things go awry. And when it comes to autoimmune disease, it can have a huge impact.

We've just seen that a controlled amount of autoimmunity is part of the body's waste disposal system. If the messages to stop are not released or can't get through, the self-antigens mistakenly identify healthy, normal tissues as damaged and start to break them down for disposal. This continues until the message to stop is received and can cause huge damage in the body. This is now autoimmune disease as shown opposite.

One way the immune system stops recognising 'self' cells and treating them as 'non-self' is thought to be due to molecular mimicry. This occurs when an antigen has a similar molecular structure to a 'self' protein. This could be a virus, bacterium or even a protein in food. Once the antigen enters the body, the immune system revs up to prevent it from creating harm. Both the innate and learned immune systems are involved, creating a full inflammatory response. In a sustained period of pro-inflammatory activity, confusion may arise, and the 'self'-cells are mistaken for the antigen and attacked. This then is molecular mimicry – invading molecules that have a similar structure to certain 'self' cells triggering an immune response to both, leading to damage in the tissues or organs where these cells are located.

Chapter 1

WHAT HAPPENS IN AUTOIMMUNE DISEASE?

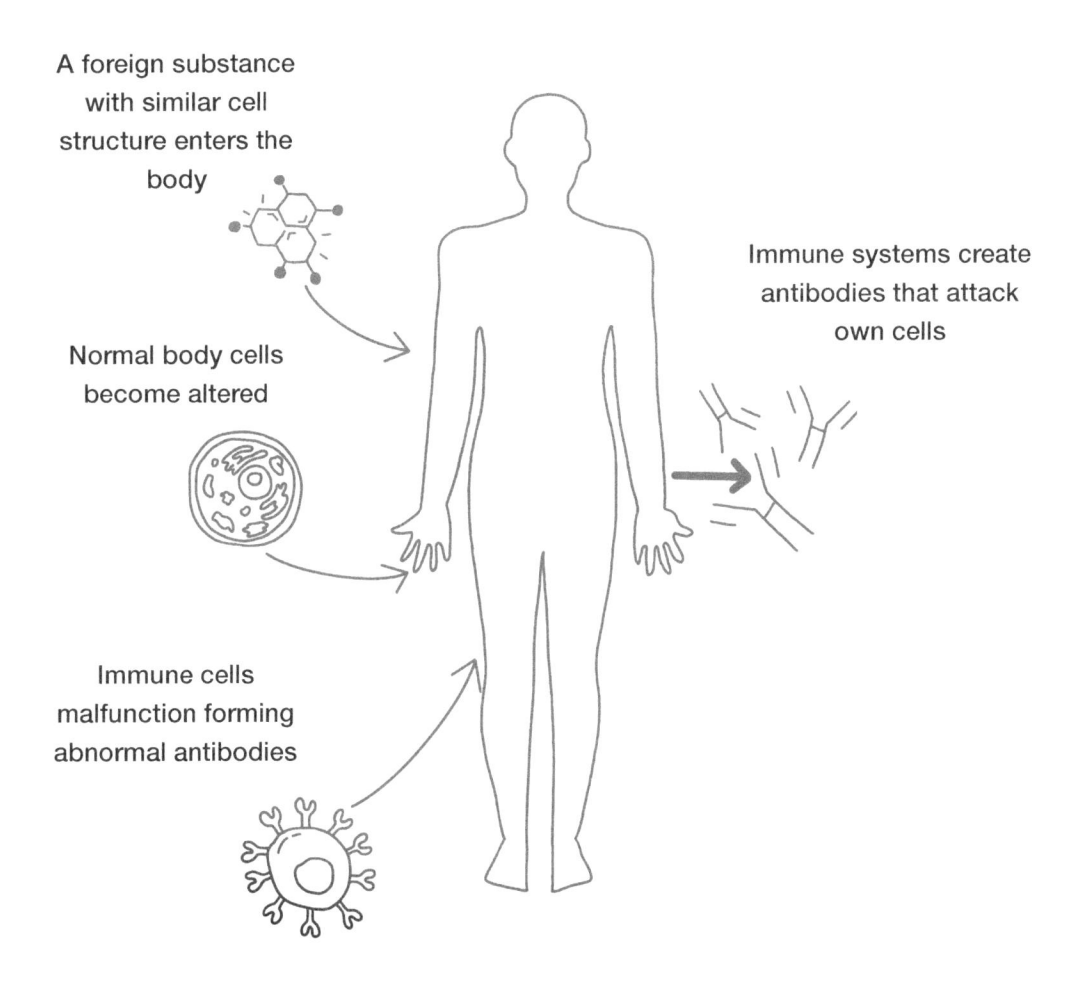

A foreign substance with similar cell structure enters the body

Normal body cells become altered

Immune systems create antibodies that attack own cells

Immune cells malfunction forming abnormal antibodies

Molecular mimicry has been identified as being a key player in many autoimmune diseases, including type 1 diabetes where insulin-secreting cells are destroyed, arthritic conditions like psoriatic arthritis where joint tissue is attacked, lupus which affects multiple organs, rheumatoid arthritis causing chronically inflamed synovial tissue around the joints and multiple sclerosis through the destruction of the myelin sheath that protects nerves.[8]

Another way things get out of control is through 'bystander activation'.[9]

This happens when T cells are activated *without* the presence of an antigen. This can occur during an inflammatory response to a pathogen. Messenger cytokines that activate the immune response mistakenly activate self-antigens, triggering an autoimmune response.

By now I'm sure you're wondering what causes all this confusion. Let's explore some causes and risk factors connected to autoimmune disease.

What causes autoimmune disease?

I wish I could give you a clear answer to this, but I can't. Much remains to be learnt about the root causes of autoimmunity and sadly a *single* cause has yet to be pinned down. For most people, there's a multiplicity of factors, some within and some outside of an individual's control, building up over time until the perfect storm hits. There may be no warning and problems appear almost overnight. Alternatively, a random collection of symptoms may be smouldering away in the background. It could be a rash here or a pain there, a sore joint or intermittent headaches – everyday grumbles that everyone gets. Except one day the body's amazing ability to adapt and cope with these inflammatory insults is overwhelmed, resulting a crisis with symptoms that can no longer be ignored.

This is what happened to me as you saw in the introduction (page 13). And it's a story I hear time after time from others. So, what nefarious factors are pushing our immune systems so far they start to bite back?

- **Genetics** – Some conditions, like MS and lupus, can run in families, but not always. Having a close relative with the condition increases your risk of developing it too. Sometimes it's autoimmunity itself that runs in the family rather than a specific condition. You could have three sisters with three different conditions. However, just because families share these genes, it's not inevitable that everyone will develop autoimmunity. These genes must be switched on to have an impact. Gene sequencing for autoimmune conditions has identified multiple genes as potential problems. You can still have the genes even if no one else in your family has become ill. The positive take-home is that, even if you carry autoimmune genes, they don't have to be switched on. There are lots of lifestyle tweaks that can be done – including diet – to keep these genes tucked away where they can't get up to mischief.

- **Infections** – Having briefly explored the complex world of the immune system, I'm sure it won't be a surprise to know that infections from viruses and bacteria can trigger an autoimmune response. We're surrounded by these all the time and they're much better at adapting and surviving than we are. We saw in the Covid-19 pandemic how the virus mutated as it spread and came up against the vaccines. Like us, pathogens do their best to adapt and survive. Sometimes we don't even know we've been infected. This is common for many viruses that have become embedded in the population over time, like the herpes virus or Epstein Barr virus (EBV), which are thought to be connected to autoimmunity. Recent research shows a highly likely connection between EBV and MS and lupus. Guillain-Barré syndrome (GBS), which weakens the peripheral nervous system, is connected to an infection caused by campylobacter, usually found in undercooked meat or contaminated water. Autoimmune gastritis is connected to *Helicobacter pylori*, also responsible for stomach ulcers. Remember, just because you get a specific infection doesn't mean you'll develop autoimmune disease, but in susceptible individuals, it can be part of the cause.

- **Medications** – Taking medications to manage acute and chronic health conditions has become the norm in Western medicine. And the rise in chronic health conditions means the pharmaceuticals market is huge. Many of these meds can be lifesaving, but unfortunately, all drugs come with potential side effects, even developing an autoimmune condition. Certain blood pressure meds, antibiotics and cholesterol-reducing statins are implicated here, particularly for lupus and autoimmune hepatitis. Treatments for one autoimmune condition can even trigger autoimmunity in another. All drugs come with risks, but if you read this and are concerned, please *do not stop* without first consulting your doctor.

- **Environmental toxins** – Clusters of people with autoimmune diseases close to chemical waste plants, agricultural chemicals and highly toxic wasteland have drawn attention to the damage toxins are wreaking on our bodies as well as the world we live in. Microplastics are yet another growing problem as tiny particles make their way into all life on the planet. Just how toxic elements and manufactured chemicals cause damage is yet to be identified, but an inflammatory pathway that negatively affects vulnerable individuals is well recognised. Some of these toxins are avoidable through choosing organic food or removing toxins from the home. Others found in the workplace, from nearby farms or just caught in the air are harder to avoid.

- **Childhood trauma** – Increasingly, research suggests autoimmunity is triggered by buried emotional trauma and difficulties. A child processes experiences with whatever knowledge they have to that point. It's difficult to understand loss, abuse or even your place in the world as a young child. Negative emotions and unprocessed trauma get buried somewhere deep in the mind; this then may contribute to chronic low (or high) level inflammation caused by stress – which is another factor. Therapies like cognitive behavioural therapy (CBT) or eye movement desensitisation and reprocessing (EMDR) can be very effective for people with autoimmune disease. I have undertaken both and believe they have had a positive effect on my MS.
- **Stress** – Ongoing, chronic stress leaves the fight-or-flight response switched on and raises cortisol levels. Both contribute to chronic inflammation, which in turn can trigger autoimmunity. Chronic stress is a common problem in the digital age. Work and financial issues, relationship problems, unsuitable housing, poor sleep, social isolation, all contribute. I now realise that working in ITU was a major contributor of stress for me, and although it was hard to leave nursing, my health benefited greatly. Stress also has an impact on gut health which can lead to the next factor in the list…
- **Leaky gut** – As mentioned earlier, the gut is a key protective barrier between the outside world and the inner mechanisms of the body. If that barrier becomes inflamed and leaky, proteins, bacteria, and chemicals can get through into the bloodstream and trigger an acute

or chronic inflammatory response. A compromised gut is thought to be a key factor in autoimmunity – so key I have dedicated a whole chapter to it (see Chapter 2).

> Many people with autoimmune disease identify a stressful life event or situation prior to their first full attack. For Rosa, it was ending a difficult relationship, for Kate it was the busy life of being a teacher, and for Tricia it was a traumatic life event. Acute stress happens to us all, but when combined with chronic stress, it can be a powerful trigger for immune system chaos.

Research continues into discovering the root causes of autoimmune disease, which is good news. Once the cause has been found then, they can hopefully not only be prevented from developing but a cure can be found to relieve the suffering experienced by so many people around the world.

Alongside potential causes, scientists have identified specific factors that increase the risk of developing an autoimmune disease. Some are lifestyle behaviours that are common in all chronic health conditions. One, unfortunately, can't be avoided!

- **Smoking** – Cigarettes contain toxins that challenge the immune system. Never smoking or becoming an ex-smoker is a positive step for your health for many reasons.
- **Being a woman** – Sorry ladies, but unfortunately, we have a four-fold risk of developing autoimmunity compared to men. In some conditions, women make up 80% of patients. It's still not clear why but hormones and child-bearing abilities are thought to be a major contributor as women have a higher antibody load than men.
- **Low vitamin D levels** – Many autoimmune conditions are prevalent in the northern and southern hemispheres where it's hard to get outside in the sun for six months of the year. Sunlight on the skin produces vitamin D which has many roles, including supporting the immune system. The risk of low vitamin D levels is increased in people with African and Asian heritage as darker skin requires

longer sun exposure. Like gender, race can be a risk factor in some autoimmune conditions. Taking a vitamin D supplement as well as getting outside whenever possible can reduce this risk.

- **Obesity** – As the number of people with obesity grows, so does autoimmunity. That doesn't mean that if you're not obese you won't get an autoimmune condition or that if you are obese, you will. However, figures show there is a higher incidence of autoimmunity in obese people, probably connected to chronic inflammation as well as an increased amount of fatty adipose tissue, which contains many immune cells. The more immune cells you have coupled with chronic inflammation, the more likely you are to have autoimmune antibodies. Key lifestyle factors like diet quality, exercise and stress management all help reduce obesity and therefore the risk of autoimmunity. Another thing to bear in mind here is that poor gut health and obesity are linked, as is chronic inflammation.
- **Diet** – Some foods are thought to increase the risk of autoimmunity in certain people. For example, the milk protein casein has been associated with the development and progression of MS. And poor micronutrient intake is associated with lupus. Fortunately (for most of us), diet and lifestyle are key activities we can have control over.
- **Having an autoimmune disease** – It might seem unfair, but having one condition puts you at increased risk of developing another – or more. Research suggests this isn't the case in all autoimmune conditions,[10] and lifestyle changes can reduce your risk of anything new taking you by surprise.

Don't despair – there is hope!

I hope that reading all of this won't add to your anxiety levels and that instead it has helped clarify why you may be feeling the way you do. The hard-nosed fact is that autoimmune conditions are difficult to live with, but the good news is there are many things you can do alongside standard medical treatment protocols to help slow down and, ideally, halt progression. Even reverse it in some cases. Small improvements can make a huge difference to how you feel about yourself and your condition. Making positive choices and taking healing actions can help you feel more in control of your life. After all, autoimmunity is you attacking yourself; understanding what changes to make can have a powerful effect. This is about self-empowerment, not self-blame.

> **Rosa's story:** Rosa and her mum were devastated by her diagnosis of sarcoidosis aged only 29. Her advice to her younger self, now? Don't despair; it's not the end of the world. There are things you can do that can make a difference, including a plant-based diet. In Rosa's case, that supports her values as well as her health.

Now we've looked at the immune system, autoimmunity and the potential causes, it's time to explore the role of the gut and look at why gut health is so important to our overall health as well as managing autoimmune disease.

Chapter 2

Why gut health is so important

Introduction

Unless you have an autoimmune disease located in your gut, like coeliac or Crohn's disease, you may be wondering why I have dedicated a whole chapter to gut health. Well, it turns out that the immune system and gut health are intrinsically linked; 70% of the immune system is found in and around the gut[1] – what goes in, through and out of the gut has a dynamic impact on the body as a whole. It's also the home of the microbiome, a huge community of microbes that have a key impact on our health, in a good way, and bad.

In this chapter, I explore what the microbiome is, how it got there, what it does and, crucially, what happens when it becomes disturbed or damaged. But first, let's have a quick look at the gut itself, how it works and the things that can create problems.

Gut 101

What do you think of as the gut? Your stomach? Maybe what's underneath your belly? Both are right, but there's so much more going on without us having to think about it – unless it starts playing up.

The gut, or gastrointestinal tract (GIT), starts at the mouth and runs all the way through the body to the anus. Approximately 9 metres long in adults, it's a mainly muscular tube that varies in size, width and wall thickness depending on its location and function. It is one of the earliest organs formed in the foetus and acts as an active transit route and protective barrier. Unlike the skin, this barrier is porous, which makes it more vulnerable to damage. And, unlike the skin, we can't easily see that damage or pop on a plaster to help it mend.

The GIT has different sections with specialist roles. This means its structure and environment vary depending on the job in hand. For example, the stomach is a large bag-like structure with thick, muscular walls. Its high acidity (pH 2–3) helps break down tough food structures and kill potentially harmful bacteria and other pathogens. Partially digested food, gastric acid and digestive enzymes mix together to form a pungent mix called 'chyme'. It's most unpleasant if any leaks out!

Acidic chyme is released into the small intestine, gradually becoming more neutral in pH as it travels through the tract. The muscular intestine walls move chyme with peristaltic waves; I imagine it looks like a caterpillar moving on the ground. It's important to keep things moving as you don't want waste products hanging around for long, irritating the gut lining. Nerve impulses and fibre-containing foods stimulate this action; a low-fibre diet will slow peristalsis, as can medications like opioid painkillers. Conditions that affect the thyroid or nervous system can also have a negative impact. Further down the small intestine, nutrients like glucose, fatty acids and amino acids are absorbed through the gut wall along with minerals, vitamins and phytonutrients. The environment here is much less acidic, almost neutral, with a pH between 6 and 7.4.

Next is the colon, the first part of the large intestine. It's taken around seven hours to get here and by now chyme consists mainly of water, undigested fibre and waste products. The colon is home to the microbiome mentioned earlier, a bespoke community of microbes that play an important role in our health and well-being. This community loves to dine on undigested fibre through fermentation. The pH has changed again, to 5.5–6.0: beneficial bacteria thrive in a more acidic environment. The gut lining is thin here, making absorption of water and nutrients easy. Peristalsis keeps things moving along still, but at a more leisurely pace. Toxic compounds like excess or secondary bile salts and unwanted cholesterol as well as cell waste and dead microbes are building up now, forming faecal matter ready for expulsion. Movement needs to be slow enough for satisfactory absorption but fast enough to prevent toxic compounds from causing localised damage. Fibre is key to getting this balance right. A daily bowel movement ensures waste products are removed in a timely manner and in a healthy person, the whole process should take 24–48 hours. Too fast and there's not enough time for nutrients and water to be fully absorbed. We all know how unpleasant and debilitating diarrhoea can be, I'm sure! A slow transit time, though, can mean toxic by-products build up, creating inflammatory compounds. Constipation is a chronic problem for many, often seen in those with a sedentary lifestyle eating a low-fibre Western diet. It makes you feel sluggish and crap – which you are literally full of! It can even become a medical emergency when someone is so bunged up their gut stops working. Not a pleasant for anyone involved.

Gut health is inextricably connected with immune health, which also means autoimmunity is involved here too. Increasingly, researchers are

ESSENTIALS FOR A WORKING GUT

- the right pH in the right place
- appropriate transit time
- absorption of nutrients, compounds and water
- removal of waste products and toxic compounds
- high-fibre diet to keep things moving
- happy and well-fed microbiome

focusing on this link and it's why this book is focused on food choices that support gut health and immune health.

The magical microbiome

Everyone's talking about it, but what exactly is the microbiome? And why is it so important?

Scientists have found our bodies play host to a huge number of microbes that live in and on us. Before you go rushing for the handwash, that's a good thing. These microbes – a selection of bacteria, viruses and fungi – play a key role in supporting our health. We are their home, and they work hard to keep it a great place to live.

Microbiomes, colonies of microbes, can be found on the skin, in the mouth and, most importantly, in the gut. Here they work hard to fight off unwanted pathogens and toxins, help develop and support the immune system and, as mentioned above, help with digestion and the release of nutrients.

It's thought humans are made up of roughly 37 trillion cells.[2] Scientists estimate there are as many microbes as human cells in the body, making us half human, half bug. Some even suggest we're 90% microbe, which is an interesting idea. It's hard to comprehend as we can't see them with the naked eye. As mentioned, while most of these microbes are bacteria, viruses and fungi are also key members of the community. Microbiomes are like any ecosystem – everything has an important role, even the worst type of microbe, as long as the balance is right. Whether we're talking about a tropical rainforest, or a gut microbiome, biodiversity and balance are essential for that environment to flourish.

Like fingerprints, everyone's microbiome is unique. Even identical twins who have the same genetic make-up have individual microbiomes, which is why you can have identical twins with different weight issues or chronic diseases; it's their individualised set of microbes that make the difference.[3]

We are not born with our microbiome; the community is seeded during birth and develops as it's exposed to the array of microbes that live around us. The make-up changes at different ages and with exposure to different environments, in a good, and bad, way. This is interesting when it comes to health problems with a genetic element, like autoimmune diseases. Many genes can take thousands of years to adapt to external influences. The microbiome, however, can rapidly respond to its environment.[4] Gut composition can alter in just 24 hours as multiple generations of microbes procreate, live and die in a single day.[5] This is why what we eat mealtime to mealtime is so important. Different foods feed different microbes; lack of diversity on the plate means lack of diversity in the gut. If a microbe is starved, it dies, and its unique role is lost. Balance and harmony start to break down and the gut heads towards dysbiosis, when gut bugs go bad.

Before we explore the problem of dysbiosis in more detail, let's look at what the microbiome gets up to when it's happy and healthy.

So, what has the microbiome ever done for us…?

If you're feeling a bit freaked out about being host to a bunch of microbes, don't be. Like anyone, they want their home to be a great place to live and are happy to work hard to keep the community strong. This symbiotic relationship has become key over thousands of years of evolution. The microbiome has even taken over some roles so we can focus on other things, and our understanding of the microbiome grows every day. Just look at the information on page 34 to see some of the amazing things we already know about.

They really are very busy! We can see from the list that the microbiome has a direct impact on key regulatory processes, including immunity, metabolism, hormone expression and cognition. By helping the body to function well and keep chronic inflammation at bay, it can positively influence gene expression, helping to prevent switching on genes that can lead to disease states.

What the gut microbiome does for us
- digests complex fibres we can't
- supports the development and health of the immune system
- produces enzymes to help synthesise vitamins, particularly B1, B6, B12 and K
- supports the health and integrity of the gut wall
- produces neurotransmitters like serotonin and dopamine
- forms part of a superhighway to the brain
- produces hormones that help control metabolism, especially appetite
- makes short-chain fatty acids (SCFAs)
- helps process drugs – this can have an impact on their effectiveness
- recycles bile (and helps get rid of secondary bile acids and cholesterol).

What influences the make-up of a person's microbiome?

As more is understood about the importance of a balanced, healthy microbiome, we can now also recognise what affects it, positively and negatively. Here are some key influences – you might like to think about how they have affected you.

- **Method of birth** – I mentioned above how the microbiome is seeded during birth, only if it's a vaginal delivery though. Caesarean section cuts out this 'seeding' opportunity.* A C-section is often an emergency intervention, although many are a choice. I had pre-eclampsia[†] with my first child who was born via an emergency C-section at 33 weeks. It all turned out well in the end but 28 years ago, we didn't know that this would affect her microbiome. Today, some healthcare systems are providing specialist probiotics for Caesarean babies. I've checked with a midwife friend and sadly this is not standard practice in the NHS. Yet. Hopefully it will change going forward.

*Currently 25% of UK births and 32% of US births are by Caesarean section.
[†]Interestingly, pre-eclampsia is thought to be another type of autoimmune condition.

- **Breast or bottle** – Mother's milk is the ideal food for babies when it comes to nutrition. Breast milk also contains a selection of probiotics to help support a baby's developing microbiome; contact with microbes on the skin helps too.[6] What about formula-fed babies? Some brands are now fortifying their formula with beneficial bacteria, but not all. And anyone who was bottle-fed before the early 2000s will have missed this essential seeding opportunity. Even a few weeks of breast feeding can make a difference to a baby's microbiome make-up.

- **What we eat** has a huge effect on the make-up of our gut microbiome,[7] in a positive and negative way, from the moment you start eating solid food onwards. The modern Western diet, high in saturated fat, refined sugars and salt, low in fibre, fresh produce and healthy fats, is known to enable 'bad' microbes to flourish whilst reducing diversity and balance. A diet high in plant foods with complex fibre from whole grains and pulses, low in refined sugars and salt, full of a range of colourful fresh produce and healthy fats, help the microbiome thrive. If you're mum to a toddler, there's no judgement here! It's hard to get some adults, let alone a toddler with developing opinions, to eat these gut-loving foods. If you've eaten a Western diet for years, don't despair. The microbiome wants to thrive. As soon as you start giving it the good stuff, things will start moving in a positive direction.

- **The environment** we live in also has an impact on the make-up of our microbiome. This is particularly pertinent in early infancy but can have an impact at all stages of life. Too clean and too dirty both have a negative impact on the gut. Children learn through touch and putting things in their mouths. Whilst it can be a bit revolting (I once found a dead daddy longlegs hanging out my son's mouth!), exposure to microbes in and around the home can help seed the microbiome. It also helps the immune system learn to distinguish between friend and foe. It's why rolling in the mud and having pets can help to form a well-prepared immune system. The 'hygiene hypothesis' – constant use of anti-bacterials and keeping children ultra clean – may be contributing to the increase in allergies and food sensitivities we see in the population. Equally, a child living in a dirty home and eating festering food or excess mould will be exposed to too many microbes and this can have severe consequences. Diarrhoea is still the number-one killer of infants in poor countries with no clean water and open sewers; of course, these conditions are not beneficial for anyone's health.

- **Environmental toxins** can negatively impact gut health, even if they're not directly ingested, and are linked to the development of autoimmune disease.[8] Agricultural chemicals can be avoided if you eat only organic food, but if you're living near a farm spraying these toxins, you can't. Urban towns and cities have their own toxin load, whether from industrial plants, exhaust fumes or chemicals used in buildings. Certain chemicals used in plastics, like BPA, are a known issue and microplastics are increasingly working their way into the food system, and therefore our bodies. In the modern world, it's hard to avoid toxins of any kind; where you live may be outside your control, but what you eat and choose to use in the home are. And don't forget that both cigarette smoke and alcohol intake are included in this list of toxins; they not only impact the microbiome but the body as a whole.

- **Prescribed and over-the-counter medications** can also have a direct negative effect on the microbiome. The most obvious one is broad-spectrum **antibiotics**. Life savers when needed, but they wipe out a colony of friendly bacteria. Even targeted antibiotics can have a negative impact. Antibiotics in food are also a big problem.[9][‡] Non-steroidal anti-inflammatory drugs (NSAIDs), like ibuprofen and naproxen, can damage the gut lining, change the pH, affect gut motility and alter the environment to make it more favourable for

---

[‡]Animal agriculture is the biggest user of antibiotics: 73% of antibiotics used worldwide are used in animal farming. In 2006, the UK and EU banned the practice of generically adding antibiotics to animal feed to promote growth but in the US and other places around the world, it's still standard practice. Even when there is some control, they're still widely used. Not only is this contributing towards antibiotic resistance in many bacteria, but antibiotic residue remains in the meat products eaten by humans. Continual, low doses of this residue negatively affect the microbiome make-up.

'bad' bacteria to thrive. Pain is a common problem for people with autoimmune disease and these drugs are often recommended, even though they can perpetuate symptoms if used for any length of time. **Antacids** or PPIs (proton pump inhibitors) also affect the microbiome by altering the pH in the stomach and subsequently throughout the gut. Finally, **immune-suppressing drugs**, including those used to treat autoimmune conditions, can negatively affect gut health. Whilst these medications may help in the short term, it's easy to see how people with autoimmune disease get stuck in a cycle of continual poor health.

- **Stress** can also impact the microbiome.[10] If you've ever had 'butterflies in your stomach', you'll have experienced the direct impact of the brain and gut communicating. Gut function and

BRAIN–GUT INFLUENCES

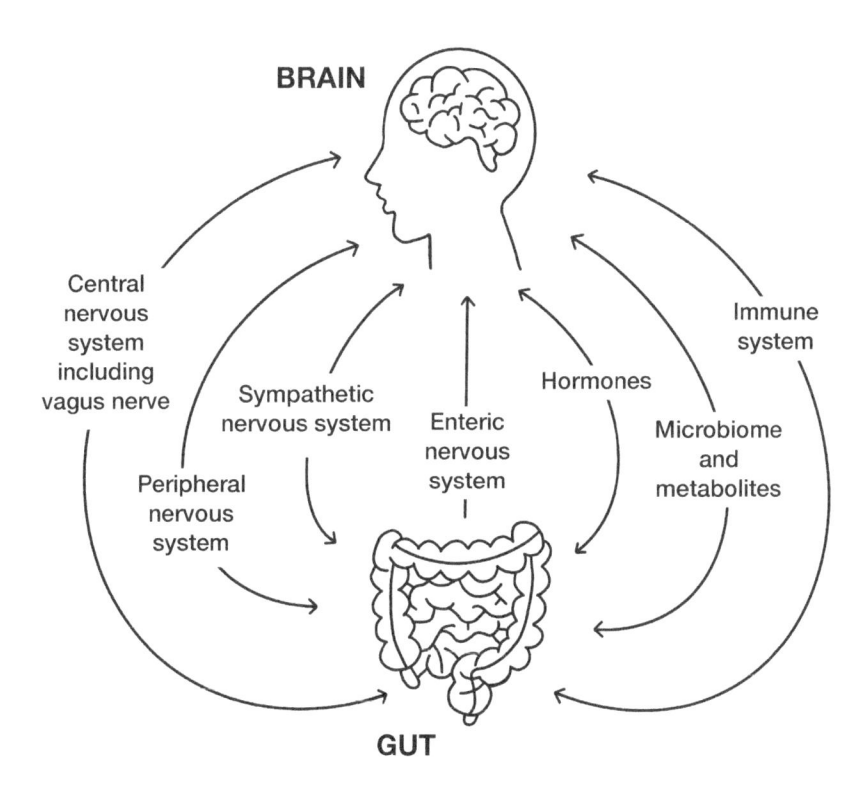

BRAIN

Central nervous system including vagus nerve

Sympathetic nervous system

Enteric nervous system

Hormones

Immune system

Microbiome and metabolites

Peripheral nervous system

GUT

activity are influenced by different nerves and nervous systems. The microbiome communicates with the brain via neurotransmitters and short-chain fatty acids (more on these shortly). The gut and microbiome are influenced by the fight-or-flight response, controlled by the autonomic nervous system and, interestingly, 70% of serotonin and 50% of dopamine, the happy hormones, are produced in the gut. Stress is a risk factor for autoimmune disease; it's also one for an imbalanced microbiome. Depression and anxiety are key features of many autoimmune diseases; emotional resilience is essential in dealing with the stress of having these conditions and a vibrant, balanced microbiome is key to this. When you adopt stress reduction practices, your microbiome benefits as much as your brain.

As you can see, there are many aspects of modern life that negatively affect the microbiome. So much so that a balanced, thriving community can rapidly change into a dysfunctional autocracy – a state known as dysbiosis.

What is dysbiosis?

Dysbiosis is a common thread that connects different types of autoimmune condition.[11] This is why clinicians feel that autoimmunity is one disease with over 100 ways of presenting. But what exactly is dysbiosis? And what does it look like?

In simple terms, dysbiosis is the loss of harmony and balance within the gut. As mentioned already, the gut microbiome is a smorgasbord of microbes including bacteria, viruses and fungi. Some are beneficial, others are pathogenic – that is, they cause disease. Microbes know how to survive – they have been around as long as life on Earth has been possible. Pathogenic ones are particularly hardy and will survive and even flourish in environments that less hardy, but friendlier microbes can't deal with.

The list opposite shows there's much in our day-to-day lives that makes it hard for friendly bacteria to thrive. Dysbiosis, or a pathogenic microbiome, is rife in the Western world. We know this through huge research programmes like the Human Microbiome Project,[12] the American Gut Project,[13] the British

Chapter 2

GUT DYSBIOSIS SIGNS AND SYMPTOMS

> Dysbiosis can manifest in many ways – one or more of these can make your gut unhappy:
>
> *Inside the intestines:*
> - Abdominal pain, cramping
> - Wind
> - Bloating
> - Food sensitivities
> - Diarrhoea
> - Constipation
> - Mucus in stool
> - Nausea
> - Indigestion or heartburn/reflux
> - Recurrent burping
>
> *Outside the intestines:*
> - Weight gain or loss
> - Fatigue
> - Brain fog
> - Difficulty concentrating
> - Fluctuating mood
> - Anxiety
> - Skin problems
> - Joint and/or muscle pains
> - Weakness and fatigue
> - Bad breath
> - Congested sinuses or wheezing

Gut Project (that's turned into the Zoe app) and, most recently, the Human Gut Microbiome Atlas[14] that maps the population's microbiome make-up through analysing poo samples from people all over the world. This data has provided new information about the microbiome and its roles. The impact of dysbiosis on population health is one possible explanation for the explosion of chronic health conditions, including autoimmune disease, over the last 70 years.

So how does dysbiosis affect the gut, microbiome and body as a whole? To answer that, let's start at the gut wall in the small intestine and colon.

The structure of the gut wall

I am constantly astounded by the remarkable bio-engineering that has led to the wonderous structure that is the human body. The gut lining in the

STRUCTURE OF THE GUT LINING

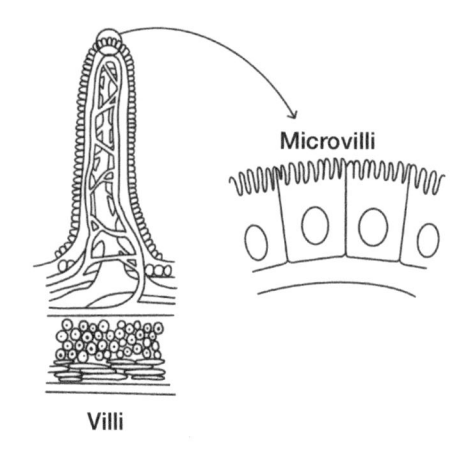

small intestine is particularly ingenious. This is the area where most of the nutrients released by digestion are absorbed into the blood system. Once in circulation, these nutrients and compounds can be sent to wherever they're needed in the body, or processed and stored for later use. To create an expansive surface area for maximum nutrient absorption, the lining of the small intestine is covered in folds. Even though this increases the surface area to a whopping 18 metres, more is needed, so each fold is covered by tiny finger-like protrusions called villi – millions of them. Each square-millimetre is covered by 30 villi, poking out of the gut lining into the watery chyme. To maximise the space even more, each villus is covered with even smaller protrusions, rather unimaginatively called microvilli, thereby creating an even larger surface area to capture tiny nutrients. To put this into perspective, it's estimated that if the whole surface area was flattened and spread out, it would cover a tennis court.[15] Incredible!

Every villus has its own capillary blood supply, and lymph vessels, 'lacteals', are found between villi. The surface of the villi is very thin, and that of microvilli even more so. This ensures tiny nutrient molecules can be absorbed into the bloodstream, but larger, less welcome molecules are kept at bay. Once in the bloodstream, all absorbed substances travel to the liver to be screened for harmful substances. These are destroyed before the nutrient-rich blood heads off to the heart for circulation around the body.

Lacteals play their own part in nutrient absorption, focusing on fats and fat-soluble vitamins (A, D, E and K). The lymphatic system is part of the overall immune system. A second set of lymph vessels are found just below the villi in the mesenteric, a layer of connective tissue just outside of the gut wall. As well as fat absorption, the lymphatic system in and around the gut is involved in immune surveillance/antigen recognition as well as fluid homeostasis (balance).

The colon, which houses the microbiome as we've seen, has a larger diameter but smoother surface compared to the small intestine. Water is absorbed here, along with electrolytes and any left-over nutrients. Its lining, the epithelial layer, is just one cell thick and whilst there are no villi, microvilli are found on the outside edge of the cells in the epithelial layer. Unlike the skin which has lots of protective layers to keep the outside out, the gut, and the colon in particular, has very few. But it does have one important feature – mucin, a thick, gloopy mucus layer that coats the gut lining throughout the gastrointestinal tract. As the stomach is so acidic, it has a double layer of mucin to protect the lining of the stomach wall. The colon also has a double layer as its wall is so thin and needs protection from microbes in the microbiome. There is only a single layer of mucin in the small intestine, though, making it more vulnerable to damage.

Made up of glycoproteins, mucin performs three main roles:
- **Lubrication:** It helps gut contents to continue moving along.
- **Protection:** It forms a barrier against microbes, including pathogenic invaders and those living in the microbiome plus environmental toxins and irritants.
- **Communication:** It contains compounds involved in cell signalling for homeostasis plus cell and immune regulation.

Because mucin is so important for protection,[16] it contains innate and adaptive immune compounds and cells that respond to pathogenic bacteria and specific antibodies. T and B lymphocytes are vital for gut homeostasis and protection against gastrointestinal diseases but can also produce excess amounts of inflammatory cytokines if left unchecked.

CELL TYPES OF THE INTESTINAL EPITHELIUM

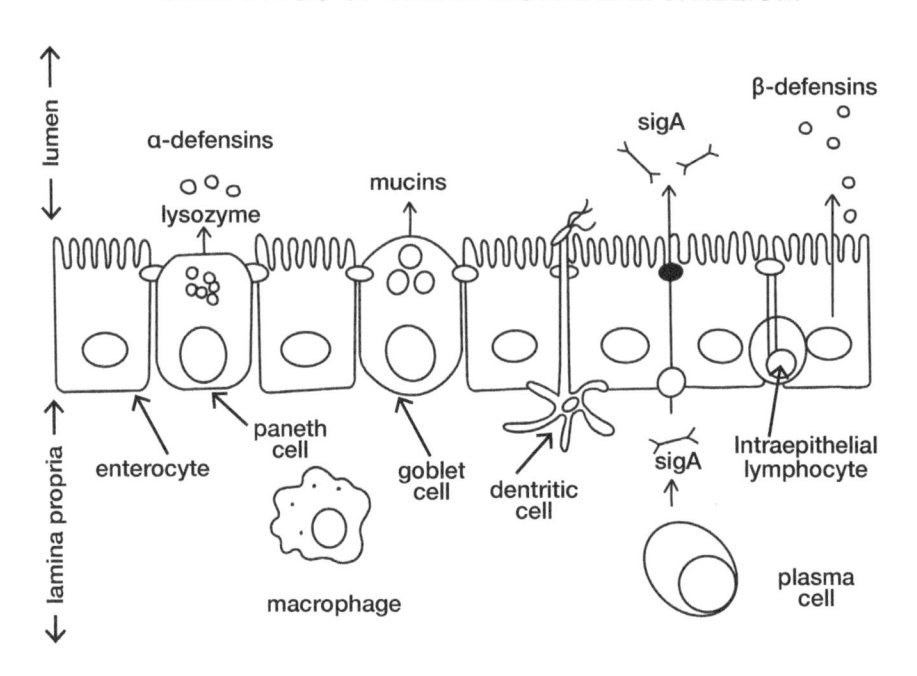

(Diagram showing cell types: enterocyte, paneth cell (with α-defensins, lysozyme), goblet cell (producing mucins), dendritic cell, intraepithelial lymphocyte (with sigA, β-defensins), macrophage, plasma cell (with sigA); arrows indicating lumen and lamina propria directions)

Type 1 diabetes and gut health

Research looking at the gut health of people with type 1 diabetes found changes in the mucin layer, dysbiosis and lower amounts of the SCFA-producing microbes required to keep mucin integrity and immune tolerance in the gut.[17]

It's hard to picture what the gut lining looks like; most of what I've described is only visible under a microscope. Try to visualise a row of cells packed tightly together. Some are lining cells; others have a specialist role such as goblet cells producing mucin or paneth cells that produce self-made antibiotics that manage microbe levels. The tight junctions between each cell are important, making sure only tiny molecules can pass through, keeping out larger pathogens or proteins that might upset the immune system that is doggedly patrolling the area.

Before we look at what happens in a dysbiotic gut, I need to briefly introduce you properly to SCFAs – short-chain fatty acids – which I have already mentioned in passing.

A brief introduction to SCFAs

In the past, nutrition experts thought that insoluble fibre and resistant starch had no nutritional value. Yes, they support gut motility, but, as we can't digest them, it was assumed this complex fibre exited the body in a similar state to how it entered. However, it turns out that this fibre can be digested – by the microbiome instead of by us. Our gut microbes love it! They break these tough fibres down through fermentation, producing tiny compounds called short-chain fatty acids, or SCFAs, and gas.[§] As the name suggests, these are very short chains of carbon atoms that form acid compounds. There are three main types – acetate, propionate and butyrate. Scientists tend to study them on their own, but in your body they work together as a team. Different types of fibre stimulate different microbes to trigger their fermentation.[18] Again, the need for variety in the diet pops up – it's so important to ensure you have a smorgasbord of beneficial microbes.

SCFAs have a range of functions; many more are being discovered. Good things really do come in small packages.[19] Here are just a few – we'll look at more once we've finished delving into the chaotic world of dysbiosis.

- Microbes love to eat them! As more and more SCFAs are produced, the happier and better-fed the microbiome becomes.
- SCFAs increase the acidity in the colon; friendly bacteria thrive in a more acidic environment, whereas 'bad' bacteria are not so keen.
- They create up to 10% of the body's daily energy requirement meaning that complex fibre is an energy source after all. Not only that, but they provide around 70% of the energy needed by colon cells to function well.

[§]Yes, fibre makes you fart! But in a healthy gut this shouldn't be in excess or noxious. If you suffer from fruity flatulence or persistent trumping, you may well have an overgrowth of bad bacteria having a party on the inside. It's a good idea to seek help from a nutritionist or dietitian who can help.

Dysbiosis and the gut lining

It can take a while for dysbiosis to develop. It's usually due to a combination of factors – for example, when beneficial bacteria die off due to lack of fibre, exposure to environmental toxins, a change in the pH caused by medications and a hefty dose of antibiotics. Pathogenic bacteria are tough, and this is the perfect environment for them to thrive in, filling the space left by microbes that have died off. These microbes still need feeding, and with fewer SCFAs being made, they turn to the next best option – the gloopy mucin layer. Goblet cells in the epithelium will try to patch up the damaged areas by secreting more mucin, but this might not be enough if the pathogenic microbes continue to run riot.

With dysbiosis, endotoxins (internally made toxins) become another problem. Lipopolysaccharides (LPS) are one example. Found on the outside wall of gram-negative bacteria, LPS communicate with the immune system, triggering an inflammatory response. In acute situations, this can be life-threatening, leading to septic shock and endotoxaemia. Persistent, ongoing low levels of LPS leaking into the bloodstream results in less dramatic but potentially life-changing outcomes. And it's not just 'bad' bacteria that influence LPS. High amounts of fat in the diet, especially saturated fat, alcohol and even excessive physiological and psychological stress can all increase levels of LPS.

Metabolites like LPS are thought to be connected to the development of autoimmune disease either via acute damage to local structures, as seen with inflammatory bowel diseases,[20] or chronic long-term systemic inflammation.[21]

LPS and inflammatory bowel disease (IBD)

IBD includes Crohn's disease, which can affect any part of the gut, and ulcerative colitis, found in the colon only. Both are autoimmune conditions where the immune system attacks the cells in the lining of the gut. This can cause abscesses, and fistulas, and often requires major surgery. It can be a very debilitating disease, sometimes life limiting. A combination of factors has been connected to the development of IBD, including genes, environment and lifestyle. It's increasingly seen in people consuming a Western diet pattern – low fibre, high fat and lots of ultra-processed foods.[22] Research also shows an increase in IBD as people move away from plant-predominant to meat-predominant diets. Elevated blood levels of LPS are often found in people with IBD, part of an ever-increasing inflammatory pathway; LPS promotes dysbiosis, which increases inflammation, which in turn increases LPS.

Short episodes of inflammation in the gut are not always bad news. It's thought they can train the immune system to differentiate between friend and foe, helping it to learn how to be tolerant to foods and other substances. It's long-term dysbiosis, or a pathogenic make-up in the

LEAKY GUT

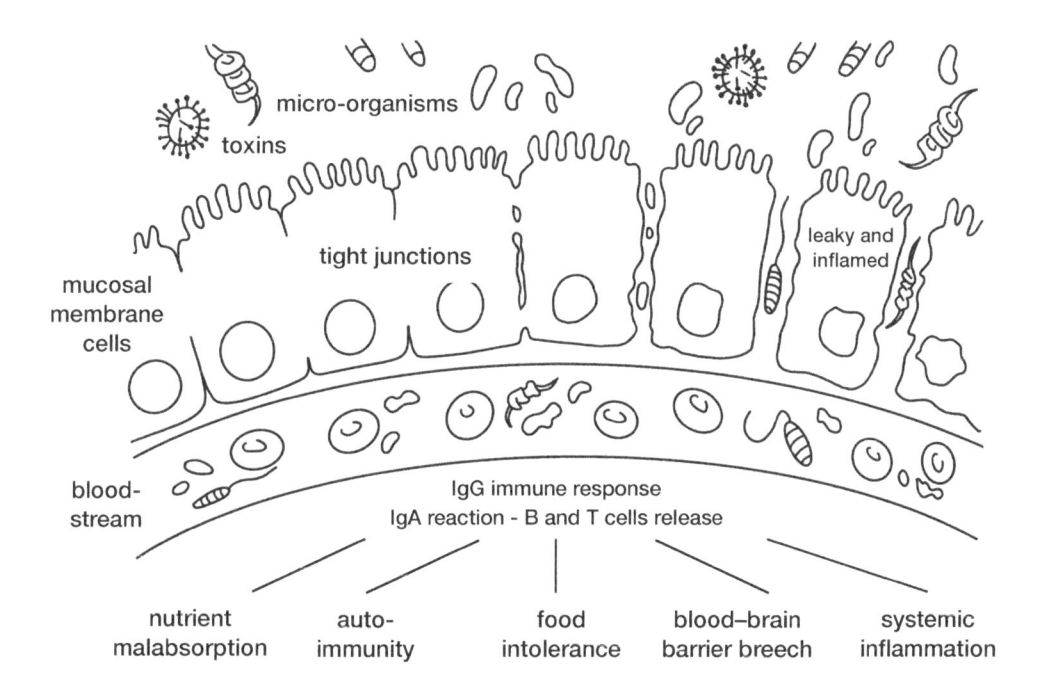

gut, that can lead to long-term issues such as food sensitivities, chronic inflammation and molecular mimicry. This is when a now confused and over-reactive immune response results in the attacks on 'self' cells – autoimmunity.

Cells in the epithelial layer are packed closely together, with tight junctions creating narrow channels that only desirable compounds can traverse. A sustained assault by toxins, 'bad' bacteria, chemicals and more starts to weaken the tight junctions, eventually making them loose enough for larger, unwanted molecules to squeeze through and sneak into the bloodstream. The immune cells directly behind the gut wall kick off an inflammatory response, putting the body on full alert. Once in the circulation, these invaders have the potential to go anywhere, triggering a localised immune response. Blood vessels become 'leaky' so the larger white blood cells can reach their target. If this assault is ongoing, and with the right influencing factors (genes, environment, stress etc), the immune system can become overwhelmed and confused and start to attack 'self'- tissues instead of 'non-self' – an autoimmune attack.

Whilst this is a very simplified explanation of a highly complex process that can take years to develop or produce symptoms, I hope you can see how the gut is inextricably mixed up with this generalised inflammatory pattern that can target anywhere.

Whilst diet is just one of the influencing factors that can trigger a condition or relapse, it can also help to calm the immune response, promote remission and even help to prevent it developing in the first place. This is good news if you have siblings or children; they are at an increased risk of autoimmunity. Knowledge is power; autoimmune disease is not inevitable if precautionary steps are taken. Personally, I find that very comforting!

SCFAs part 2

We have explored how a balanced microbiome is integral to gut health, and therefore overall health. We've also seen that it can be hard to achieve this balance when there are so many different factors that can disrupt it. However, a multitude of microbes *can* enjoy a happy and harmonious existence when there's a diverse community that can keep each other in check. When all is well, these microbes keep the gut lining healthy and strong and continue to produce compounds, hormones and signalling agents to ensure their hosts (us) are healthy, strong and resilient too.

A variety of foods needs to be eaten to ensure this diversity in the microbiome is maintained. Just like you and me, microbes have preferences for the type of food they like to eat, so eating a range of foods keeps everyone happy. Insoluble fibre and resistant starch are particularly important for creating SCFAs.[23] We've already seen how important they are for the microbiome, but that's not all. Here are a few more benefits we know about.

SCFAs:

- act as a mediator between the microbiome and the immune system, sending signals when the immune system needs to be ramped up to deal with a problem, and helping to calm it down again.
- help regulate the metabolism of glucose and fats as well as controlling blood sugar levels by influencing insulin and glucagon release (through the metabolite GLP-1, the 'new' breakthrough drug for obesity).
- participate in gut-brain communication, especially our emotions and mood.
- play a role in metabolic homeostasis and even weight control through hormone signalling.
- support heart health.
- improve skin conditions like psoriasis (another autoimmune disease).
- help improve the absorption of minerals.

And that's just what we know today! Research continues to reveal more about SCFAs as well as the fascinating symbiotic relationship between microbiome and host.

Whilst there's much we don't know, there is one glaring fact we do. Fibre, essential for the microbiome, is only found in plants. That is why a diet packed full of different types of plant foods is key to gut health, and therefore key to overall health. Limiting plant foods, or certain types of plants, can lead to a reduction in the microbes that rely on it as their food source, in a very short period. According to Dr Will Bulsiewicz, every single meal has an impact on the microbiome as the microbes procreate so rapidly the food eaten in 24 hours can affect 50 generations of microbes![24]

Summary

How do we know that dybiosis and autoimmune disease are connected? The simple answer is that research tells us so. A review in 2020 looked at previous and ongoing studies of the gut health of people with autoimmune disease.[25] Whilst the conditions were different, they summarised that all the studies demonstrated a common problem: dysbiosis in the microbes in the colon.

Hopefully you're now up-to-speed regarding the importance of the microbiome and how our diet can have a huge impact on whether it thrives or not. We know that fibre is a crucial ingredient to keep it well nourished. But what else in our daily diet is causing havoc? That's what we're going to explore next.

Chapter 3

Inflammatory foods

Introduction

In the last chapter, we explored the importance of gut health, how the immune system is triggered and the importance of a balanced microbiome. The gut must deal with everything we eat, from breaking it down into constituent nutrients to then absorbing them and dealing with the waste products ready for removal. Food is more than just a mechanical and chemical process, as any foodie will tell you! From reading about it to making it, from private indulgences to communal social events, food is a subject we all have opinions on.

There's much that can be discussed about food and the food industry, about clever marketing and what is, or isn't, 'healthy' food. There are just not enough pages to cover it here, but if this is something you're interested in, I've added a few good books in the Resources section (page 321). For the sake of simplicity and page allowance, these next two chapters (3 and 4) focus on foods that trigger inflammation, and those that help calm it down – otherwise known as inflammatory and anti-inflammatory foods.

So how do we know which food goes in which category? Fortunately, nutrition researchers developed a very handy tool called the Food Inflammatory Index (FII), sometimes also known as the Dietary Inflammatory Index (DII).[1] Focusing on foods and food groups rather than individual nutrients, the system enables scientists to identify foods and dietary patterns implicated in promoting inflammation, and those that calm it down. This makes nutrition information more accessible and helps people make healthier choices. For example, everyone knows vegetables are good for us, but this covers a huge range of options. Vegetables could mean deep-fried white potatoes and yams – they have a high score on the FII. But steamed or boiled potatoes or yams served in a salad of four or five other colourful vegetables is a different matter – with a very low FII.

It's not a perfect tool, but using the FII has enabled researchers to identify the best anti-inflammatory foods as well as diet patterns. For example, the Mediterranean diet pattern which is high in fruit, vegetables, wholegrains, legumes and nuts, has a negative DII/FII score (which means it's anti-inflammatory). This pattern of eating consistently comes out on top in dietary research.[2] You probably won't be surprised to hear that a high-fat, high-sugar, high-animal-products and low-fibre Western dietary pattern carries a very high score. As more research is done, more is understood; in the short term though, there are often conflicting results with other dietary patterns that are promoted as healthy, like the ketogenic-style diet that features high-fat, low-carbohydrate foods. The FII score is high and therefore inflammatory, but other researchers have concluded it's anti-inflammatory. It's fair to say nothing is black and white and it's definitely nuanced. One thing all the research agrees on is that the most common eating pattern in the Western world, with its high FII score, is closely related to chronic health conditions including autoimmune disease.[3]

I am not a researcher, but I do believe that whole plant foods which carry a low FII are the best option, particularly for those of us with an immune system that's on fire and needs calming down. Before we look at the foods and ingredients that fan the inflammatory fires, I just want to give you a few thoughts about the body's relationship with food.

1. **Our bodies are amazingly complex** which is why scientists are still discovering new information about how they 'work'. Every function requires a combination of compounds and a complex cascade of chemical reactions.
2. **Change is constant.** Each cell, tissue and organ is going through a process of renewal, with old, possibly damaged cells dying and new ones being created in their place. The speed of this varies throughout

the body. It's calculated that an incredible 330 billion cells are replaced every day. And although some cells, like bone, take decades to regenerate, others like blood and gut-lining cells take days. This means we can influence this change in both a good and a bad way.

3. **Humans (and all animals) are programmed to survive.** Each process and function in the body has at least one back-up in case the first fails. The body can also heal itself. Raw material for these processes is taken directly from food eaten every day, or from stores in the body. When these options are unavailable, resources are scavenged from areas of the body deemed less essential for survival. This is important to consider when it comes to healing and health. The body will work hard to survive, but at what cost?
4. **The more stress the body is exposed to, the harder it must work.** Psychological and emotional stress are increasingly common as is environmental stress. Stress is also triggered when the body struggles to function effectively.
5. **The body likes to be safe.** It has an optimal internal environment (homeostasis) with quite narrow parameters; it does not like to be pushed outside of these. There are optimal levels for blood sugar, potassium, iron and sodium. An ideal blood temperature, carbon dioxide and acid level, and many more. Go outside these parameters and cellular processes become less efficient or may even stop completely. Our bodies work hard to stay safe; extra work requires more nutrients and produces higher inflammatory by-products.

Hopefully you can now see just how amazing our bodies are. Wellness is an inbuilt setting. We just need to provide the right nutrients and environment to enable it to work effectively and efficiently. Which is why every time we eat, it's an opportunity to heal, or to fuel chronic inflammation. Please keep that in mind as we now have a look at foods and ingredients that stoke the inflammatory fires.

Fat and saturated fat

Fat has many roles. It's a dense source of calories that can be stored in specialist cells for times of scarcity. This was important in the past for survival when little or no food was available during long winters, drought or other natural phenomena. Fat is also the base structure for many hormones, required for adequate absorption of some essential nutrients, a key part of cell membranes and plays an important part in switching on an immune response, and switching it off again.

So, what is fat? You may visualise it as lard, a solid white lump, or cooking oil, a yellowy-clear liquid. Both are forms of fat. The consistency changes depending on the type of fatty acids it contains. These are chains of hydrogen and carbon molecules that vary in length with a 'methyl' group at one end (this makes it an acid). Fatty acids are often found in groups of three – triglycerides – in food. During digestion, enzymes break down the bond holding them together (glycerol) and they are absorbed into the bloodstream as fatty acids. Once in circulation, their first stop is the liver. Here, fatty acids are either sent off wherever they're needed, converted to glucose for energy if no other source is available or converted back to triglycerides and stored in muscles and adipose tissue, mainly found around the belly, bum or thighs.

> **Fat as a source of energy**
>
> Fat is a secondary energy source. When glucose and glycogen stores are depleted, it's released from cells and converted to glucose in the liver. A less efficient process, it requires more nutrients and co-factors which, if not available in the diet, will be scavenged from other areas of the body. Ketone bodies are a by-product of this process, formed in the liver, and can be used as a secondary fuel source when glucose is not available, particularly in the brain which is a hungry organ. When ketone bodies are produced over glucose (due to lack of supply), the body is said to be 'in ketosis'. Creating this state through fasting and a high-fat, low-carb diet is the basis of a ketogenic diet.

Chapter 3

There are two main groups of fatty acids – saturated and unsaturated. They both contain carbon and hydrogen molecules, with carbon forming the backbone of the chain and hydrogen hanging on via little 'docking stations' either side. The diagram below shows it more clearly than I can explain it!

saturated fatty acid

unsaturated fatty acid

There's much to say about fats; here's a headline summary:
- Saturated fat has all the docking stations filled with hydrogen. This makes it solid and stable at room temperature, like a block of lard.
- Unsaturated fat is missing one or more docking stations as well as the hydrogen molecule that should be there.
- Monounsaturated fatty acids (MUFAs) are missing just one hydrogen atom.
- Polyunsaturated fatty acids (PUFAs) are missing two or more, making these fats more flexible but less stable.
- MUFAs are liquid at room temperature but can become solid at lower temperature (like olive oil in the fridge).
- PUFAs are liquid in any condition, more volatile and can become rancid and unpalatable.
- Triglycerides can be made up of the same type of fatty acid or a mixture, depending on the excess found in the diet.

Saturated fat is found in most foods, even whole plant foods. That is fine as we do need some. High intakes, however, are bad news for the body, particularly the immune system.[4] For example, fat is a key component of every cell membrane, the thin outside layer of each cell, including all types of immune cell. Formed of fatty acids, the body uses the fats that are available when new cells are formed. This should be mainly unsaturated fatty acids with a small amount of cholesterol for structure.

Cell membranes contain channels that allow nutrients and compounds in and waste products out, supporting cell function. Unsaturated fats are perfect for this. If saturated fats are dominant though, the cell membrane becomes clogged up, reducing the cell's ability to function adequately.[5] In immune cells, this can negatively impact immune cell activity, gene expression and the formation of precursors for pro- and anti-inflammatory compounds. Everyone needs healthy immune cells; even more so when managing a chronic health condition like autoimmune disease.

Fats and gut health

When it comes to gut health, a high intake of saturated fat has a direct negative effect on the gut lining and increases the amount of lipopolysaccharides (LPS – see Chapter 2) in the gut and circulation.[6] Microbiome make-up is also impacted by high amounts of dietary saturated fats, increasing the pathogenic microbe population. This also affects the gut lining, triggering both the innate and learned immune responses, making an acute immune response chronic over time. For example, palmitic acid, one of the most common saturated fats in the Western diet, increases the expression of the pro-inflammatory cytokines TNF and interleukins and reduces the capability of macrophages, the cells that attack pathogens. It also activates T-cell signalling involved in autoimmunity.[7] Other types, like lauric and stearic acid, also promote inflammation via different signalling routes. This is why scientists suggest people with autoimmune disease eat less saturated fat.[8]

Chapter 3

Essential fatty acids

The body can make most fatty acid chains itself. There are two it can't make – omega 3 and omega 6, 'essential' fatty acids we must get from food. The name comes from the position of the first double bond (or missing hydrogen) in the chain from the omega end.

Omegas 3 and 6 are polyunsaturated fatty acids that have a range of important roles throughout the body, such as brain health, skin and eye health, pain control, heart health and, most importantly for autoimmune conditions, immune signalling. This is a complex cascade of chemical reactions using compounds like vitamins, minerals and omega fatty acids. In general terms, omega 6 is involved in the 'danger' trigger, initiating an immune response while omega 3 is required for the 'danger over' signal, so the immune reaction can stand down. Without this second message, the immune system remains in 'attack mode'; this is chronic low-level inflammation. Therefore, it's important to consume equal amounts in the diet, ideally an omega 6 to 3 ratio of 1:1 or 2:1. Unfortunately, the ratio in the Western diet pattern is over 15:1.[9]

Highly refined oils found in the Western diet contribute to chronic inflammation.[10] The refining process uses high temperatures and chemicals to alter the structure of natural fats whilst removing all nutrients and flavour, creating a flavourless, colourless oil devoid of anything other than fat, and dominant in omega 6. The body doesn't like it and responds accordingly. The process for producing cold-pressed oil, like extra-virgin olive oil or flaxseed oil, is different and whilst many nutrients are still lost, it retains some healthful properties like polyphenols and lignans. Flaxseed oil is particularly high in anti-inflammatory omega 3 fats, with a ratio of 4.5:1 omega 3 to omega 6 in cold-pressed flaxseed oil.

Most oils consumed in the Western diet contain high amounts of omega 6 compared to omega 3, making this an essentially pro-inflammatory way of eating. For example, sunflower oil has a whopping 40:1 ratio and even avocado oil, which is being touted as healthy, has a 12:1 ratio. These oils, and saturated fats, are contained in most chilled and ambient (stored at room temperature) food in our supermarkets. Sometimes it's only in low amounts, but if it's in everything you eat throughout the day, a small amount soon adds up.

The downside of heating oils and fats

If you've not been put off these fats and oils yet, there's one more thing to mention here – the toxins created when these oils and fats are exposed to high heats. Cast your mind back to food tech classes and you might remember learning about the Maillard reaction. When food is exposed to high heat, it changes the structure of the fat, forming the golden brown, crispy texture of fried food along with the compelling rich, savoury aroma and flavour. The smell, flavour and texture tick all the boxes in the pleasure centres of the brain; we love them! However, not only has the oil, already damaged by processing, been absorbed into the food, but it now contains new inflammatory compounds created by the high heat, like acrylamide and polycyclic aromatic hydrocarbons (PAHs).[11] Neither sound good – and they're not.

Acrylamide is a known carcinogen (it causes cancer) and a nerve toxin. PAHs are created when food, particularly meat products, are cooked on a flame. They're the same toxic compounds that make smoke inhalation from house fires so dangerous, just in smaller amounts. Frying food also forms compounds like trans fats and pyrazines, volatile compounds that produce reactive oxygen species (ROS) often known as free radicals. ROS are a normal by-product of cellular processes and play a key role in cell signalling. However, in excess they have a negative impact on important structures, even on our DNA.[12] The body cannot heal if it is constantly firefighting the effects of these harmful chemicals.

Heating and cooking in oil just once creates these problems, but how many catering establishments change cooking oil every day? The average restaurant reheats cooking oil between 5 and 10 times before changing it. If you eat there on day 10, you're getting a huge ROS dose alongside your fries. You can tell if the oil is old – it stinks! The rancid aroma hangs in the air and seeps into your clothes. If you smell it, turn round and leave. Or just avoid eating deep-fried food altogether, as even if the oil is fresh and pristine, all the above issues still apply!

What about pan frying? Does this have the same effect? The contact point of the oil in a metal pan still rises to high temperatures; fatty foods pan fried still release ROS, PAHs and other volatile compounds. So, whilst you may ingest less oil than deep frying, the high heat itself is still an issue. This is why I recommend frying with water. The temperature in the pan is much lower and, as water evaporates at 100°C, it can't go any higher. Baking in the oven or using an air fryer is better. The heat is ambient, not direct, meaning your food avoids these excessive heats.

> **Kate's story**: Reducing her saturated fat intake by following a vegan diet had a great benefit for Kate, although she still had flare ups and needed medication. This changed once she moved to a whole-food plant-based diet, replacing refined and saturated fats with nuts, seeds, whole grains and fatty fruits like avocado. Autoimmune disease requires a highly nutrient-dense eating pattern – the effects can be remarkable.

It's important to remember that fat is not the enemy. It's an essential, healthy dietary component as long as it's eaten in its natural, whole form. High-fat foods like nuts and seeds are an essential and tasty component of a health-supporting plant-based diet and of course contain a whole range of nutrients, not just the fat.

Sugar

Sugar, or rather glucose, is the key energy source for our bodily functions. Easy to process, it's readily absorbed into the bloodstream, travelling to wherever it's needed. Our brains require a lot of energy to function and utilise 25% of the sugar we consume. This is why we have evolved to love it. There's plenty available in our food, either as natural sugars found in whole foods, or, increasingly, refined rapidly released sugars found in processed foods. A Western diet contains too few of the first and way too many of the second, making the body work harder to keep blood sugar levels at the right level – high levels can cause all sorts of damage around the body, often seen in people with poorly controlled diabetes.

Natural sugars in whole foods are bound up in complex carbohydrate fibres. Digesting these foods takes some time, resulting in a slow, sustained release of sugar (and therefore energy) in amounts the body can manage. These foods contain simple sugars like glucose and fructose, or a compound of both called sucrose. There's a lot of fearmongering and confusion around these sugars, even though they are naturally found in whole fruits, vegetables and wholegrains. Many food processing methods refine natural sugars, removing the fibre and other healthful nutrients that are in the whole food, leaving just the simple sugar compounds. This is the type of sucrose and fructose added to processed foods and drinks, often with extra fat or salt to replace some of the flavouring lost from the original ingredients, making it ultra-palatable and pinging dopamine receptors so we want to come back for more.

THE POWER OF COMBINING FAT AND SUGAR

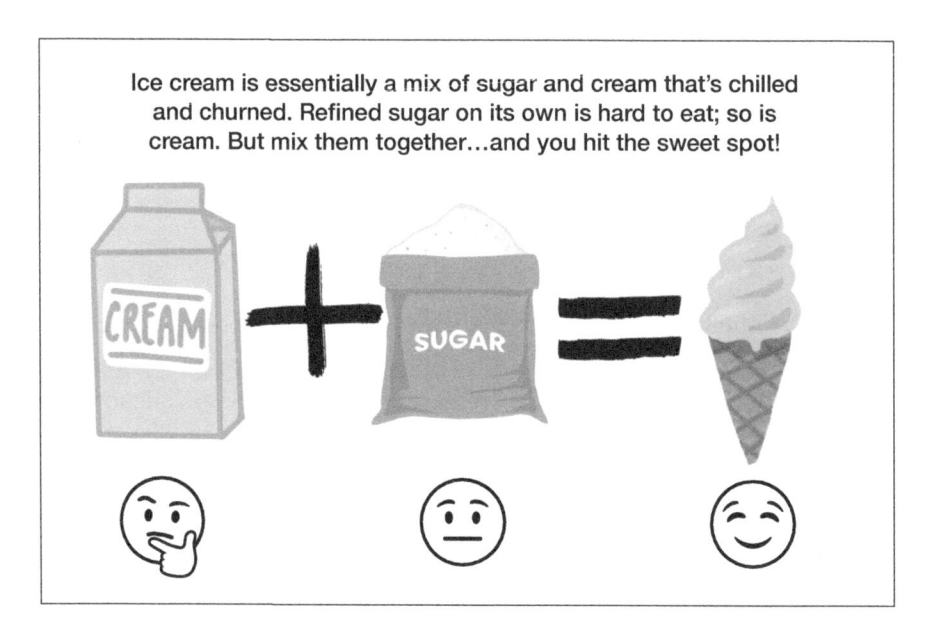

Ice cream is essentially a mix of sugar and cream that's chilled and churned. Refined sugar on its own is hard to eat; so is cream. But mix them together…and you hit the sweet spot!

The problem of added sugar

It's this **added** sugar that's a real problem in the Western diet. Along with refined fat and salt, added sugar is behind the burgeoning obesity epidemic and continual rise in chronic health conditions, including autoimmune disease.[13] Obesity creates chronic, low-grade, systemic inflammation and is now a risk factor for fuelling many types of autoimmune disease. Here's a quick summary of the processes involved.

1. Excess sugar in the bloodstream is first converted to glycogen for quick storage. These stores are only small, so the rest is converted in the liver to stable, saturated fat and stored in adipose tissue around the body, particularly the abdomen, bum and thighs. We have already explored how excess saturated fat fuels low-grade inflammation.
2. Adipose tissue expands to manage increased storage requirements. However, this tissue also excretes hormones involved in signalling like leptin, which in turn creates inflammatory cytokines like IL6, IL12 and TNF.
3. Excess refined sugar reduces gut microbiome diversity, promoting harmful microbes and reducing SCFA production, resulting in increased gut permeability and circulating LPS along with the associated inflammatory cascade.
4. Excess sugar and saturated fat increase platelet production, making blood and other cells 'sticky' and less efficient, increasing systemic stress and subsequent inflammation.
5. High levels of refined sugars accelerate cell ageing and reduce resilience.

As you can see, there's lots going on that's making the body work super hard, increasing the metabolic load and the chance of the immune system becoming confused. You don't have to look overweight to carry excess fat stores either. Fatty liver disease is an increasing issue for people eating diets full of ultra-processed foods.[14] Instead of fat from excess sugar being stored in adipose tissue, it ends up surrounding the liver and other abdominal organs, unseen and silently fuelling inflammation.

I'm not saying that foods that contain sugars should be avoided – far from it. For example, whilst whole fruit and vegetables contain some sugar, they also have a whole range of essential nutrients including fibre, vitamins, essential oils and wonderful phytonutrients which we will explore in a while. One of those groups are polyphenols which the microbiome just loves to feast on,[15] as we discovered in Chapter 2. In the polarised carb vs fat debate, 'carbohydrates' have become demonised in popular media. Complex carbs are great for health; it's the refined carbs that cause the problem. It's a shame there's not another name to clearly differentiate them.

Salt

The final nutrient in the addictive triad, salt (or sodium chloride) has an essential role in homeostasis and fluid balance (osmosis). Maintaining ideal blood sodium levels is so important that we evolved to store any extra dietary salt for when it was scarce. Animal products and fish are naturally higher in sodium but were not that easy to obtain. Potassium, which is the other important element in this balancing act, would have been readily available in plant foods foraged through the day – so much so that our bodies excrete excess amounts rather than storing it. And that was just fine until our diets changed to include more high-sodium foods, like animal products and processed and ultra-processed foods. Even adding salt to home-cooked food, especially if it includes fish and meat, is a problem, although not as much as in food cooked outside the home. Fast-food contains 100 times the amount of salt compared to home cooked. 100 times!

High-salt diets are linked to high blood pressure, which increases the risk of heart disease and stroke; people with autoimmune disease are known to have an increased risk of these other chronic health problems. There was limited research specifically on salt and autoimmune disease until recently when we have seen that salt directly influences the immune system. It's not clear for all conditions, but research studies into multiple sclerosis, rheumatoid arthritis and other inflammatory joint conditions, plus lupus, have all shown a correlation with high salt intake since the first studies on this relationship were published in 2013.[16]

What is going on? It appears that high salt levels cause osmotic stress, releasing pro-inflammatory cytokines. Increased sodium also seems to increase T cell production at a cellular level in specific tissues that then become damaged. This inflammatory response can have a knock-on effect on regulatory hormones, releasing glucocorticoids and cortisol in excess, which compounds the damage. Unsurprisingly, the gut is involved too. A high-salt diet activates Th17 cells in the gut lining, promoting inflammation. Th17 cells are found in much higher numbers in people with autoimmune disease. A high-salt environment also negatively impacts the friendly gut bacteria, changing the balance of the gut microbiome to a more inflammatory profile.[17]

A little added salt won't do us harm, but the high sodium content of many commonly eaten foods will. Tastebuds that detect salt flavour become less sensitive the more you eat. This can make whole-foods without added salt taste bland to start with. Don't worry though, as tastebud cells have a rapid turnover; after two to three weeks, the natural food flavours are no longer masked by the lack of salt, and you start to discover a whole new and tasty world of food.

Dairy

Discovering I had a strong intolerance to milk was a pivotal moment in my life. I ate a lot of it – it was in all my favourite foods. Creamy desserts, ice cream, cake, cheese. Oh, cheese! Looking back, however, it had always been a problem for me. As an adopted baby I was never breast fed, had real difficulty keeping milk down and experienced what would now be called a 'failure to thrive'. Eventually I was prescribed 'some drops' and things settled down. In spite of my mum's best efforts, I still struggled with food. I regularly vomited after meals, or when anxious or overexcited. This just became part of 'normal' for me, as did severe headaches and migraines. Nowadays I would have been diagnosed with a dairy allergy, but back in the early 1970s it wasn't really a 'thing'.

It took 40 years for me to finally discover I had an issue with dairy. Removing it from my diet was hard but life changing. The headaches eased, my very noisy guts calmed down and, after years of yo-yo dieting, I lost weight – and kept it off. Moving over to a mainly whole-food plant-based diet also helped. Unfortunately for me, I believe the damage was already done. Dairy is commonly connected to a range of autoimmune diseases.[18] I had random symptoms rumbling around for years before my MS diagnosis following acute optic neuritis and the (temporary) loss of sight in my right eye.

What is it about milk, particularly cow's milk, that triggers an autoimmune response? It's hard to know definitively, but there are several things about consuming the breast milk from another animal that are more than a bit odd, particularly as adults.

There's no doubt that milk from all mammals is nutritionally rich. Baby mammals all need mother's milk before they have developed enough to tolerate solid food. This is the time of rapid growth and development. Higher amounts of protein, fat and sugar are needed along with vitamins, minerals and other compounds like growth factors, along with the microbes that seed the microbiome. It's all good stuff. The makeup of mother's milk is ideal for each species' offspring.

Is cow's milk ideal for humans?

Cow's milk has three times the amount of protein and twice the amount of fat that human breast milk has. It's needed for calves to reach their adult size and weight (roughly 250 kg) in two years. Dairy products like cheese and cream contain high amounts of saturated fat, which we know fuels inflammation. If human babies don't need such high amounts of protein and fat, why do we think human children and adults do? Essentially, the dairy industry is huge, with a strong influence on governments and policy making, ensuring milk products appear on healthy-eating guidelines. Some countries, however, are being led by the science. Despite a strong dairy lobby, Canada has side-lined milk products, removing dairy as a group on its own from their healthy-eating guidance and adding it to options for protein choice.[19] We just don't need it.

It's not just the nutrient balance in animal milk that might be an issue.

There are other inflammatory factors involved, like pus secreted by cows with mastitis. If you drink pasteurised milk, I guess you assume that all the bad bacteria have been destroyed. They haven't. Some hardy microbes are unaffected by high temperatures. Pasteurised milk has an allowable amount of pus that can be left in. And these are not the friendly microbes that support the microbiome, but pathogenic ones out to cause harm. Dairy cows are milked twice, even three times, a day and mastitis is a huge issue; this is where the pus comes from. Yuck! Not only that, but traces of the antibiotics used to prevent or treat mastitis are also found in milk; we saw earlier on how antibiotic residue in food affects gut health and contributes to the rise in antibiotic resistance.

Dairy also contains high levels of oestrogen and other pregnancy hormones as well as growth hormones and TNF, a cytokine that promotes inflammation by stimulating both the innate and learned immune responses. Certain proteins, like butyrophilin, are also found in high amounts. Present in cell membranes, this protein has a co-signalling role in molecules that regulate T-cell activation. It's been identified as a potential trigger in autoimmunity, particularly in people with multiple sclerosis.

Finally it's worth considering that around 70% of the world's population is intolerant of lactose,[20] the sugar found in milk, causing bloating, diarrhoea and generally feeling awful. Even those who can digest lactose as a child, often lose this ability during adolescence and into adulthood. Continually consuming foods you react to has a serious impact on gut health and the microbiome. Maybe this is why people of African descent, who tend to have lactose intolerance, also have higher levels of autoimmune disease? It certainly could be a contributing factor.

Should people with autoimmune disease avoid dairy?

Research into dairy and autoimmune disease continues. The link with some conditions is clear, whereas for others it's less clear or even unknown, which is not that helpful for the autoimmune community. There is one process connected to dairy that's common in all autoimmune diseases – molecular mimicry.[21] This occurs when the immune system is consistently triggered and confuses different but very similar molecules with one another. In a bid to deal with the threat, the immune system becomes overwhelmed and identifies 'self' protein on cell walls and tissues as 'non-self'. For example, butyrophilin found in dairy milk is very similar to oligodendrocytes found in the cell wall of the myelin sheath. This is the protective fatty layer surrounding nerves in the brain and spinal cord. In an acute response, the adaptive immune system (T cells) mistakes these self-proteins with non-self (dairy) and this essential protective layer is broken down, resulting in the symptoms and limitations associated with multiple sclerosis.

Casein, another dairy protein, has the same effect in type 1 diabetes, particularly in children.[22] And interestingly, whilst gluten has the same effect for the development of coeliac disease and other inflammatory bowel diseases, dairy is also culpable, particularly in people who have not received any disease specific treatments. Indeed, molecular mimicry and dairy is connected to autoimmune conditions affecting all parts of the body including rheumatoid arthritis, idiopathic nephropathy, uveitis and Behçet's disease, a genetically based AID that affects multiple systems.

The nutrients found in dairy are readily available in other foods. As there are many other issues related to the dairy industry, such as pollution, ethics and carbon footprints, ditching dairy to reduce inflammation makes perfect sense.

Meat

I recently saw an autoimmune Facebook group thread about eating a carnivore diet to manage their condition. The carnivore diet is a meat-only diet that has been popularised by influencers and a few doctors, without any research backing. Someone claiming to be a 'qualified nutritionist' stated that meat wasn't inflammatory. They couldn't be more wrong! Claims like this concern me as it can lead desperate people to exacerbate their problems, even it if may alleviate symptoms in the (very) short term. Even small amounts of meat can trigger an inflammatory response, especially cheap, intensively farmed meat that is commonly used in fast and processed food.[23]

Chapter 3

> **Rosa's story**: Rosa was brought up vegetarian but started to eat meat as a teenager and in increasing amounts into her 20s. At the same time, she always felt tired with low energy and frequent stomach aches. When she stopped meat and started a plant-based diet, she immediately felt clearer mentally, had more regular bowel movements and noticeably fewer stomach aches.

'But humans have always eaten meat,' I hear you cry. And it's true; meat has been an important nutrient source for thousands of years, from animals that would have had space to roam and left to forage for themselves. Or at least until relatively recently. The breeds have changed too; modern farmed animals are selected for rapid growth or weight gain to meet the rising demand for chicken wings, steak or a joint for the Sunday roast. This 'progress' in animal farming creates several issues when it comes to health and specifically autoimmune disease.

1. The omega 6:3 balance is skewed. The ratio for wild meat (i.e. hunted wild animals) is generally 1:1 – the perfect balance. In farmed animals, it's around 15:1. The issue lies in animal feed, particularly in industrially farmed grain-fed animals. Even 'grass-fed' animals can have their diet supplemented with grains which pushes the ratio into a more inflammatory ratio. Meat from 100% grass-fed animals left to forage all year round and wild meat is expensive and therefore unaffordable for most people, and unsustainable.

2. Meat contains high levels of saturated fat, even traditionally low-fat options like chicken or turkey. And don't forget this fat forms volatile, toxic compounds when cooked at high or direct heat, particularly on a BBQ.

3. Viruses and bacteria from the animal can linger, especially if the meat is not kept hygienically or well cooked. In theory, these pathogens should be killed by stomach acid during digestion, but many people in the Western world have low stomach acid or take antacid medication, increasing the number of bad microbes in the digestive tract. This can lead to an overgrowth of pathogenic bacteria in the

microbiome and dysbiosis. We've already seen that people with autoimmune disease tend to have a leaky gut; meat is not helping to address this but is perpetuating it.

4. There's no fibre in meat to support the microbiome.
5. Meat contains stress and growth hormones as well as residues of antibiotics. This is a big problem for the microbiome as repeated low doses reduce gut diversity, favouring only the hardiest pathogens which then flourish. It is also fuelling the rise in antibiotic-resistant microbes, a threat to everyone's health. Over 70% of antibiotics sold globally are used in farm animals to treat infections caused by cramped, unhygienic conditions. Some countries also use them to promote animal growth despite a ban on this practice in the EU and other countries.
6. The haem-iron in meat can trigger inflammation. Iron is essential for many body functions, and low levels can lead to anaemia – characterised by lack of energy and strength, and maybe breathlessness. Iron is so essential that the body evolved to store excess amounts rather than excrete it, saving it for times of scarcity. This was important when most of the iron available came from plants – non-haem iron is harder to absorb than haem-iron from meat. But the slower absorption of iron is helpful, as excess amounts of stored iron become toxic, which then triggers inflammation. Some autoimmune conditions are specifically related to raised iron levels, like AIHA (autoimmune haemolytic anaemia) where red blood cells carrying haemoglobin are attacked, releasing excess iron into the blood. Whilst treatable, this can be a life-limiting condition. And excess iron can exacerbate joint pain and swelling in rheumatoid arthritis (RA) patients.
7. Arachidonic acid (AA), a polyunsaturated fat, found in meat, particularly poultry, is another problem for autoimmune disease.[24] It's a key part of eicosanoids, pro-inflammatory messengers. Helpful in small amounts, it's made by the body and found in low levels in many foods. A high-meat diet provides excess amounts and is known to be one of the drivers of chronic inflammation, particularly

in autoimmune diseases such as MS, type 1 diabetes, psoriasis, IBD, lupus, RA and Graves' disease. Scientists are looking at AA inhibitors as a treatment option. Why not just stop eating meat?
8. Meat contains Neu5GC, a specific sugar found in animals.[25] Humans can't synthesise it but it's easy to absorb. This alien compound triggers the immune system, which should identify and label it with a correct antibody. However, we know that an overwhelmed and confused immune system can misidentify 'self' as 'non-self', and this can occur with Neu5GC – molecular mimicry again, particularly with MS.

Kate's story: On reintroducing meat after an elimination diet, Kate found her body strongly reacted to red meat, bacon, sausages, cheese and eggs, illustrating that these products really can fuel inflammation.

Meat has been marketed as being good for us for decades, if not centuries. We're told it makes us strong and tough. In times of scarcity, a small amount is no doubt a concentrated source of essential nutrients. However, high-quality meat is expensive and not accessible to most people – nor could this be sustainable. Plants contain all the nutrients available in meat at a much lower cost.

Principal cause of deforestation of the Amazon rainforest: Cattle ranching is responsible for 80% of deforestation in the Amazon rainforest fuelled by demand for grass-fed beef. Human and planetary health are intertwined; we cannot continue destroying nature without destroying the future health of everyone and everything living on this planet.

Summary

I've covered a lot of negative information in this chapter – sorry about that! We've explored how the Western diet is full of foods that stoke inflammation and focused on specific nutrients, food groups and compounds involved and how this can trigger autoimmune reactions. I hope you're not feeling too despondent, wondering 'what in the world can I eat?'

Don't despair. From now on we're heading for the bright side. Eliminating inflammatory foods is a great start. Next, we'll be exploring the wonderful world of plant-based eating. We'll look at how whole plant foods can support the body, help reduce inflammation and autoimmune attacks and, most importantly, help your body heal.

Chapter 4

What is a whole-food plant-based diet and why does it help?

Introduction

If you're left wondering what's left to eat, don't worry! There's an abundance of super-tasty, nourishing nutrients readily available in (most) supermarkets ready for you to start exploring. I said 'most' as there are areas where healthy food is hard to access, particularly in low-income and deprived communities. If this applies to you, have a look for community kitchens and food groups in your local area. There are many dotted around with a mission not only to reduce food waste but to improve accessibility to healthy food. With free cooking classes, community fridges and 'pay what you can' shared community lunches, they are an invaluable resource for everyone. I've listed a few in the Resource section at the end of the book (page 321).

A whole-food plant-based diet is exactly as it sounds. It includes whole or minimally processed plant foods that fall into five main groups:
- Fruit
- Vegetables
- Whole grains
- Beans and pulses
- Nuts and seeds.

Packed full of essential nutrients, powerful, anti-inflammatory properties, flavour and vitality, they can also be less expensive than many animal products and processed foods. And yes, this way of eating does involve more preparation and cooking than popping a ready-meal in the microwave, but it doesn't mean you have to be a slave to the kitchen; there are plenty of super-quick meals to make. I'll also share some cooking tips and short cuts later in the book.

In this chapter, we'll focus on how nutrient-dense whole plant foods will help nourish our bodies, promote healing and help us to flourish. Even though an autoimmune condition is there for life, it doesn't mean we can't live well by eating excellent food.

First, let's have a quick look at why whole foods are key when it comes to nutrition.

Why we need whole foods

Much of the discourse around food and health focuses on individual nutrients, usually around the problem of too much fat or sugar or whether there's enough protein in the diet. I've done this myself in the last chapter when exploring the issues around saturated fat or excess salt. I'm going to do it again in this chapter as we look at specific nutrients for health. Sometimes this is important to understand the underlying issues, but let's remember we eat food, not nutrients. Focusing on constituent parts of food causes confusion, something the food industry is quite happy about! That way they can market products as 'low fat', 'low carb' or 'high protein' without many people questioning whether they're 'healthy' or 'real'.

I'm a big fan of whole foods in their natural form, or as close to it as possible. These foods retain their powerful micronutrients more readily and of course are full of gut-loving fibre. Once a natural food is processed, the nutrient balance is lost, and it becomes easy to consume more than nature intended.

Apples are the perfect example. How many can you eat in one go? Most of us, just one, or two if they're tiny. Sweet and tasty, they have lots of sugar wrapped up in complex fibre. It takes time to bite, chew and digest an apple; the sugar is released slowly along with the vitamins and phytonutrients. When you drink apple juice, however, the whole biting, chewing and digesting processes are bypassed. With the fibre removed, the sugar is readily released and absorbed into the bloodstream in higher than ideal amounts. Fresh apple juice retains many of the other micronutrients, but you still tend to drink more juice than you'd get from just one apple – most glasses contain two to three apples. Long-life or juice made from concentrate loses most of the nutrients, making it a glass of apple-flavoured sugar drink.

This same process can be applied to most foods; whole-food derivatives, or foods that are processed, concentrate the larger nutrients, lose the micronutrients and fibre and, once out of their natural form, become easy to over-consume. One way to understand this is to make almond or peanut butter at home. It's easy if you have a food processor. You'll be amazed just how many nuts there are in it and how easy it is to eat way more than a normal portion.

The importance of whole foods for the body

Eating whole foods provides the body with the full range of nutrients it needs to work effectively. It works hard 24 hours a day just supporting us to be 'alive'. Whilst we sleep, 30 trillion or so cells are still busy at work supported by energy, oxygen, nutrients, enzymes, co-factors and other tiny compounds. Demand is high, even when someone is healthy and disease free. These nutrients are also involved in cleaning up all the chemical reactions going on; for every reaction, there are always left over compounds that must be stabilised before they go rogue.

Continual supply of raw materials for the thousands of complex processes going on inside of us can never be guaranteed so resources need to be used efficiently and effectively. Many of the core processes in the body, like body temperature, blood sugar control and energy creation, are kept within tight parameters. Just like Goldilocks' porridge, our internal temperature mustn't be too hot, or too cold. The body works hard to keep us 'just right' as long as there's an ongoing availability of raw materials to work with, like glucose for energy, minerals and other micronutrients that act as co-factors or enzymes.

Of course, this is the ideal – reality can be somewhat different. A lack of raw materials, and/or an increase in stressors in the body, makes it work harder. This increases demand for certain nutrients and creates more waste that needs dealing with. If these are not readily available, nutrients are redirected from less important areas, meaning certain functions become compromised. Alternatively, back-up systems kick in until normal service is resumed – we're programmed for survival, so we're used to adapting. However, these back-ups are not for regular use as they're less efficient, demanding more nutrients and energy. This increases stress elsewhere in the body and eventually we move into the disease state - chronic low-level inflammation. We are no longer at ease!

Eating foods that supply the whole range of nutrients the body not only requires but thrives on is important for all; even more so for those of us already in that unbalanced, disease state. This is why *what* we eat is so important. And why I love eating whole plant foods. Packed full of all the tiny nutrients the body needs to function and heal, every meal is a chance to refresh our nutrient stores and support cell health. It's not just me – meta-analyses of published research show that plant-predominant diets packed full of colourful and healthy whole foods are key to disease prevention and recovery.[1]

> **We really are what we eat:** The turnover of cells in our bodies is constant. Some only have a life span of three days, others much longer, but even tough structures like bone turn over every eight years or so. All new cells, and the tissues and structures they form, use the raw materials we supply. We literally are what we eat!

A brief exploration of nutrient groups

You may have heard that it's hard to get all the nutrients required on a plant-based diet, or they're difficult to absorb. Whilst it's true there are a few nutrients which need supplementing, like B12 and vitamin D, this applies to many people eating the regular Western diet. Others, like calcium and iron, are abundant in plant foods but can still be a problem for some. Again, this applies to many people – anaemia due to low iron levels is just as common in meat eaters as non-meat eaters.[2]

Despite negative messaging in the media, a well-planned plant-based diet is suitable and healthy for all stages of life. That's not just me saying that. This is the statement from the British Dietetic Association.[3] That well-planned bit is important and should apply to all dietary patterns, not just plant-based. We've already seen how the regular Western diet doesn't reach this standard. If it sounds like hard work, don't worry; eating a range and variety of foods during the day has you well covered.

Whole plant foods are packed with nutrients the body needs to be well, and to flourish. Table 4.1 gives a very quick summary.

Table 4.1: Nutrients provided by whole plant foods

Macronutrients	Micronutrients	Other
Carbohydrates – for energy, fibre **Protein** – chains of amino acids **Fatty acids** – saturated, mono-unsaturated, polyunsaturated	**Minerals** – potassium, sodium, magnesium, iron, zinc, phosphate, calcium, selenium, boron, manganese, copper **Vitamins** – water-soluble: B complex, C – fat-soluble – A, D, E and K	**Phytonutrients** – in their thousands! Includes carotenoids, flavonoids and polyphenols **Fibre** – insoluble and soluble fibre which includes resistant starch and prebiotics

Nutrition has been studied for years and scientists are still making new discoveries about how foods and their nutrients work in the body. Looking at nutrients separately is important, but getting bogged down into exploring the minute detail can blur the overall picture. Nutrients interact and impact each other. They might compete for absorption, or enhance absorbability, work together to maximise effectiveness or combine to form building blocks required for other compounds and co-factors essential for cellular processes.

We need carbohydrates for energy and to fuel cellular processes. Proteins, made of chains of amino acids, are the building blocks of all body structures. Fat insulates our bodies and is used for fuel, essential compounds and transporting fat-soluble nutrients. But the macronutrients are not the whole story. Minerals are essential co-factors for all bodily functions and, whilst they're required from food, less essential functions can release their minerals in times of scarcity. This doesn't happen with vitamins though, particularly water-soluble vitamins B and C.

> **Fun fact:** What do humans, apes, bats and guinea pigs have in common? They are the only mammals that can't make vitamin C.

Currently, 10% of the world population suffers from undernourishment and subsequent malnutrition.[4] Whilst this has reduced in some areas due to world food programmes, famine due to adverse weather or war and conflict affects millions of people. Opposite that, though, is another type of malnutrition – over-nutrition. This is not just seen in the Western world, but also in developing countries where populations move away from traditional diet patterns towards a Western diet pattern. Ultra-processed and fast foods, loaded with higher-than-needed macronutrients (fat, protein and sugar) and devoid of healthful micronutrients, phytonutrients and fibre are leading to populations that are overfed but undernourished.

It's not a wonder therefore that this rapid change in dietary patterns lies side by side with increasing levels of chronic health conditions including autoimmune disease which, as we saw in Chapter 1, affects a massive 10% of the Western population.

Having established the importance of eating whole foods, and the absolute basics of nutrition, let's have a brief look at how food processing impacts this nutrient balance and the challenge of ultra-processed foods. So prevalent in everyday eating, they can be hard to avoid and sometimes even to identify as they're often hidden in plain sight.

Chapter 4

Levels of processing and ultra-processed foods

The system of food production has radically transformed in the last 80 years or so. Home-cooked meals made from raw, whole ingredients are becoming a rarity. In the UK alone, around 60% of food eaten is classified as ultra-processed. This rises to a whopping 80% in children and adolescents[5] – a future health crisis in the making?

Ultra-processed foods are so embedded in modern food systems it can be hard to spot them. Facsimiles of traditional foods, they present as easy, time-saving and cost-effective meals. In today's busy world, time, energy and money are at a premium. Ultra-processed foods are portrayed as costing less in all these areas.

Whilst there is still no universally agreed definition of ultra-processed foods, they can be described as 'formulations of ingredients, mostly of exclusive industrial use, typically created by a series of industrial techniques and processes'.[6] Yum, tasty. Not! In a nutshell, they are packaged foods where the ingredients have been industrially altered from their original state, containing additives, preservatives and emulsifiers.

Rosa's story: Rosa notices a big reduction in her energy levels and increase in brain fog when she eats ultra-processed foods, so she sticks to whole foods whenever she can.

These foods tend to contain high amounts of altered fats, often stable saturated fats, sugar and salt – the triad of flavours that pings our dopamine receptors and makes us want more. They are often cheap by-products of other food products, like high-fructose corn syrup, a highly concentrated sugar, extracted from corn kernels. In many countries, these crops are also used for animal feed and supported by government subsidies. This supports the production of cheap food, with a high cost.

> **Subsidies for animal agriculture:** Farmers working in animal agriculture in the UK and elsewhere receive a number of subsidies and other support from government. Most of the animals involved are grain-fed to some extent, often because the animal breeds are not hardy enough to live outside to graze all year round. Meat from grain-fed animals has an inflammatory imbalance in omega 6 to 3 fatty acids. It's also an inefficient use of resources: 40% of crops grown are fed to animals and animal agriculture uses 85% of farmland in the UK, but meat only produces 30% of dietary calories. These subsidies are supporting the rise in chronic health conditions, at a cost of billions. The government (and therefore our taxes) are financing this! Why not support the farmers financially to grow crops for direct human consumption that in turn help to support rather than hinder health?

Levels of food processing

Processing food has always been a key part of the human diet. From the discovery of fire to the establishment of farming, nutrient-dense food was key to the success of our early ancestors. Processing raw produce promoted human development as well as access to food all year round. With our modern food system though, understanding what is and what is not ultra-processed can be tricky. Fortunately, a nutritional scientist in Brazil – Professor Carlos Monteiro – developed a classification system called NOVA which is summarised in Table 4.2.[7] As food processing is a normal process that humans have always undertaken in some form, this system starts with whole or minimally processed food at level 1 down to ultra-processed at level 4.

This classification is still open to nuances, but is a useful, simple guide to follow. Essentially, if you pick up a product with a long list of ingredients that includes words like mono- and diglycerides of fatty acids, gum, maltodextrin or lecithin, it's best to put it straight back on the shelf.

Table 4.2: The NOVA classification of food processing levels[7]

Level 1	Unprocessed or minimally processed foods like whole fruit, vegetables, beans etc
Level 2	Processed culinary ingredients used to extend shelf life or flavour like herbs, fats, vinegar etc
Level 3	Processed foods that are a mix of levels 1 and 2, like cooked tinned beans, traditionally made bread, preserved fruit etc
Level 4	Ultra-processed food (UPF), formulations of multiple ingredients that include additives, preservatives, modified starch, emulsifiers, hydrogenated nutrients etc

Kate's story: Although Kate's condition greatly improved on a vegan diet, a fundamental healing shift only occurred once she removed refined grains and ultra-processed foods after being inspired by a fellow vegan runner.

Avoiding ultra-processed foods is imperative if you want to start along the healing process or prevent it developing if you are at risk. As we have already explored, saturated and refined fats, sugar, meat, dairy and salt can all contribute to inflammation as well as disrupt the gut lining and the microbiome. Ultra-processed foods are calorie dense but devoid of many beneficial micronutrients, phytonutrients or fibre. What's been taken out is not the only issue – the chemicals added in are a big problem too. Many disrupt the beneficial bacteria, and some can actively damage the lining of the gut wall, particularly chemicals like emulsifiers.[8]

Emulsifiers: Fat and water don't mix, which is not a problem in whole foods as fibre keeps everything together. Once processing has removed it, though, fat and water separate, which can be a problem in ultra-processed foods. So, chemicals called emulsifiers, like polysorbate 80, guar gum, carrageenan and lecithin are added. This reduces or prevents this natural separation, creating creamier, more palatable products. However, research has now linked these additives to inflammatory bowel disease and other chronic health problems. It seems that emulsifiers promote the pro-inflammatory molecules that contribute to a leaky gut, a key underlying cause of autoimmune disease. There is some evidence that soya and sunflower lecithin don't have the same impact, but as eminent gastroenterologist Dr Alan Desmond suggests, it's best just to avoid them all whenever you can.

It is, however, a challenge to avoid additives in foods that have been stored and packed, even level 1 and 2 foods. Reading ingredients labels can help identify them. Ultimately, cooking at home is the only way to ensure you know what is in your food. The recipes found in the second half of this book (see page 169) are a great way of ensuring you are nourishing your body and avoiding many of these toxic chemicals. Once your body has reduced its inflammatory load and your gut health has improved, you might be able to tolerate a tiny amount of ultra-processed food. But by then, your tastebuds will have tuned in to eating fresh, wholesome food, so you might well find it's just a big, disappointment.

'Processes and ingredients used to manufacture ultra-processed foods are designed to create highly profitable (low-cost ingredients, long-shelf life, emphatic branding), convenient (ready to consume) hyper-palatable products liable to displace freshly prepared dishes and meals made from all other NOVA food groups.'

Dr Christian van Tulleken, Ultra-Processed People[9]

Essential fibre

Whilst exploring gut health back in Chapter 2, you may have noticed a small but important word kept popping up – fibre. Found in complex carbohydrates, fibre is found in all – and only – plant foods. Sometimes called 'dietary fibre', or 'roughage', unlike sugars and starches, fibre reaches the large intestine mainly undigested.

If you remember, fibre plays many important roles in the gut. It:
- slows the breakdown and absorption of sugars into the bloodstream.
- helps stimulate the gut to keep waste products moving along.
- prevents constipation and moderates transit time.
- acts as nature's 'Brillo pad', cleaning the gut as it moves along, collecting inflammatory debris like LDL cholesterol and secondary bile salts.
- feeds the microbiome.
- provides the raw ingredients for short-chain fatty acid (SCFA) production.

> **Differentiating 'good' from 'bad' carbs:** Carbs have been demonised. Many people are fearful that a 'high-carb diet' will lead to weight gain. It seems such a shame that there's not better terminology to separate refined, unhealthy carbs from whole, healthful carbs. Food is complicated as soon as processing and refining are involved. Ironically, you can find 'low-carb' products with different types of fibre added back in. Fearmongering is rife, particularly online. And it's not the end user who seems to be benefiting; someone is making a lot of money somewhere!

Different plants contain different combinations of fibre. When you eat a variety of whole foods, you naturally get a combination of them all; this is what the gut needs to thrive. There are three main types of fibre found in whole foods – soluble, insoluble and fermentable fibre, which has characteristics of the first two. The box on page 80 gives a short summary. If you want to know more, see Appendix 1.

The next big question is how much fibre should we eat? The current government guidelines state 30 g a day.[10] Unfortunately, only 4% of the UK population hit that target.[11] No wonder there's such a surge in chronic health problems. If 30 g sounds a lot, don't worry. It's surprisingly easy when you eat a variety of whole plant foods throughout the day; many people happily consume around 50 g a day.

If that's making your stomach rumble and groan, you're not alone. A sudden big increase in fibre can cause bloating or lots of wind if you're

DIFFERENT TYPES OF FIBRE

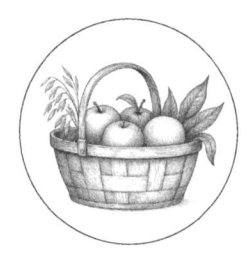

① Soluble fibre:
- Dissolves in water, forming a gloopy gel
- Found in the cell wall of plants: fruit, veg, pulses, grains like oats and seeds
- Can help lower cholesterol levels, manage blood sugar levels and provide food for friendly gut microbes.

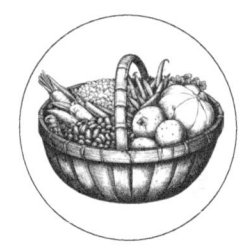

② Insoluble fibre:
- Does not dissolve in water
- Found in skins and outer husks of grains, nuts, seeds and some vegetables and in the outside skins of pulses and beans
- Promotes gut motility/bowel movements
- Supports immune function.

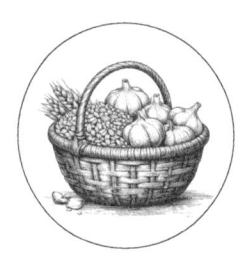

③ Fermentable fibre:
- A soluble fibre with some insoluble fibre
- Found in oats and legumes in particular
- Undigested in the small intestine, feeds the microbiome
- Sometimes called 'prebiotics'.

used to a low-fibre diet. That's your gut microbes having a party on the extra raw materials you've just given them. If your dominant microbes are pathogenic varieties, they can produce particularly explosive gas, especially if they have moved up into the end of the small intestine. This may make you wary of increasing fibre intake; you may have even been told not to.

The problem of FODMAPs

We saw in Chapter 2 that abdominal bloating, excess gas and pain are all signs of dysbiosis, as is a leaky gut that can lead to food intolerances or sensitivities. We also saw how fermented fibre helps the microbiome form short-chain fatty acids that can in turn help heal a leaky gut and support a healthy balance of microbes. However, if eating fibre produces such bad side effects, it can be hard to know what to do. One solution is to avoid FODMAPs – fermentable oligosaccharides, disaccharides, monosaccharides and polyols. Such a long name; it's obvious why an acronym is essential!

FODMAPs are simple chained, fermentable carbohydrates found in plant foods. The microbiome loves them and readily converts them to short-chain fatty acids. Unfortunately, in dysbiosis, this process goes haywire, and the gas produced causes pain, bloating and severe wind. FODMAPs are found in some super-healthy foods, which creates a real dilemma: what to do?

Low FODMAP diets are often suggested for people experiencing uncomfortable gut symptoms. This means eliminating highly fermentable foods for between four and eight weeks followed by slowly reintroducing them one at a time. It was never designed to be a permanent way of eating as the removed foods are also the ones that readily support gut health. Not only are they prebiotics (gut microbiome food), but many of the fruit, vegetables, whole grains and beans contain polyphenols and other compounds that benefit our health. Unfortunately, these foods have gained a bad reputation and, without the right support, many people never reintroduce them. Never eating these foods focuses on the symptoms, not the underlying problems.

UNDERSTANDING FODMAPs

Lactose: the simple sugar found in milk and the sugar that 70% of the world's population can't digest.

Galacto-oligosaccharides (GOS): complex sugar chains mainly found in beans and legumes which are well known wind machines!

Polyols: sugars like mannitol and sorbitol found in artificial sweeteners as well as some fruit and veg.

Fructose: the simple sugar found in many fruit, some veggies like asparagus and Jerusalem artichokes, and sugar syrups ranging from ultra-processed high-fructose corn syrup to honey.

Fructans: saccharide chains made of three or more carbon atoms, otherwise known as oligosaccharides; found in whole grains, some fruit and veggies including garlic and onions.

Plus, only eating low-fibre foods is known to be bad for gut health; dysbiosis will never be resolved; it will only get worse.

Eating a low-FODMAP diet is often the advice given to people with inflammatory bowel disease (IBD) even though plant fibre should be encouraged, not avoided. Research has shown that, once in remission, 92% of patients eating a plant-predominant diet stayed in remission compared to 33% of omnivores.[12] A treatment plan featuring a low-fibre diet may seem to make sense if diarrhoea is a problem, but in essence it continues to starve the microbiome of short-chain fatty acids. Fibre can not only reduce chronic diarrhoea in IBD, but, by feeding the microbiome, it helps to heal the gut lining as well as send signals to the immune system to prevent further localised attacks in the gut.

> **Tricia's story:** After doing some research, Tricia put herself onto a low-fibre diet for 3–4 months during the acute stage of her Crohn's disease flare up. Even though she found her diet bland and pretty tasteless, her symptoms not only stopped getting worse but started to improve. Feeling better, she was nervous about introducing more whole foods. Listening to her body, she gradually introduced higher-fibre foods, including wholegrain bread and pasta, before upping the variety of vegetables on her plate. This slow but steady method meant her body had time to heal. Now her gut has improved, and her microbiome has re-established, she can enjoy all types of high-fibre foods.

The same has been specifically shown for rheumatoid arthritis, MS,[13] psoriasis, lupus,[14] Hashimoto's and Graves' disease and type 1 diabetes, and there appears to be a consensus that complex fibre and the subsequent production of SCFAs is beneficial for autoimmune disease overall.[16] The microbiome is totally dependent on us to provide the fibre it needs to help calm the immune system, to ensure that it works for, rather than against, us.

Everyone's microbiome is unique and at first you may find eating more fibre a challenge. You don't have to do it all at once though; a gradual increase works well for most people and there are ways to help reduce the windy after-effects. If you are someone who really struggles with FODMAPs though, please get advice from a specialist dietitian or nutritionist who can create an individualised programme for you.

Healing nutrients

Apart from macronutrients, micronutrients and fibre, there's another group of tiny compounds in whole plant foods – phytonutrients. Found abundantly in fruit and vegetables, as well as other whole plant foods, these compounds have a strong anti-inflammatory effect on the body. And they look good too, as phytonutrients are stored in colourful pigments, making those foods enticing to our human eye.

Currently over 25,000 phytonutrients have been identified with new ones being discovered all the time. It's an exciting area of research and, for me, makes eating a whole-food plant-based diet even more enjoyable, knowing that each mouthful is packed with the goodness my body needs to heal.

Phytonutrients are involved in several roles in the body, including signalling pathways, supporting the immune system, metabolic processes and stress responses. Along with vitamins A, C and E, phytonutrients also have a strong antioxidant effect in the body, which protects us from oxidative stress and reduces inflammation and subsequent chronic health conditions, including autoimmune disease.

> **Oxidative stress** can be caused by excessive amounts of highly reactive molecules called ROS – reactive oxygen species. Released as by-products of cell metabolism, they are involved in a variety of processes including signalling. High levels can increase inflammation, damage healthy cells and even lead to cell death.

Antioxidants neutralise pesky ROS, or 'free radicals', by connecting to them, forming stable compounds that don't cause harm. It's important to ensure the body is provided with a good amount of these helpful compounds throughout the day, particularly during times of stress or ill-health. At these times, the body must work harder; this increased effort creates even higher levels of free radicals. If the supply of antioxidants is low, there won't be enough to quash them all, creating oxidative stress which damages cell membranes, proteins, fats and even our DNA. If continual, cells can even die, and their functions will be lost.

Phytonutrients help our bodies to work efficiently, effectively and effortlessly. Isn't that fantastic? It makes sense to consume these foods that help support the immune system, as our bodies needs all the help available. (You can find out more about antioxidants, free radicals and telomeres on my website: https://thesensitivefoodiekitchen.com/antioxidants-and-free-radicals-how-do-they-impact-health/.)

Every type of plant eaten contains a plethora of phytonutrients. Some have been well researched, like lycopene found in tomatoes, which can help reduce prostate cancer; or curcumin, found in the bright yellow root turmeric, highly effective at reducing pain and swelling, particularly in joints. Much of this research is aimed at discovering new medications or supplements; there is a lot of money to be made in chronic health conditions. However, isolating or concentrating these compounds alters how they work naturally and may not provide the positive effects hoped for if no other diet or lifestyle changes are made. Indeed, in some cases, supplementing with certain phytonutrients can cause harm. For example, studies examining the supplementation of concentrated amounts of beta-carotene for reducing lung cancer found it *increased* the risk in those who continued to smoke.[15] This wasn't an issue when beta-carotene-containing foods were eaten, though.

This reductionist approach of focusing on just one compound in food misses out on the positive effect of all the others. There are multiple phytonutrients in every food and, alongside minerals and vitamins, they work together as a team to support cellular function, protection and overall body health.

There is just too much to write about phytonutrients in this book – many people have got there before me too! You can find a summary of the main ones in Appendix 2. There's one group I want to have a deeper look at though as our microbiome loves them as much as our cells – polyphenols.

Polyphenols

There are currently over 8000 known polyphenols; these largely fall into four groups with slightly different structures and roles. These colourful compounds protect plants from oxidative damage, like excess UV rays from the sun, and resist attacks from pathogens. They can do the same for us. Food processing, like cooking, can cause the loss of some polyphenols but enable the release of others, so eating a mix of raw and cooked foods throughout the day gives you the best of both worlds.

Polyphenols are becoming recognised as essential for preventing certain health conditions, especially neurodegenerative diseases like Alzheimer's and ageing cognitive decline. A group called anthocyanins, found in purple or blue foods, are particularly effective at reducing oxidative stress in the brain,[17] which is great news although there are many more elements to managing and maintaining brain health.

What about autoimmune disease? Polyphenols contain immuno-modulatory agents, compounds that positively influence inflammatory signalling pathways – they can turn inflammation down. Equally exciting is that they also positively impact our genes. In a process called epigenetic modulation, these tiny compounds help to switch off the genes connected to autoimmune conditions and even help prevent them being switched on in the first place. That is certainly something to celebrate!

Research into polyphenols has found positive effects in a range of autoimmune conditions, including vitiligo, ulcerative colitis, Sjögren's, MS and more. One paper concludes that when taken together, polyphenols make 'promising candidates for novel therapeutics in autoimmune disease'.[18] In other words, they could be made into a pill sometime in the future. Why not get ahead of the game by making them a key feature of every meal so you can start experiencing those beneficial effects right now?

Polyphenols are good for gut health too. These colourful compounds have a direct impact on the cells lining the gut wall, helping to switch off inflammatory signalling that initiates attacks on the tight junctions and protective layer of mucin. They are also a favourite dining option for friendly microbes, promoting the growth of beneficial bacteria and reducing pathogenic ones. Polyphenols also help form short-chain fatty acids. As we saw earlier, these not only form a smorgasbord of dining options for the microbes but act as signalling molecules when abundantly available, helping to reduce the inflammatory response. Short-chain fatty acids create a more acidic environment, perfect for beneficial bacteria to flourish, but not pathogenic ones, transforming the make-up of the microbiome.

The multi-positive impact of gut healing, microbiome transformation and direct action at cell level throughout the body means polyphenols, along with all types of phytonutrients, are highly beneficial for everyone, especially those of us with chronic inflammatory conditions like autoimmune disease.

Healthy fats

In the previous chapter we looked at different types of fat and how saturated and adulterated fats contribute to chronic inflammation. Now it's time to explore the types of fat we want to include, particularly those found in whole plant foods.

No one can avoid saturated fat 100%. Nor do we want to, as we need small amounts for various functions. Saturated fats are found in variable amounts in whole foods alongside mono- and polyunsaturated fat. A few plant foods contain high amounts of saturated fat, particularly coconut and its products. Palm oil is also sourced from plants but worth avoiding wherever possible.

Coconut oil is often celebrated as a healthy saturated fat, often focusing on the medium-chain triglycerides (MCT). These make up around 60% of the fats in coconut. They are promoted as being good for heart health and inflammation as these types of fat are more readily burnt for energy. MCT oil is now available, at a premium price. Is it beneficial for people with autoimmune disease? One trial in people with rheumatoid arthritis compared patients taking MCT oil supplemented with added fibre with others taking a standard triglyceride/saturated fat supplement.[19] The MCT group showed a significant reduction in their inflammation score compared to the control group. This looks like a great win for MCT oil. There's a big question over this result, though – was it the MCT oil or the added fibre that made the difference?

Other trials in mice with MS found that MCT oil (along with a ketogenic diet) can calm inflammatory cascades and the destruction of myelin.[20] However, we are not mice and react differently, so I would say this is not a green light yet. One other thing to point out is the process to extract MCTs is complex, requiring fractionation, esterification (adding to glycerine to make triglycerides), filtration, deacidification, bleaching and finally deodorising – all the processes used for highly refined and ultra-processed oils. You don't need any of that for whole foods!

Essential fatty acids again

Earlier on we looked at the essential fatty acids and how omega 3 is involved in anti-inflammatory pathways and omega 6, whilst having a small part in reducing inflammation, mainly operates in the inflammatory pathway. Plants are a great source of essential fatty acids. Highly processed oils, however, contain high levels of omega 6; the Western diet is packed full of them in processed foods, fast foods and margarines, not to mention the imbalance in meat and dairy products from grain-fed animals.

Omegas 3 and 6 are both absorbed through the same channels and, although the body doesn't favour one over the other, they compete for absorption. If one is available in higher amounts than the other, it's more readily absorbed. This means if you are eating a Western-style diet, omega 6 is dominant, contributing to chronic inflammation. Eating whole plant foods can redress this balance. Omega 3 fatty acids are found in all sorts of whole plant foods including wholegrains, green vegetables and some nuts and seeds.

Alpha lipoic acid (ALA) is the main form of omega 3 found in plants. It needs to be converted to DHA and EPA, the bioactive forms of omega 3 used in metabolic processes, a reaction that requires various compounds and co-factors. If someone has poor nutrition, these may not be readily available; the benefits of ALA have been questioned if it is not properly converted.[21] A nutrient-dense diet, however, can overcome this, which makes a whole-food plant-based diet well positioned to support the conversion of ALA to DHA and EPA, although this can take time. To start with, additional supplementation is usually a good idea.

When it comes to omega 3 supplementation, fish oil usually comes to mind. Take a step back from that; oily fish as part of the diet has always been promoted as a great source of essential fatty acids. Many dietary programmes for autoimmune disease include oily fish as a cheap and readily available option. They provide a direct source of DHA and EPA (as they have already done the conversion), it's cheap and readily available. So why don't I include it in my book?

Sadly, fish is no longer as healthy, or sustainable, as it used to be. Fish numbers are severely depleted due to overfishing, contaminated with heavy metals dumped at sea and polluted with plastics leading to a compromised food source that contains increasing levels of toxins like mercury and microplastics.[22] In the past, only larger fish like tuna and swordfish were affected, but now even small fish, like mackerel and sardines, are being contaminated. Recent research has identified microplastics in food triggering inflammation, disrupting the microbiome and provoking immune responses, all the things we are trying to avoid. Fish farming is just as bad, if not worse. Poor standards of care and the overuse of antibiotics create problems for the fish and their consumers whilst polluting local waterways.

Supplementing omega 3

This all takes us back to fish oil. Consistently promoted as healthy, high demand is contributing to the problems. Krill, the perfect whale food, are being overfished for krill oil, causing a problem for whales, the guardians of our oceans. Larger fish contain contaminants, so smaller fish, like mackerel and herring, are being sourced as cod is at dangerously low levels. These are being caught before they are fully developed, further reducing stocks. Human demand is too high; sustainable options are needed instead.

Algae oil is one. After all, this is where the fish get their omega 3 from! Algae farms are popping up to meet the demand; these also help to sequester carbon dioxide, making them more sustainable too. Algae oil carries a higher price tag than fish oil; hopefully this will come down as supply increases. Algae food sources like nori, spirulina and chlorella powder also offer reasonable amounts of omega 3 and can be incorporated into daily smoothies, plant-based recipes or sushi.

Seeds like chia, flax and hemp contain good amounts of ALA; including these in your diet every day will help. They are also great sources of plant protein, and fibre, so increase the amount gradually whilst your gut gets used to them. Cold-pressed flaxseed oil provides a concentrated amount of omega 3 fatty acids – adding a tablespoon or two to your food during the day gives you a hefty dose of ALA for your body to work with. This is a highly volatile oil and rapidly goes rancid if not prepared or stored correctly. The plus side is that there's no way you will consume 'bad' oil as it's so foul it's intolerable. You can only tell this in oil, not capsules, and you should never use it for cooking. Add it as a garnish before eating your meal or in dressings or smoothies. In the UK we have some fantastic flax farms that provide high-quality flaxseed oil – the details are in the Resources section (page 321).

When it comes to nuts, walnuts contain the best amounts of omega 3; most other nuts contain some, but omega 6 dominates. Nuts are great for other nutrients though, so still play an important role in a balanced plant-based diet.

Summary

This chapter has explored the wonderful benefits of eating a whole-food plant-based diet as it's packed full of gut-loving fibre, body-loving phytonutrients and fabulously healthy fats.

I hope by now you are feeling confident that eating whole plant foods is going to support your body to heal in a natural and sustainable way. You may still have some niggling questions at the back of your mind about whether plants are actually good for you, or, as one US doctor has declared, the concern that 'plants are trying to kill you'. I'll address this in Chapter 6 (page 107) where I'll do some myth-busting. By now, you might be raring to make some positive changes, so next let's look at ways to start your healing journey.

Chapter 5

Starting your healing journey: Seven steps to healing from the inside out

Introduction

The hardest part of making changes that last is to start. It can be overwhelming, especially when it's a profound shift, like changing the way you eat. Having a roadmap of simple changes can minimise the overwhelm whilst making a big difference. Before I share my Seven Steps to healing from the inside out, I do have a proviso. Please remember that **everyone is different**. What works for one person may not be so effective for another. This particularly applies if you:

- have food allergies or sensitivities; your body may respond differently, particularly if you avoid key food groups. Leaky gut is so common in autoimmune disease, most of us have at least one.
- take prescribed medications; these may interact and interfere with progress. If you are doing so, please see the footnote below.*
- your gut microbiota are unique (and that's true for all of us) and will respond differently to others. Even genetically identical twins won't have the same microbiome.
- have nutrient deficiencies or absorption issues. This is common in

---

*Please don't stop taking any prescribed medications without first discussing doing so with your doctor or specialist nurse; they can advise if it's safe to do so. Some medications, particularly antidepressants, blood thinners and some painkillers, must be reduced gradually to avoid unpleasant side effects or potentially dangerous reactions. Some plants interact with pharmaceuticals – please see Chapter 8 (page 153) for more information.

autoimmune disease. For some, additional supplementation may be needed in the short term. A plant-based nutritionist will be able to offer personal advice.

> **Kate's story:** Kate laughs at how bad her food tasted when she first moved to a whole-food diet. Being used to added sugar, salt and oils, her taste-buds took time to adjust. Once they had, and she'd learnt how to create tasty meals, there was no thought of going back to her old ways of eating.

Eating a whole-food plant-based diet is not a magic pill that makes everything disappear overnight, although that would be a wonderful thing for sure. It takes time: patience is key. You may even feel a little worse to start with as your body adjusts, so listen to your body and what it's able to do. It's working hard, with all those trillions of cells jostling with each other for the right combination of nutrients. It can take time to clear out the waste and push your body towards healing. With luck, you will start to feel the benefits within a few days, more so over the following weeks and months. It may be a bumpy ride, but your body knows how to heal. It just needs the right materials to do it.

Ready to get started? Okay, let's go.

Step 1 – Eat more fresh vegetables and fruit

This may not seem like rocket science, but only a third of adults in the UK hit the five-a-day target.[1] This means a scary two-thirds are not getting the bare minimum required to support health, even though five is itself a number chosen as an achievable target, one that helps reduce the risk of *dying* from chronic health problems. So, what is the optimal amount?

A meta-analysis of published research by scientists at Imperial College London in 2017 showed that 10 portions of fruit and vegetables every day is a healthier target and that more is even better.[2] If you're struggling to eat two or three, don't be put off. The key really is the more you eat, the better it is for your body. So, whatever your starting point, look to have more.

If you are already eating plenty of fresh fruit and veg but not feeling the benefits, other elements of your diet might be the issue, or even other aspects of your lifestyle, like stress or lack of exercise. Everything has an impact. It could just be a simple tweak though, so here are a few ideas to help you troubleshoot.

- Are your portions big enough? Each portion should be approximately 80 g – an easy measure is roughly a handful.
- Do you eat a variety or limit yourself to a handful of products? You need to eat different fruit and vegetables to get the whole range of nutrients and their benefits. Eating a huge amount of just one vegetable has the potential to negatively impact your microbiome rather than help.
- Are you eating just cooked fruit and vegetables? Heat can deplete some nutrients so eat a mix of raw and cooked during the day.
- How is your gut health? You may not be able to absorb all the available nutrients right now. This should improve over time. If you have ulcerative colitis or Crohn's disease, you may need some additional support from a qualified dietitian or nutritionist.

As always, gut health is key. We have already seen that people with autoimmune disease have dysbiosis. The polyphenols packed into fresh produce will help to support and restore the microbiome, but it will take time. Check out the Resources section at the end of this book (page 321) if you feel you need professional guidance.

If you're below five portions a day, 10 may well be overwhelming. Aim to get to five as soon as you can and just carry on increasing the amount. If you're wondering how to do that, here are some ideas:

- Add extra portions to your main meal. This is a simple yet effective way, especially for leafy green veg, like steamed broccoli, cabbage or kale.
- Make soup full of veggies (see recipes on pages 188 to 201) – tasty, filling and an effective way of eating more veg without realising.
- Eat a fresh salad every day. It doesn't have to be fancy, but make sure

you vary the ingredients. Not only is this a great way to up veg and fruit intake (as I enjoy apple, pear or grapes in a salad), but it helps increase the variety too.
- If you need a quick snack, have a piece of fruit or some carrot sticks instead of a biscuit. I know that doesn't sound very exciting, but you'll feel great – and angelic too! One of my favourite snacks is a walnut stuffed inside a date. Three of those will vanquish any hunger pangs for me.
- Add fresh fruit to your breakfast, like frozen raspberries, blueberries or mango. Or grate an apple or pear into your porridge. If you have a cooked breakfast, add in tomato, mushroom and/or a good portion of leafy greens like spinach or kale.
- Green smoothies are a great way to increase your raw food intake. Be bold and brave with a mix of kale and spinach with some lemon juice (to help you absorb the nutrients) and a banana or chunks of pineapple to make it more palatable.

All the recipes in the second half of this book are packed full of different ways to enjoy lots of fresh produce throughout the day. When fruit and veg fill up half of your plate, you know you're heading in the right direction.

Step 2 – Eat healthy fats

Many whole plant foods contain healthy fats, including whole grains, soya beans and even cruciferous vegetables like broccoli and Brussels sprouts. Fruit like avocado and olives have mono-unsaturated fats mixed up in the fibre too.

Nuts and seeds provide the most concentrated form of essential fatty acids. The ratio of omega 3 to 6 varies within both groups so it's important not to stick to eating the same type all the time. Walnuts have the best ratio of omega 3 to 6. They're good for brain health – they even look like a brain! All nuts also contain minerals, fibre and other healthful compounds.

Flax, chia and hemp seeds are all excellent sources of omega 3 fatty acid in the form alpha-linoleic acid (ALA). As mentioned in the last chapter, ALA must be converted to the bioactive forms of omega 3, DHA and EPA. Whilst at first this may seem a poorer source, consuming ALA daily can still bring the body back to a better balance of omega 3 to 6 over time. These seeds contain much more than just ALA of course, including protein, minerals and lots of fibre.

Flaxseeds have a tough outer coating that can't be digested. If eaten whole, they'll come out looking the same as they went in, so make sure you grind them before consumption. The oils in flaxseed are highly volatile and, once ground, they should be kept in the fridge and used up within a month. I prefer to buy whole flaxseeds, grind them myself and store them in a jar in the fridge. Buying ready-ground flaxseed means you're never sure how old it is, or how well it's been stored.

Chia seeds can also be ground or left to soak for a few hours. As the water is absorbed, the seeds swell, making the omega 3, protein and other nutrients available for absorption. Soaked, they do look a bit like frog spawn, but don't let that put you off. This gloop is the mucilaginous fibre which is fabulous for the gut. I add chia seeds to overnight oats or chia pots to eat for breakfast, or in a custard-like dessert with summer fruit making them super-tasty, not just healthy.

Hemp seeds must be shelled before eating. Buying them hulled is a convenient option. They contain the least amount of omega 3 compared to chia and flax, but have a fantastic array of other nutrients, including protein, magnesium, iron and zinc. Some people find the fibre of hemp seeds more tolerable than that of flaxseeds, making them a good alternative.

Omega 3 fatty acid is also found in edible seaweed and algae. These foods are eaten in different amounts around the world. Laverbread, a type of seaweed, used to be commonly eaten in the UK as a cheap and nutritional food source, but is not popular today. Japanese cuisine is a tasty option, with nori commonly used. You can also find edible seaweed snacks or powdered chlorella and spirulina to add to green smoothies. I'm not a fan – they taste too much like pond water to me.

> **There is a note of caution with seaweed and algae**, especially in powdered form. It's good to check out the provenance as some products are poorly produced and can contain toxins and bacteria, something you certainly want to avoid. Chlorella also contains iodine and can be contraindicated if you have thyroid issues. It's advisable to avoid during pregnancy and breastfeeding too, just as a precaution. If you are not sure, check with your healthcare professional or dietitian, if you have one, to check if it's right for you.

Whilst this Seven Step programme is focused on eating whole plant foods, research has suggested that people with autoimmune disease should supplement with omega 3. To avoid fish oil, the plant-based options are cold-pressed flaxseed oil and algae oil. Both are an acquired taste. Algae oil contains DHA and EPA – it's where the fish get omega 3 from after all. Price-wise, it is more expensive than fish oil but the environmental cost is much lower. Cold-pressed flaxseed oil contains ALA so has to be converted to DHA and EPA by your body. It is highly volatile and goes rancid if not properly prepared or stored. You'll know for sure if flaxseed oil has gone off – it's foul – and smells foul too! I recommend buying it direct from a good producer, not from a store, so you can guarantee quality and freshness. I've added a couple of options in the Resources section (page 321).

Remember whilst increasing your intake of healthy fats, you also need to lower your intake of unhealthy ones to push your body into a more balanced omega 6 to omega 3 state. Reducing and ultimately cutting out all those inflammatory foods mentioned in Chapter 3, and increasing your intake of whole plant foods, will make all the difference.

Step 3 – Eat the rainbow

We all need a bit of colour in our lives. In our food too. Every colour found in fresh fruit, vegetables, nuts, seeds, wholegrains, beans and legumes provides different chemical compounds that the body needs to function well. Eating a rainbow assortment of food every day can make a huge difference to how we feel.

Whilst I use the term 'rainbow', colours in food are usually split into five main groups. All are important, but the blue/purple group are particularly magical. The phytonutrients found in produce like blueberries, blackberries, purple sweet potatoes, red cabbage, purple sprouting broccoli and aubergine have specific antioxidant properties that support the brain and heart. This strong anti-inflammatory effect is super-important for those of us with autoimmune disease.

Table 5.1 is a summary of the foods in each colour group, the nutrients they contain and their healing effect. It's not exhaustive; there are just too many different foods to include.

Foods like red cabbage and purple sprouting broccoli are doubly powerful. As well as strong anti-inflammatory water-soluble phytochemicals called anthocyanins, they're also members of the cruciferous family which are equally powerful (we cover this in Chapter 7), making 'eat your purples' as important as 'eat your greens'.

Eating the same food in different colours maximises your intake of colours. Red apples have different phytoactive properties in the skin to green apples, as do yellow bell peppers compared to red or green ones. Tomatoes can come in a full rainbow array if you can find them and dwarf beans come in yellow, brown and purple varieties as well as green. Rice is the same. Whilst white or brown is more common, red and black varieties are delicious options found in health food shops and online.

Mindfully eating the rainbow every day ensures you benefit from nature's healing power whilst enjoying a plate full of technicolour beauty.

Table 5.1: The colour groups of foods

Colour	Found in:	Star nutrients:	Body benefits:
Red	Tomatoes, red peppers, beetroot, radishes, red potatoes, red chillis Red apples, grapefruit, cherries, strawberries, raspberries, watermelon, red grapes	Vitamins A and C Manganese Beta-carotene, quercetin, lycopene	Reduces inflammation and improves immune function Reduces risk of cancer and heart disease Good for eyes, skin and hair
Green	Broccoli, cabbage, Brussels sprouts, spinach, kale, seasonal greens, peas (all types) and peas shoots, asparagus, green beans, courgette, avocado, lettuce, rocket Green grapes, kiwi fruit, green apples, green figs	Vitamins A, B complex, C and K Potassium Chlorophyll, Carotenoids, leutein, zeaxanthin	Good for immune health, cell regeneration Supports the liver, blood pressure and clotting, Good for eye health
Yellow/ orange	Carrots, orange/yellow peppers, squash, pumpkin, sweet potatoes. Bananas, apricots, melon, nectarines, peaches, pineapple, yellow plums	Antioxidants – beta-carotene, lutein, alpha-carotene	Reduces inflammation Reduces risk of cancer, heart disease Good for hair, eyes and skin
Blue/ purple	Aubergine, red onions, red cabbage, purple sweet potatoes, purple sprouting broccoli. Blueberries, blackberries, dark plums, figs	Vitamin B Antioxidants – anthocyanins, resveratrol, flavonoids	Reduces risk of cancer, heart disease Protects cells from damage Improves memory Anti-ageing
White/ brown	Cauliflower, garlic, onion, mushrooms, parsnips, celeriac, turnips, swede, potatoes. Cocoa, dates	Vitamins C and K Folate Antioxidants – allicin, quercetin, anthoxanthins	Protects against cell damage Improves immunity Reduces cholesterol Reduces risk of cancer and heart disease Good for eye, bone and skin health

Step 4 – Variety

Your daily dose of rainbow eating ensures you eat at least five different plant foods during the day. However, eating the same five every day means you're not getting any variety.

Variety matters, not just when it comes to ensuring you have the full range of nutrients your body needs. It's essential for gut health; a variety of foods providing polyphenols and fibre results in a diverse, health-promoting microbiome. Lack of diversity leads to an unbalanced and unhealthy ecosystem.

Anthropologists and archaeologists have found that a diverse diet was key to human evolution. Our ancient ancestors ate whatever was available season to season, area to area. Modern humans, however, despite the overall higher availability of food, generally consume a diet limited to a narrow range of products. Rice, wheat, corn, meat and dairy are the foods eaten in the largest amounts around the world. Sometimes these foods are just part of a wider diet, whereas for others, it forms the bulk of the meals consumed every day, as with the Western diet. Information collected through large research programmes like the American Gut Project reveals that those with the least diverse diet have the least diverse microbiome, high in pathogenic microbes. It's also been found that the microbiomes of immigrants from countries with traditional, highly diverse diets quickly change to a less diverse, more pathogenic make-up after changing to the Western diet. That's a big worry.

Fortunately, microbiomes move in a positive direction as well as negative. Increasing the variety of food eaten day to day automatically increases diversity in the microbiome, helping move the body from an inflammatory, degenerative state into one that promotes healing and health.

You may be wondering how much fibre and variety a human body can tolerate as our environment has changed so much. Answers come from the Hazda tribe, one of the last hunter-gatherer tribes located in Tanzania, Africa.[3] These nomadic people have a highly diverse microbiome make-up. Whilst the food they eat can be placed into five groups, there's a large variety of foods in four of them (the last is honey on its own). Eating seasonally, they consume different types of berries, tubers, leaves and grains. They do eat meat on occasion, but as they must hunt, capture and prepare it, the amounts are much smaller compared to their plant intake.

Each type of plant seems to support different types of microbes. The turnover of microbes is rapid, going through three or four generations a day, so it doesn't take long for some to starve and die off if the right food is not provided. We see the same in ecosystems around the world as in the human gut – monoculture killing biodiversity.

As heading out to forage is not an option for most of us, we can opt to use a practical guide instead. Aiming for 30 different plant foods in a week will improve gut health and diversity in a relatively short period of time. These are whole plant foods, containing lots of fibre. By upping your variety, you'll naturally increase your fibre intake without really thinking about it, as well as all the healthful nutrients and phytonutrients we have already discussed.

Eating 30 different types of plants a week may be a huge challenge to you. Just start increasing your intake of plants and view 30 as a target, aiming to get closer each week. Even herbs and spices count. If you hit that magic number, you don't have to stop. If variety is suiting you, keep exploring and adding new foods to your diet. Every day can be a new adventure in food if you let it.

> **Tricia's story:** Too much of one food can cause problems, even if it's a healthy food. Just before Tricia had her major IBD flare up, she had eaten copious amounts of kale grown in her garden; she really feels she overdid it. Now she eats a huge variety of different plants every week but still can't quite manage much kale.

Step 5 – Minimally processed

All life on earth performs some form of food processing. Whether from accessing a nut from a shell, removing pips from a fruit or sucking the innards out of a grub (eww!), processing goes on all the time. Indeed, our whole digestive system, from the first bite to the elimination of waste, is our innate way of processing food. Some foods like fruit can be plucked from a tree and eaten, but most need some form of processing and preparation, including meat and dairy.

We looked at different levels of processing in the last chapter. Ideally, we want to retain as much of the fibre and nutrients as possible, so eating minimally processed food is important. That means eating an apple rather than drinking the juice, wholegrain rice instead of white or tomatoes instead of ketchup. Creating tasty recipes can often mean ingredients are mashed or processed, but as long as the ingredients haven't had anything taken away, you still get the whole food. You could start with chickpeas, sesame seeds, onion, garlic and coriander – all super-tasty on their own – and turn them into falafels. Nothing has been removed so the nutrients and fibre remain, just in a more interesting form.

Processing becomes a problem when nutrients are removed or chemically altered. These are the foods to avoid. White rice is still rice after all; it's lost fibre and lots of nutrients though, leaving just the starchy, energy-full core, fine for short-term fuelling only. Many veggie burgers contain hydrolysed soya protein instead of soya beans. This might increase the protein content but in a concentrated form not found in nature, without the fibre and unsupported by the other nutrients normally bound up in soya beans.

To maximise your nutrient intake through minimal processing, it's better to prepare food yourself with whole ingredients. That doesn't mean you can never eat out. Nor that you must be a slave to the kitchen. Rather, it gives you control over the food you eat – as much as possible anyway. Remember, each meal is the opportunity to support your body to heal.

There are plenty of short cuts that can help in cooking whole foods. Tinned beans and lentils are a great staple, cutting out the time needed to soak and cook dried beans – just rinse and drain them well. Chopped frozen vegetables cut out the prep time and retain nutrients, sometimes providing more than fresh produce that has travelled far or been stored for months. Gluten-free pseudo-grains like quinoa and millet take less than 15 minutes to cook and can be batch-cooked at the beginning of the week if needed.

All the recipes in the second half of this book use whole, minimally-processed ingredients and can mostly be made in less than 30 minutes.

Many can be batch-cooked and kept in the fridge or frozen for another day, although you may need to double the ingredients if you have a hungry family after them. When my children were at home, a meal destined for the freezer rarely made it there.

Step 6 – Fill up with fibre

Hopefully you are becoming a big fan of fibre. Apart from supporting gut health, fibre helps to manage energy levels by releasing sugar at a slow and steady rate. It also fills you up. The combination of fibre and plant protein improves satiety, that comfortable, satisfied feeling post meal that lasts for a good few hours before the next meal, triggered by hormones like leptin and GLP-1 sent from the gut to the brain. That's the same GLP-1 now being prescribed for people with obesity; a healthy gut can send those signals without medication.

As the Sensitive Foodie, I've given many talks, workshops and classes. I regularly experience scepticism when saying whole plant foods are filling, understandable if your only experience of eating plants is through dieting, limp lettuce leaves or soggy tomatoes. Eventually, I realised the food needed to speak for itself and included a meal as part of the event, a type of experiential learning. No one leaves with an empty stomach!

One time I invited a group of people to lunch; none were plant-based but they were all happy to eat my food. I served a rainbow mix of dishes and everyone left fully satiated. A few days later, a guest confessed her post-lunch plan was to head for Burger King, thinking she'd be hungry. Imagine her surprise when lunch filled her up so much, she wasn't hungry for the rest of the day. Everything served was so packed with fibre, it took a long time to digest.

Can you eat too much fibre? Yes, it's possible, especially if you have a gut disorder. Excess fibre increases gut motility, reducing the time taken for food to be digested and absorbed. We do have a much higher capacity than we think, though. The Hazda tribe, mentioned earlier, can consume between 100 and 150 g of fibre a day. That's almost five times the amount of the daily target set by the government, and I am not suggesting you consume this much right away. People who have been eating a whole-food plant-based diet for some time can comfortably consume 50 g a day. If you have IBD and are in an acute inflammatory phase, this will be way too high. This is a time for low fibre, not high – in the short term. Once the acute stage has passed, building up your fibre content can help prevent future relapses as Tricia found.

> **Tricia's story:** Tricia found following a low-fibre plant-based diet key to starting her recovery and pushing her gut towards healing. White rice and pasta, well cooked vegetables, tofu, blended soaked cashews, ginger, turmeric and tinned rather than fresh fruit all helped to calm down her highly reactive gut. Whilst boring and bland, she started to improve after just 3–4 months and could slowly start to introduce higher-fibre foods that supported her microbiome. Tricia recommends listening to what your body has to say and be guided by it. Don't be afraid to try something you've excluded, or you'll get stuck in boredom. Little and often worked best.

Some plant foods can have a gassier effect than others, particularly if they are high in certain types of fibre, like inulin. Found in some tubers, fruit, oats and the onion family, it's a powerful prebiotic, a food microbes love. If you have an unbalanced microbiome, however, pathogenic bacteria will break down inulin with gusto, producing lots of gas as a by-product. Great for the microbes, not so great for you if it results in bloating and severe abdominal pain.

Jerusalem artichokes are a particularly powerful source of inulin, as I found out to my detriment before I changed the way I ate. My family already teased me about my ability to fart for England; this was before I knew about the microbiome and just how much mine was struggling. Jerusalem artichokes caused absolute havoc after I ate some before going on a night shift. I was doubled up in pain, farting like a trooper all night long. Fortunately I was away from colleagues looking after a well-sedated patient so hopefully only disturbed myself!

What I didn't realise at the time was the 'fartichokes' were not the main issue.

At the time, I considered my diet to be healthy. Unaware of my intolerance, I still consumed dairy, a small amount of meat, a reasonable intake of fresh produce and lots of refined sugar in cakes, desserts and alcohol. I have always had a sweet tooth and craved sugar constantly. I also had a yeast overgrowth which just fuelled my cravings and contributed to increasing dysbiosis. No wonder I was so gassy and overreactive to prebiotic fibre.

Increasing your fibre intake is certainly essential for improving gut health and reducing systemic inflammation, but not advisable to change overnight as you might well run into trouble. You might experience benign but uncomfortable bloating and noxious wind but also potentially serious levels of constipation, especially if you don't increase your fluid intake. Very occasionally, this can cause an obstruction, which is a medical emergency. An extreme and rare outcome, for sure, but worth taking note of, particularly if you are an 'all or nothing' person.

Instead try my **top tips** to help your gut microbes calmly adjust to an increase in fibre:

- Drink a glass of water before you eat as the additional fibre will absorb more water. Avoid fizzy drinks though.
- Swiftly remove UPFs and refined sugar products from your diet. This will stop feeding the 'bad' bacteria that thrive on them and help you tolerate more whole foods.
- Gluten-free whole grains are less fermentable than whole grains so start increasing these straight away. Swap to whole-grain rice, buckwheat flakes, flour or groats, quinoa and millet grains.
- Oats contain a lot of soluble fibre, so if you're not used to eating them, start with a small amount and increase over a couple of weeks.
- Eat fruit at the start of, or between, meals. Sugars contained in whole fruit tend to be more rapidly released in the gut. It's best to let them have free passage rather than get caught behind harder to digest foods. Microbes in the small intestine can start fermenting these sugars and producing the gas by-product that results in bloating and trapped wind if it has nowhere to go.
- Cruciferous vegetables like kale, sprouts and broccoli contain amazingly healthful compounds but lots of sulphur. This can

produce additional, rather 'eggy' gas, especially in dysbiosis. Eating lots of these vegetables is a great goal but increase amounts slowly if you are prone to excess wind.
- Ginger or mint tea can help to relieve painful wind or bloating. Even a cup of hot water can help.

Filling up with fibre reduces the desire to snack and eat ultra-processed foods. Being in tune with your body, recognising how it responds to certain foods, becomes easier the more whole foods you eat. Whilst caution is sensible, do keep increasing your fibre intake every day, even if it's a tiny amount. As gut microbes rapidly turn over, it doesn't take long before a healthier population is established. If you do suffer extreme bloating and pain, however, please seek advice from a health professional. Finally, if you are an 'all or nothing' person, you can change overnight if you wish. Just be aware that the people around you might not appreciate it quite as much, to start anyway.

Step 7 – Feel empowered

Being diagnosed with autoimmune disease can rock you to the core. I believe that post diagnosis is one of the most stressful periods, filled with a roller-coaster of emotions. Having spoken to others with a similar diagnosis, or any autoimmune disease, this is common, often overwhelming. I consider myself to be so fortunate to have had access to great information about actions I could take straight away to support my health, as well as the financial ability and spousal support to change my lifestyle, including giving up my job as an intensive care nurse. I appreciate that not everyone is in the same situation.

Equipped with my knowledge about eating well, and access to information about other lifestyle modifications, my grief gave way to a deep determination that I was not going to be defeated and give my power away to others. I had looked after too many patients with long-term health conditions living a disempowered and severely limited life, bereft of knowledge about changes they could make to improve their health themselves, in conjunction with their medical care.

Knowledge is powerful – as long as you put it into action. Embracing this knowledge is also part of the healing process. That's not just my belief; research has shown improved outcomes when patients feel knowledgeable and empowered to take action, preferring to work in partnership with their healthcare team rather than have a top-down approach.[4]

> **Kate's story:** Kate worked with her doctors to reduce her medications but also empowered herself to keep learning and exploring the connection between food and inflammatory arthritis. A whole-food plant-based diet is essential to her everyday life, and she now wouldn't eat any other way. She believes without it she would have ended up in a wheelchair, old before her time, like her mum who also has the condition.

Feeling empowered helps reduce anxiety. This slows the stress response and therefore inflammation. It also helps us to make more healthful decisions in everyday life. Understanding that each meal can help your body to heal makes food choices easier. Being told to avoid certain foods, especially your favourites, is hard, and rarely successful in the long term. *Choosing* to avoid these previously favourite but less healthful foods is different. Knowing that every meal can help you heal, and experiencing the positive benefits of those changes, is truly empowering. Even if there are times when you decide to go for the less healthful option, the knowledge that it's your choice makes a huge difference too.

Autoimmune disease is for life; the changes you make need to be for life too. Feeling empowered and inspired to make those changes enables you to head towards wellness, whatever that may look like for you. Others may not like it. They might even try to sow doubt or confusion, especially if they don't understand the changes. Be adventurous, and don't get put off by others. This is your journey to wellness, one that not only benefits you, but the world around you. That is truly empowering.

Chapter 6

But what about...?
Myth busting

Introduction

The internet provides us all with a wealth of information - and disinformation. With polarised viewpoints and opinions carrying more weight than science, it can be hard to sort fact from fiction. Social media is the go-to source of health support and information; beneficial if the source is based in sound research and experience but not when the information is not only bad but dangerous.

Having been diagnosed with an autoimmune disease, I empathise with the feelings of anxiety and desperation that overcome many people. Autoimmune conditions are still not well understood, particularly less common ones, and treatments and support can be scant. Suffering in isolation, searching for a clear route to recovery or just something to make it go away, makes us vulnerable to unresearched or misinterpreted 'facts'.

When I first investigated dietary changes for autoimmune disease, I kept coming across the same advice – eat grass-fed or wild meat, fish, vegetables, only certain fruit and avoid dairy, whole grains, beans, nuts, seeds and nightshade vegetables. As I was already plant-based, this set off alarm bells – was everything I knew about food wrong? Digging deeper to find the research studies to back this up, I couldn't find much except the theory behind it that genes take a long time to adapt, and our bodies haven't yet evolved to tolerate products from 'modern' farming. Therefore, eating a paleo-style diet – called the Autoimmune Protocol – in line with our hunter-gatherer ancestors, will solve the problems created by autoimmunity.

The connection between modern farming techniques and industrial food production and health is sound. Monoculture, the overuse of fertilizers and pesticides, and plastic pollution in the oceans and waterways around the world are causing harm to human and planetary health. At first, the Autoimmune Protocol was a theory adopted as proven science. Since my first investigations, some small scientific studies have been undertaken in the last few years with favourable results. Which is great news, until you investigate it a bit more.[1, 2] The studies I found had 20 or fewer people, often included other lifestyle changes or personal support, the outcomes re-shared as evidence of effectiveness were often slightly different to the research article. For example, a 2019 study on 17 people with Hashimoto's following the protocol as part of a wider lifestyle programme found their inflammatory markers reduced – great news – but no change in their thyroid function.[3] There are so many nuances here. Changing to a diet with lots of vegetables could have helped those inflammatory markers. Or eliminating gluten, which *is* connected to Hashimoto's. This research also points out that the autoimmune protocol is an elimination diet not a long-term programme.

We saw back in Chapter 2 the importance of gut health in autoimmune disease and how it's supported with complex fibre found in whole grains, beans, legumes, nuts and seeds. So how can a programme that eliminates all of these be helpful for autoimmune disease? The Autoimmune Protocol is researched as a short-term elimination diet, with the gradual reintroduction of grains, beans etc to help identify potential issues through personalised nutrition. This is not how it is promoted by many doctors and nutritionists in the Western world, though. Instead, many gut-loving whole foods have become demonised as containing 'anti-nutrients' and grass-fed or wild meat touted as the panacea of good health.

What did our ancestors eat?

Let's consider the paleo diet for a moment. Eating like our ancestors makes sense in terms of eating fresh, unadulterated food. Often described as hunter-gatherers, the latest anthropological studies reveal the opposite.[4]

Like the Hazda people, most of the diet consisted of foraged plants, with meat, eggs and fish eaten on occasion. The structure of our digestive system backs this up too; if humans evolved to eat mainly meat, the digestive tract would be shorter, teeth would be much sharper and jaws would move differently. In 2010, archaeologists found evidence of ancient grain consumption 30,000 years ago,[5] disproving the theory that humans only ate grain *after* farming was established 14,000 years ago. Admittedly, the grains commonly farmed today are different to their ancestors, but then so is the meat, which is important due to the change in omegas 3 and 6 content, as we saw in Chapter 3. The cost of grass-fed and wild meat is high – for humans, animals and the environment – and unattainable for most.

Achievable health solutions must be accessible and sustainable, for the individual and the world in which we live. I don't see this paleo approach ticking either of those boxes. Even if you remove the environmental and ethical issues, the price tag of grass-fed meat makes it elitist; the 2025 Food Foundation 'Broken Plates' report[6] found that the poorest 20% of the population would have to spend 45% of their income to follow the UK government's healthy eating guidelines, rising to a whopping 70% for families with children. Choosing expensive cuts of meat is not going to be plausible when even the affordability of fresh produce is a challenge.

Dietary intake in many parts of the world, including the poorest, is mainly beans and other legumes, rice and seasonal vegetables. Meat or dairy may feature in small amounts or for celebrations. Indeed, the Mediterranean diet pattern, the most researched and accredited diet, is based on these food groups. In the original Blue Zones research,[7] these whole foods were identified as being abundantly consumed by a healthy yet aged population. Chronic health conditions, including autoimmune diseases, were much less prevalent.

An 'anti-nutrient' conspiracy?

I was very curious about why an approach without a well-grounded evidence base was more recognised than a plant-predominant one supported by one of the most researched dietary patterns in the world.[4]

And whilst I could come up with all sorts of conspiracy theories, there is a strong narrative that many plants are full of 'anti-nutrients' that are harmful to health whereas animal products are essential for human health. Which is an interesting argument when the World Health Organization has classified both processed meat and red meat as class 1 and class 2 carcinogens (cancer causing, or high risk of causing).[8] But no plants. And let's not forget that many modern pharmaceuticals will have originated from plants.

Many people have real concerns about the presence of 'anti-nutrients' in plants or plant families. This is why I've written this chapter, to explore each one. To avoid bias as much as possible though, it's important to point out once again that we are all different, as are our microbiomes. How I respond to one food might be different to how you do so. Everyone with a leaky gut is at risk of reacting to food badly. A dietary pattern needs to be an adaptable framework to accommodate these individualities. There are also autoimmune conditions like coeliac disease that can make people particularly vulnerable to nutritional deficiencies, so great care needs to be taken – a well-planned diet is important.

Let's now explore the issues around the 'anti-nutrients' discussion so you can see if they affect you. As protein is always the first question I get asked about a plant-based diet, we'll sort that question out too. Hopefully, by the end of this chapter your concerns will be allayed.

Lectins

As a teenager, I had a summer job working in a local vegetarian café. I loved it and it triggered my interest in healthy food, alongside a love for carrot cake. To be a bit fancy, we served baked potatoes with mixed beans instead of the standard baked beans – it was the 1980s! One lunchtime, an anxious customer kept asking about the kidney beans in the mix – had they been properly cooked? I had no idea but suggested as they had come from a tin, they'd be fine. He left without any lunch, muttering about food poisoning.

At the time I just thought he was a bit of an odd bod. How could a tiny bean make you ill? It turns out they can, or at least kidney beans can. White and red kidney beans contain a toxin called PHA (phytohaemagglutinin) that causes gut issues if eaten raw. Cooking neutralises it, making them safe to eat. There are several documented cases of food poisoning connected to kidney beans, a total of 50 between 1976 and 1989 in the UK.[9] (I couldn't find more recent figures.) It looks like a big problem until you look at cases of salmonella poisoning from chicken: 220 cases in 2022 alone.[10] Poorly prepared kidney beans are an issue, but perspective is important.*

Beans contain a family of glycoproteins called lectins, which are what are known as anti-nutrients. Lectins are found in plants, animals and even micro-organisms and play a role in development and defence. Plants contain hundreds of different lectins that protect against insects, disease and fungus. Beans, pulses and whole grains contain the highest amounts, influenced by the season, where they're grown and susceptibility to disease. Human digestive enzymes find it hard to break down lectins without some form of processing which is why they can cause some intestinal issues if eaten raw. Proper food preparation is key here – soaking well and then boiling for at least 30 minutes eliminates lectins from all beans and pulses, even those pesky kidney beans.[11]

What about reports claiming lectins damage the gut lining, triggering an inflammatory response? At first glance, this might appear true as some studies have shown high doses of isolated lectins and flour made from raw legumes can damage the gut wall, increasing gut permeability and inflammation.[12] A couple of things to consider here – these experiments were in animals, not humans, and the experiments used concentrated lectins or *raw* bean flour, not cooked beans as we know cooking neutralises lectins. Of course, there are always going to be some people particularly sensitive to certain foods, including beans and pulses. Hopefully this will only be a short-term problem until a leaky gut is healed, but for an unlucky few, molecular mimicry could make them an issue . For everyone else, whole foods like beans, pulses and whole grains are a great source of amino acids, fibre, minerals, vitamins and anti-inflammatory compounds,

---

*For balance, there were also 16 cases of salmonella from eating cucumber in 2022. If salads have contact with water or soil contaminated with animal waste (like manure) and are not washed properly, it can make you ill. It's not the cucumber that's the issue but the way it's been cultivated.

and are associated with lower inflammatory biomarkers in those who eat them. There is even some evidence that lectins can be used in diagnosing and treating cancer, although human trials are needed to verify this.

Oxalates

If you've ever had a kidney stone, you'll probably remember one thing – pain! Once passed, you may have been given advice to avoid high-oxalate foods like spinach or rhubarb to prevent stones reoccurring. This seems good advice, although it's always the plants that get the blame. Eating lots of meat, UPFs and salt also increases the risk of kidney stones, especially if you have a genetic risk of developing them.[13]

Kidney stones are made by oxalic acid binding with minerals like calcium and magnesium to form crystals – oxalates. Oxalic acid is made by the body and is involved in the metabolism of vitamin C and collagen. It's also a waste product of other processes and is expelled in the urine, hence the kidney stone connection. Oxalic acid is also found in plants, sometimes in high amounts, once again binding with minerals to form oxalates as a form of protection. It's this binding of minerals that's the area of concern for some – nutrient availability. A plant may be high in calcium, for example, but if it's bound up in a crystal that can't be absorbed into the bloodstream, you're at risk of calcium deficiency. Or that's the argument anyway.

And in some cases, it's a reasonable one if you only eat one type of plant raw as a mineral source. However, cooking, sprouting and fermenting plant foods greatly reduce oxalate levels, making the nutrients more available for absorption.[14] Eating a diverse range of plant foods also ensures there are plenty of sources of nutrients available if you struggle with one, and if your microbiome is balanced, certain microbes can break oxalates down too.

Interestingly, scientists are beginning to recognise that oxalates have a protective effect. Oxalic acid can act as an antioxidant,[15] especially in fat metabolism, plus binding up minerals like iron that can contribute to inflammation when eaten in excess is a good thing. Foods containing oxalic acid like leafy greens not only contain minerals but lots of vitamins and phytonutrients like polyphenols that have been found to protect *against* kidney stones whereas a diet high in meat, ultra-processed foods and salt *increases* the risk.

What about people with autoimmune disease? Some conditions where nutrient absorption is already an issue like coeliac disease and IBD, avoiding eating raw high-oxalate foods is a good idea, especially as the gut microbes that digest oxalates tend to be absent in these conditions.[16] Eating a plant-based diet will help with dysbiosis, but attention must be paid to ensuring a variety of foods are eaten cooked, sprouted or fermented. If you have an autoimmune thyroid issue, it's worth being mindful about the amount of raw high-oxalate foods you consume. Calcium oxalate compounds have been found in thyroid tissue of people with Graves' disease and sarcoidosis and there are some connections between coeliac disease and Hashimoto's.[17]

If this is you, hopefully you are already receiving nutritional advice; you may need to use supplements during acute flares of your condition if it's hard to absorb enough from your food.

All plant food contains oxalates; eating an appropriately prepared, diverse diet full of fibre and antioxidants throughout the day moderates any potential issues (in most people) whilst providing a wonderful balance of nutrients and compounds that support the body.

Nightshades

Everyone with autoimmune disease should avoid nightshades, right? Especially if your joints are affected. Well, maybe not. Nightshade vegetables, which are actually types of fruit, contain some of the most antioxidant-packed foods available, like tomatoes and peppers, and are readily consumed as part of the Mediterranean diet, the most researched and highly ranked dietary pattern in the world. So why do they have such a bad reputation for autoimmune disease?

Nightshades are part of the Solanaceae family that has around 2000 members. Some, like belladonna, which has rightly earned its popular name 'deadly nightshade', are poisonous. Tobacco plants are also in this group. Many, however, are a staple for many people worldwide, like potatoes, aubergine (eggplant) and chillis, alongside tomatoes and peppers mentioned above. Putting potatoes to one side, they contain plenty of healthful antioxidants like vitamin C, and powerful phytonutrients including beta-carotene and anthocyanins. There's plenty of research showing how these foods help reduce inflammation rather than fuel it. Lycopene, found in tomatoes, can help prevent and reduce prostate cancer[18] as well as heart disease.[19] The dark purple skin on aubergine contains powerful anthocyanin compounds known to help reduce inflammation. Capsaicin in chilli peppers, has been found to help reduce pain and bloating in people with IBD[20] (although you should check how you respond before eating lots) and it's a well-known topical treatment for joint pain.

However, nightshades do also contain other compounds that can cause problems, including glycoalkaloids and alkaloids, like solanine and nicotine. Yes, you read that right! Aubergine contains nicotine. But don't worry – the amounts are minimal compared to tobacco so it's unlikely you'll get addicted. Glycoalkaloids, like solanine, found in potatoes, work as another defence mechanism against pests and diseases. If you eat green or raw potatoes, solanine is poisonous. So if you discard green potatoes and always eat them cooked (heat neutralises the toxin), you shouldn't have a problem.

I've been curious about the research connecting nightshades and autoimmune disease for a long time, but studies are scant. Most reports are anecdotal rather than evidence based. Whilst learning from lived experience is important, this may not be reflected in a larger group. One study on mice fed a fried-potato-only diet resulted in a damaged gut lining and increased gut permeability.[21] Was it the potato or the oil that caused the damage, though? Gut damage and inflammation were seen in other experiments feeding concentrated amounts of raw potatoes to rodents.[22] We've already established that raw potato is poisonous and concentrated amounts are certainly not part of the human diet. Plus, we are not rodents, and a potato-only diet isn't good for anyone. Reassuringly, a report for the European Commission found no evidence of health problems connected to the glycoalkaloids in (cooked) potatoes. There were not enough data available for tomatoes and aubergines, both in experiments but also in 'occurrence data' – that is, there aren't enough records to analyse.[23]

> **Kate's story:** Once diagnosed with psoriatic arthritis, Kate was told she would need to avoid nightshade vegetables but doesn't have any reaction to them so happily eats them on a regular basis.

We already know that people with autoimmune disease have dysbiosis and with that come food sensitivities, so there are bound to be some people who can't tolerate tomatoes or peppers. That doesn't necessarily mean everyone should avoid them, and if you react to one it doesn't mean you will do the same with others. I tried to find a figure for the percentage of people who react to nightshades, but failed. The only commentary featuring a number was from Dr Klapper, a US physician who estimates around 10% of people he's treated with an inflammatory condition react to *a* nightshade. Which means that 90% don't. There are so many healthful anti-inflammatory compounds in (most) nightshades that you could miss out on their healing properties due to fear they might harm you.

> **Nightshades and histamine:** Two nightshades, tomatoes and aubergine, are high in histamine. This is a problem if you are one of the unlucky few who have a histamine overload that fuels inflammation and manifests in diverse ways like digestive issues, headaches, skin reactions and fatigue. Doesn't this sound like many autoimmune issues? Histamine is present in all foods in varying amounts. It's difficult to manage, so if you think this is an issue, please seek out a specialist for professional advice.

Phytates

Like lectins and oxalates, phytate is another compound that has been given the 'anti-nutrient' label. Also known as phytic acid or IP6* it stores phosphate required for the germination of edible plants like grains, nuts, seeds, beans and pulses.

Phytate binds to minerals like calcium, zinc, iron and copper, which can then make them less available for us to absorb once eaten as we do not naturally produce the enzymes needed to break them down. It's not all bad news, though; this binding effect (called chelation) means they have protective antioxidant properties. However, phytates can be an issue in countries where a limited, very basic diet is available. Variety is key; if we don't eat the same two or three foods every day, they shouldn't be a problem.[24]

Culinary processes like soaking, fermenting, germinating and boiling significantly reduce the phytate level in grains, beans, lentils, nuts and seeds. Soaking in water stimulates a chemical reaction within the seed, destroying the phytate.

> **Top tip:** I always soak wholegrain rice and then just use the same water to cook it in, so the minerals get reabsorbed. I check where the rice I use has come from first as rice grown in certain areas, like parts of the US, India and SE Asia, contains raised levels of arsenic due to pollution – I don't want to introduce that back into something I'm eating!

Fermentation creates a more acidic environment. A sourdough ferment will neutralise the phytates in flour used in bread making. Fermenting soya beans to produce tempeh or miso does the same. Finally, adding lemon juice or vinegar just before serving beans or grains will also help remove phytates and make the minerals and other nutrients more absorbable in the gut. It can also make the dish taste even more delicious.

*IP6 stands for 'myo-inositol-hexaphosphate', which is bit of a mouthful so no wonder it was shortened!

Gluten

Whilst there are many disagreements about foods to eat or avoid with autoimmune disease, gluten tends to be the one ingredient where there's consensus. And for conditions like coeliac disease, dermatitis herpetiformis and gluten ataxia, there is sound evidence to back this up. Autoimmune thyroid diseases like Hashimoto's and Graves' disease also have a strong connection. For other conditions, however, the evidence is less clear. People with coeliac disease have an increased risk of developing type 1 diabetes, and vice versa; gluten is the suggested trigger. That's not all. The risk of developing rheumatoid arthritis, MS and Sjögren's syndrome also increases if you have coeliac disease, especially when diagnosed later in life.[25] Table 6.1 summarises these relationships.

Table 6.1: The most common autoimmune diseases with clear negative connections to gluten.

Coeliac disease	Dermatitis herpetiformis	Graves' disease
Hashimoto's disease	Addison's disease	Autoimmune chronic active hepatitis
Myasthenia gravis	Pernicious anaemia	Raynaud's phenomenon
Scleroderma	Sjögren's syndrome	Lupus

Gluten is not a food in itself; it's a protein found in wheat, and barley and rye to a lesser extent, that stops baked goods from falling apart – that is, it binds and gives structure to bread and cakes. Modern varieties of wheat have been cross-bred to contain higher levels of gluten compared to ancient grains, important particularly for modern bread-making methods using fast-acting yeast which require minimal proving.[†]

[†] 'Proving' is an essential part of the bread-making process that develops the gluten, making it more elastic and able to form a strong structure as the gas from fermentation causes the dough to rise. The bacteria involved also break down gluten, reducing the amount present in the final product. It takes 12-24 hours for gluten to perform its magic and be reduced, which is why traditionally-made bread like sourdough is more beneficial than supermarket bread; more expensive too.

In coeliac disease, the body identifies gluten as an antigen and creates antibodies to destroy it. Unfortunately, it misidentifies an enzyme called transglutaminase as gluten and starts to attack that too. Found in humans, plants and animals, transglutaminase acts as a binding agent that connects proteins, a type of 'biological glue'. It's found throughout the body and is used for multiple processes. This is why coeliac disease can be such a debilitating condition.

Gluten and transglutaminase are just two of the binding agents used by the food industry for processed and ultra-processed foods. The rise in the number of people with gluten-related autoimmune diseases has increased in line with the rise of processed foods, including bread, cakes and pastries. Farming practices have also changed, not just with fast-growing varieties of wheat. Fertiliser, pesticide and fungicide use has also increased massively with industrial production.

Studies suggest that gluten has a pro-inflammatory effect on the gut wall,[26] increasing permeability, increasing 'bad' bacteria in the microbiome and creating increased oxidative stress. This strongly suggests that everyone with an autoimmune disease should avoid gluten. Or that everyone at risk of one should. The research, however, has been done on animals using concentrated amounts. Unless you are eating pure gluten, which is rare, then does that have the same effect? There's no clear answer to that.

Should everyone avoid gluten?

Putting aside those conditions with a clear link, does gluten impact everyone with autoimmune disease? Is it the gluten, or the toxic chemicals causing the problem? Or the ultra-processed foods? Is it poor quality food? Studies looking at people with autoimmune disease who have chosen to go gluten free report a positive effect which is great news.[27] What other changes did they make though?

Nutrition experts are concerned that removing gluten-containing products puts people at risk of nutrient deficiencies unless it is a well-planned diet full of high-nutrient foods. Whole grains contain complex fibre as well as anti-inflammatory omega fats, both known to support the gut and overall health. Plus, shop-bought gluten-free products are often highly processed and contain lots of chemicals – not ideal for supporting health. They are often expensive too.

So, what's the answer? I'm going to say that's up to you! Sorry, a cop out but unless you have a condition that has a direct connection with gluten, then you might not need to avoid it. If you're eating a healthful, whole-food plant-based diet that is. I suggest you go for more ancient grains like spelt or emmer and avoid chemicals by choosing organic whenever you can. Homemade sourdough bread is more affordable than shop bought. That way you know exactly what has gone into it and, once you've sussed the process, it doesn't take up too much time.

Having said that, I have chosen to include only gluten-free recipes in this book to make sure everyone is covered. However, gluten-containing flour can be used too – in a little ironic twist of exclusion.

But protein…?

The world of nutrition is obsessed with protein. Important for a huge range of bodily functions and structures, protein is involved in growth and repair, and is a key part of cells, tissues and organs. Its status as king of nutrients continues whilst the polarising debate about fat vs carbohydrate for energy rages. We can even convert it to glucose when other energy sources are scarce. Connected to perceptions of strength, power and manliness, the role of meat as the main source of protein is embedded in the Western world's dietary patterns. This is now being reflected in developing countries too, areas that traditionally ate a more plant-based diet.

Protein is made from chains of amino acids, tiny compounds made up of nitrogen, hydrogen, carbon and oxygen. There are 20 amino acids in total, eight of which are termed 'essential' – they must be obtained from food because we can't make them. All proteins are broken down in the stomach and small intestine, absorbed into the body as peptides, smaller amino acid chains, or single amino acids. Once in circulation, the body can change these amino acid combinations to form the protein structure that's required at that moment. These processes are constant throughout the body, with proteins being broken down, recycled, built up again and excreted.

Protein is readily available in all foods, whether they are from a plant or animal. Plant proteins contain all the essential amino acids but not always in the exact same amounts as meat. This is where the 'problem' with plant proteins comes up. Labelled 'incomplete' proteins, and therefore inferior, by a sociology professor in the 1970s, this reputation as being inferior has been hard to shake off, even after the same professor retracted her theory a few years after publishing it. She introduced the idea of combining certain food groups to create 'complete protein' in meals, like eating beans with rice, or lentils with bread.[28] Even though it's been well known for decades now that all the amino acids we require are gained from the food we eat throughout the day, not just a single meal, the necessity of food combining is still taught in many nutrition curricula to this day.

The myth of incomplete proteins only becomes true if you eat only one or two different foods every day. This is why people who are starving and relying on meagre rations of plant-based foods become protein deficient. If they ate animal products, it would be less of an issue, but these are not so readily available in famine-struck regions or for those living in poverty. Interestingly, traditional diets eaten for thousands of years before proteins and amino acids were discovered tend to include combinations of beans, rice, lentils and flatbreads along with fresh fruit and vegetables. These dietary staples contain so much more than just protein of course, but a smorgasbord of nutrients that the body requires to thrive.

> **Tricia's story:** How do you eat enough protein when your body doesn't retain the food you've consumed long enough to absorb it? This was the problem Tricia faced during the acute phase of Crohn's disease. She found consulting a dietitian very helpful, following her advice of small but frequent meals to ensure she took in enough calories, with tofu becoming her main source of plant protein. Once the acute phase had passed, Tricia found she could slowly tolerate beans, lentils and whole grains too, slowly regaining the weight she had lost along with her strength.

The body knows what combinations of amino acids it needs and where to get them from. If a varied diet containing enough calories is eaten, there should be enough protein to meet your needs. That's not just me saying that. The British Dietetic Association in the UK states that a well-planned vegan diet is healthy for people of all ages and can support healthy living.[29] Remember, protein is in everything we eat, even the dairy-free milk in a cup of tea.

HOW MUCH IS 'ENOUGH' PROTEIN?

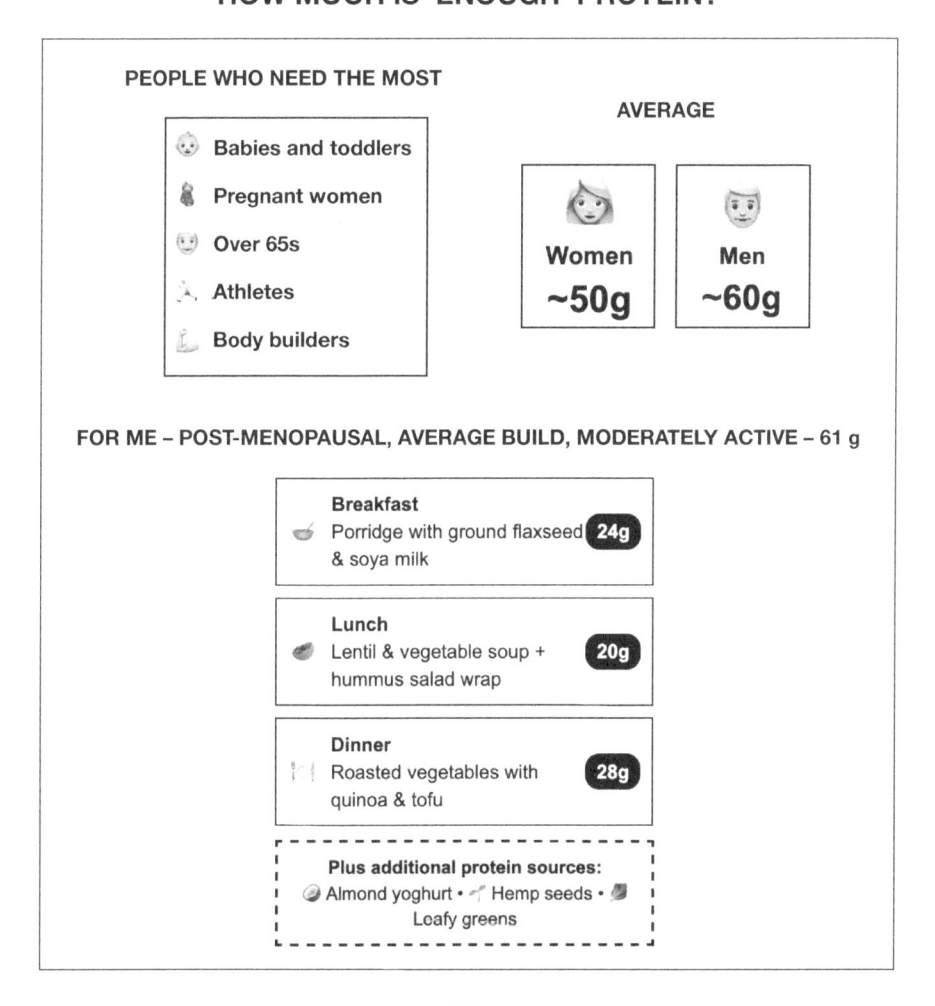

PEOPLE WHO NEED THE MOST
- Babies and toddlers
- Pregnant women
- Over 65s
- Athletes
- Body builders

AVERAGE
- Women ~50g
- Men ~60g

FOR ME – POST-MENOPAUSAL, AVERAGE BUILD, MODERATELY ACTIVE – 61 g

Breakfast
Porridge with ground flaxseed & soya milk — 24g

Lunch
Lentil & vegetable soup + hummus salad wrap — 20g

Dinner
Roasted vegetables with quinoa & tofu — 28g

Plus additional protein sources:
Almond yoghurt • Hemp seeds • Leafy greens

All of the foods mentioned in the box on page 121 contain so much more than protein, of course – healthy fats, minerals, vitamins and phytonutrients along with gut-loving fibre. This is the deficiency that huge numbers of people suffer from, not protein!

'You must take lots of supplements'

Critics of plant-based diets love to claim certain nutrients are only available in animal foods. I'm not going to say that's not true; there are a few issues for sure, but they're not unique to plant-based eaters. Most people who eat animal products don't realise that they too are supplementing these nutrients, not directly but second hand through the produce they consume.

The key nutrient issues are vitamin B12, vitamin D and iodine, although any nutrient has the potential to be an issue depending on gut health and autoimmune disease process. In acute phases of chronic health conditions, supplements can certainly provide additional support, but with a high nutrient-dense whole-food plant-based diet these requirements should drop to the bare minimum. Let's have a quick look at the three mentioned above.

Vitamin B12 is essential for nerve conduction, red blood cell formation and energy production. Unlike other vitamins, B12 is not found *in* plants but from certain bacteria found *on* them. Improved food hygiene means these microbes are destroyed before we eat them. B12 is released from food in the stomach and absorbed in the small intestine only, so although we have the capacity to make it lower down in the gut through fermentation, it just won't make it into the body. Meat is seen as a good food source of B12 as grazing animals either consume the B12-producing bacteria directly, or, in the case of ruminants like cows and sheep, gain it from bacteria in their stomachs. Industrial farming techniques mean many animals must have B12 supplemented in their feed as they are not exposed to natural sources. Meanwhile, increases in industrial food production and its knock-on effect on stomach acidity have led to a drop in many people's ability to break down protein and absorb B12 from it. Not only that, but the rise in the long-term use of proton pump inhibitors like omeprazole also reduces people's ability to access B12 in food, meaning it's not just vegans who need to supplement.

Vitamin D: Apart from mushrooms exposed to sunlight, there are no plant sources of vitamin D. Animal food sources include oily fish, egg yolks and red meat, although again industrial animal agriculture means supplemented feed is used as many animals are not exposed to sunlight. For this is how all mammals make vitamin D – skin exposure to sunlight. Our modern lifestyles mean we don't get as much exposure as our ancestors. I've already explored the importance of vitamin D in autoimmune disease (see page 25), but it's important for everyone, which is why many food products from orange juice to breads to breakfast cereals are fortified with it. Department of Health guidelines advise everyone to supplement during the winter months irrespective of dietary pattern.

Iodine is important for thyroid health and only needed in small amounts. Dairy is often promoted as being the best source, but this is due to modern farming practices, not the milk itself. Iodine supplements are added to feed and antiseptic iodine washes and sprays used on cow's udders to manage mastitis. This is what ends up in the milk – nice, huh? Iodine is often added to plant-based milks and can be found in seaweed (the next chapter has more information on this – see page 138). If this is not a regular part of your diet, a small supplement is a good idea. If you have thyroid disease, please take direct guidance from a health professional.

The need to supplement these essential nutrients can apply to anyone no matter what they eat. Don't be taken in by agendas or clever marketing – eat a wide range of whole plant foods and you will be exposed to all the nutrients you need and more.

Summary

This chapter has explored the main myths around certain groups of plant foods, or the inadequacy of a plant-based diet. Hopefully, any worries you had have dissolved and you're feeling confident about the benefits you will gain from eating a diet full of colourful foods packed with fibre and anti-inflammatory properties.

There is a proviso though. A completely whole-food plant-based diet is not right for everyone, or at least not all in one go overnight, especially if you tend to eat a limited number of foods. Going forward, hopefully, but if you have an inflamed, leaky gut, you may well have food intolerances that include certain plant foods or have an overgrowth of bad bacteria that make the consumption of FODMAPs impossible to tolerate.

Sometimes healing with food means you must do some detective work, identifying what does and doesn't work for you. One of the benefits of eating a whole-food plant-based diet is that there are so many options to explore that your choice doesn't have to be too limited or boring. The key to making positive effective change is an open and inquisitive mind. Of course you'll make mistakes, but don't be discouraged by them. They're learning opportunities on your healing journey.

You may need to do an elimination diet by cutting out foods you feel you're reacting to. It might involve removing a lot of different foods and eating a very simple diet, but it's only for a few weeks and it can really make a difference. After a few weeks, or when your gut feels more settled, reintroduce foods, one at a time, and see how you react. Keep a diary and soon you will have a record of what you can comfortably eat, and what needs to be avoided for now. After a few months, you can try introducing these foods again; with luck your gut will be in a much healthier state and be much less reactive. If this process seems too laborious or you struggle on your own, please find a nutritionist or dietitian for support.

Chapter 7

What am I actually going to eat?

Having absorbed all the information covered so far, you may be wondering what on earth you are going to eat. A most reasonable question and one I hope to answer in this chapter as we're going to dive into the gorgeously tasty foods that make up a whole-food plant-based diet. I'll also share my top tips for preparing, processing, cooking (or not) and enjoying these delightful natural foods.

As we eat food, not individual nutrients, the focus now is on the whole foods served up as part of a meal. Don't forget that when you eat a variety of foods during the day, these come with all the nutrients and fibre the body needs to heal and thrive.

Way back in Chapter 3 we looked at the five food groups that make up a whole-food plant-based diet. Here they are as a reminder, along with a couple more.

- Fruit
- Vegetables
- Whole grains
- Beans and pulses
- Nuts and seeds
- Herbs and spices
- Fermented foods.

All the foods in these groups will help you heal from the inside out. Let's now explore each group and discover what's included.

Fruit

Maybe it's our monkey genes, but humans tend to be drawn to fruit. The colours, textures and wonderfully sweet flavours tickle the taste-buds and ping the pleasure centres in the brain. The ideal snack, fruit has sugar for energy plus vitamins and other antioxidants all wrapped up in complex fibre. The sugar in fruit is fructose, but a very different type to the concentrated one in ultra-processed foods and high-fructose corn syrup associated with the rise in fatty liver disease and obesity. Natural fructose in fruit is found in much lower amounts. Fruit contains so much more than the sugar too, although sadly it has been demonised by some schools of thought. It is also hard to eat too much in one go; the high-fibre content makes fruit very filling. It can also lead to stomach-ache and multiple trips to the toilet when eaten in excess – a natural deterrent!

The sugar in fruit is released once the fibre has been broken down, ideally through eating it whole. If fruit is added to a smoothie, the blender releases some of the sugar by breaking down the fibre. This can cause blood sugar spikes in some sensitive people, making the body work harder, something we want to avoid as much as possible when supporting it to heal. A single fruit in a green smoothie to make it more palatable is usually not an issue whereas a smoothie packed with more fruit than you would normally eat in a day is worth avoiding. Fruit juice has most if not all of the fibre removed, even when juiced at home. This makes the sugar readily available and just how much you're consuming difficult to measure. Fresh home-juiced fruit will contain more vitamins and phytonutrients though, much more than shop-bought which are best avoided.

Fruit eaten in season is best. The fresher the fruit, the better the nutrient content. It's also usually more affordable than out-of-season produce shipped halfway across the world and tastier too. Force-fed, out-of-season strawberries are nothing but a disappointment. Living in the UK, berries are very seasonal so enjoy them at their best and use frozen when the season has ended. Tropical fruits are always a dilemma as they must be shipped long distances and come with an environmental cost.

Packed with their own wonderful flavour and nutrients, try to include them when they're in season in their home country, or go for frozen.

> **How much fruit should I eat?**
> Two to three portions a day is a good guideline to go on. At least one of these should be berries. Dried fruit counts too. A small handful is a good guide for one portion – remember they're whole fruits with a much-reduced water content. They're super-easy to overeat as they're lovely and sweet.

Berries

Plump, sweet, juicy berries have been a favourite of humans for thousands of years. Our ancestors would have foraged for seasonal fruit, something many of us still do today. I love exploring the local hedgerows and picking blackberries and sloes, sometimes a wild raspberry or strawberry too.

Our love of berries means they are cultivated all around the world. Polytunnels have enabled farmers in the Northern Hemisphere to extend the growing season, providing warmth and shelter from inclement weather. Cultivated berries are sadly prone to moulds; birds and bugs love them too. To maximise their crops, farmers often use high amounts of chemicals, with residue remaining even after washing, particularly in the US where strawberries and blueberries feature in the 'dirty dozen',[1] a list of the most contaminated fruits and vegetables. Berries don't appear in the top 12 in the UK,[2] although I would always recommend the organic option wherever possible, or if you have space, grow your own.

Berries are packed with vitamin C as well as a range of powerful phytonutrients, including flavonoids and polyphenols – powerful antioxidants that help to calm down inflammation and support healing.[3] In particular, dark blue/black-coloured skins contain concentrated amounts of anthocyanins that are known to support immune and brain health. Fresh, frozen and even freeze-dried berries retain these nutrients. Cooking deactivates most of them but releases pectin, a fibre loved by the microbiome, so not all is lost.

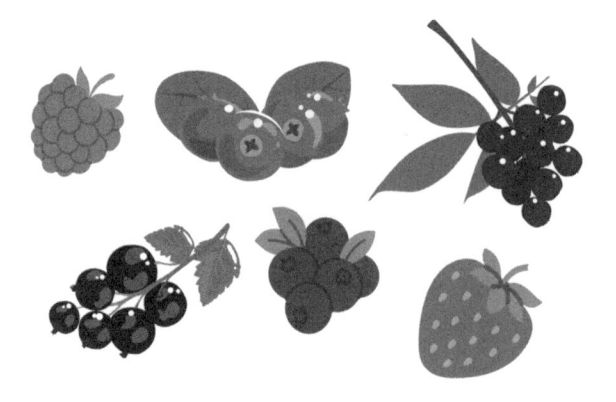

With their sharp and sweet flavours, berries can be used in salads, on cereals and to form part of tasty desserts. They make a great snack during the day and can even be blended frozen into tasty 'nice cream', a delicious and healthful alternative to ice cream. Aim to include at least one portion a day, mixing up the types and colours so you benefit from the variety of healthful properties. One portion is roughly 15–20 berries (small ones) or 80 g in weight.

Other fruit

Aside from berries, there's a smorgasbord of different fruit to choose from; stone fruit like apricots and peaches, traditional orchard fruits like apples, pears and plums, juicy grapes, citrus fruits offering segments of sharp juice and essential oils in the skin, through to beautiful exotic fruits like mango, pineapple, passion fruit and super-sweet melon.

> **Top tip:** Eat fruit with breakfast, at the beginning of a meal or between meals. The sugar and fibre content are more easily released than other foods so if they follow up a heavy meal they may create excess gas that can lead to bloating and flatulence, especially if less helpful microbes have migrated into the end of your small intestine and start chomping down on the polyphenols and fibre before you're ready.

Each fruit carries its own powerful concoction of antioxidants and fibre, all helping to support the body to reduce inflammation and heal. For example, **apples** are high in vitamin C and potassium as well as fibre, including pectin which the microbiome loves. They contain antioxidants like quercetin, a powerful flavonoid that can inhibit the production of inflammatory enzymes and cytokines, as well as help neutralise the free radical compounds that damage cells.

Grapes have a big reputation for being healthy as they contain another powerful flavonoid in their flesh, called resveratrol. Often connected to heart and brain health, research indicates that resveratrol is also beneficial for autoimmune disease, with studies noting benefits for people with RA, lupus, psoriasis, IBD and type 1 diabetes.[4] Red and black grapes contain the highest amount of their anti-inflammatory, antioxidant and anti-ageing benefits, which is why red wine is promoted as healthy.

Pineapple has been popular since the 16th century and rightly so as these gorgeously juicy fruits contain powerful compounds beneath their hard, fibrous skin. An excellent source of vitamin C and manganese, they also contain various B vitamins, magnesium and lots of insoluble fibre plus bromelain, a compound with digestive-enzyme properties that not only digest other food but can help reduce inflammation too, particularly in joints.

> **Kate's story:** Stone fruits can be a problem for some people with dysbiosis. After her elimination diet, Kate discovered she reacted to stone fruits so avoided them for a while. Now her gut has healed, she can enjoy them once more. Once again, listening to your body then helping it to heal should mean most foods can happily be included over time.

There are just too many different fruits to cover in this book. Be rest assured that each one comes with its own nutritional powerhouse that will support your body in so many ways. In times of abundance, pick or buy and freeze for dark winter days. Some fruits like citrus are in season during the winter, providing a vitamin C boost. Add the peel to hot drinks or baking as it contains beneficial oily compounds. Just make sure the fruit you are using is unwaxed – you don't want the extra chemicals that have been added to prolong shelf life.

> **Grapefruit** can interfere with some prescribed medications. Find out more in Chapter 8 (page 161) or talk to your pharmacist if you have concerns about interactions.

Aim to eat one or two portions of other types of fruit every day. A portion is a medium-sized apple or pear or around 80 g in weight. Always wash fruit well before eating and keep bananas out of the fruit bowl as they will hasten the oxidation of any fruit surrounding it.

Vegetables

There are just so many vegetables to choose from, there's always an option. I've split them into six groups for this section. Some have a tarnished reputation, like the nightshade family we discussed in Chapter 6, and white potatoes, the most consumed vegetable in the Western diet. The problem is the cooking method rather than the potato itself. There's a big difference between deep-fried chips and a baked potato. Aim to have at least one from each group every day; you'll benefit from a wonderful array of powerful antioxidants and other nutrients, as well as different textures, colours and flavours that you, your taste-buds and your microbiome will all enjoy.

Cruciferous

Cruciferous vegetables are rightly praised for their health benefits – they contain sulphoraphane, a sulphur compound with powerful antioxidant properties (and the source of their distinctive cooking smell). Although mainly green, some bright-coloured veggies are found in this group, like red cabbage, yellow swede and even purple cauliflower.

Chapter 7

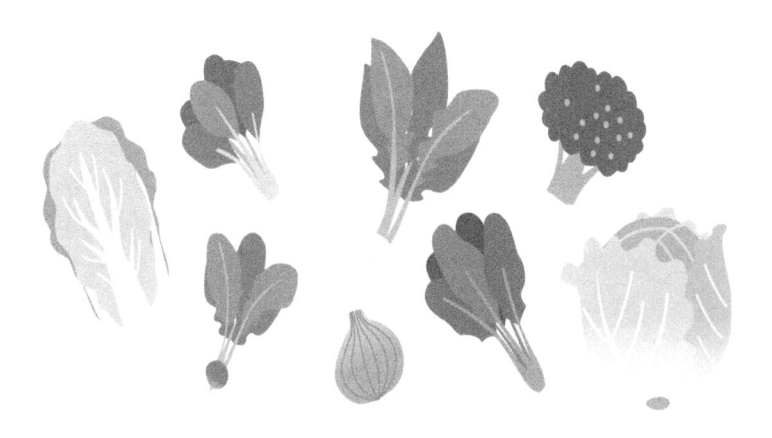

Apart from sulphoraphane, cruciferous vegetables contain an amazing array of vitamins, minerals and, of course, anti-inflammatory phytonutrients. You'll find vitamins A, C, K and B9 (folic acid), the minerals iron, calcium, copper, selenium, zinc and a plethora of polyphenols, flavonoids and glucosinolates. All these amazing compounds work together to reduce inflammation in the body.[5]

To get the maximum benefits from these vegetables, eat a mix of raw and cooked; cooking can make some nutrients more available for absorption, especially if your digestion is rather delicate to start with. Chopping vegetables like kale, broccoli and cabbage releases an enzyme called myrosinase that releases sulphoraphane. Myrosinase is destroyed by heat, but not sulphoraphane, so once chopped, leave 30 minutes to enable the enzyme to do it's magic before popping it in the steamer or oven.

Tricia's story: Tricia had been eating copious amounts of kale grown in her vegetable patch leading up to her IBD flare up. Could this have been a trigger? She'll never know, but she avoided it for some time afterwards as it can have a strong impact on a struggling gut. Nowadays, she eats small amounts only.

> **What about goitrogens?** If you have autoimmune thyroid disease, you may have been told to avoid cruciferous vegetables as they contain goitrogens, a plant compound that might affect iodine uptake and thyroid function, mainly in people already low in iodine. However, human studies suggest they're safe and even beneficial for those with thyroid disease when eaten as part of a varied diet.[6] Plant-based iodine sources include sea vegetables, green beans, potato skins, and iodised salt. Unless you're eating kilos of raw kale daily, there's little cause for concern.

Aim to include one or two portions of cruciferous vegetables, cooked and/or raw, into your diet every day. There are so many to choose from, you won't get bored.

Leafy greens

We've always been told to 'eat your greens' and rightly so. This group includes spinach, chard, all types of lettuce, endive, bok choi, pea shoots, dandelion leaves, celery leaves and fresh green herbs like parsley, mint and coriander (cilantro). Again, there are lots to choose from, providing a variety of flavours, textures and beneficial nutrients.

The green in leaves comes from chlorophyll, the compound that reacts with sunlight to create energy (photosynthesis). Previously thought to benefit only plants, humans can also utilise chlorophyll once it's been absorbed into the bloodstream and we get out in the sunshine.[7] Powerful ultraviolet waves penetrating the skin can activate circulating chlorophyll, enhancing its antioxidant and antitoxic properties. Isn't that amazing?

Leafy greens are also a great source of vitamins A, C and some of the Bs plus other minerals like iron, calcium, zinc and selenium, in differing amounts. Spinach has twice the amount of iron of other greens. Adding lemon juice or vinegar not only lifts the flavour but improves absorption too. Swiss chard contains good amounts of calcium but is high in oxalates (see page 112). You can still eat it if you have issues with kidney stones, just in moderate amounts and mixed with other types of vegetable.

Phytonutrients are abundant in all types of leafy greens. Spinach, the most researched, has at least 13 different flavonoids with antioxidant effects as well as different beta-carotenes, great for anyone trying to reduce chronic inflammation and promote healing. Some benefits are lost in cooking, so raw, wilted, lightly steamed or briefly stir fried are all preferable to cooking for any length. Serving a meal on a bed of raw leaves or adding greens at the end of cooking a stew, soup or curry allows them to wilt without losing their goodness.

Leafy greens also contain vitamin K, a fat-soluble vitamin needed for blood clotting and bone health, important for all ages, particularly post-menopausal women at risk of osteoporosis. It can interfere with some blood-thinning medications, particularly warfarin. A moderate intake should be fine, but no more than two portions a day. Please check with your pharmacist or GP if you are concerned about interactions or see if your GP will titrate your warfarin dose with your leafy green intake – you might find that greens are so powerful your clotting normalises.

Aim to eat one or two portions of leafy greens every day, mixing up the types so you get the benefits of them all.

Roots and tubers

A key staple for many populations around the world, humans have been eating roots and tubers for thousands of years, both foraged and farmed. Grown underground, tubers are a modified extension of the stem, and root vegetables are enlarged taproots. Both contain the plant's nutrient store; those benefits come to us when we eat them.

Roots and tubers make up the main energy source for many populations around the world. High in carbohydrate, most are great sources of fibre, vitamins and minerals. Not all though, particularly white potatoes and cassava. Colourful beetroot, carrot and sweet potato contain powerful anti-inflammatory compounds like vitamins A and C, carotenoids and flavonoids. Most of the beneficial nutrients are found in or just under the skin, with the energy bound up in the flesh. Radishes are different. Their powerful antioxidants are found in the flesh and colourful skins, making them pungent and peppery. Some radishes are so strong it sometimes feels like they're biting back!

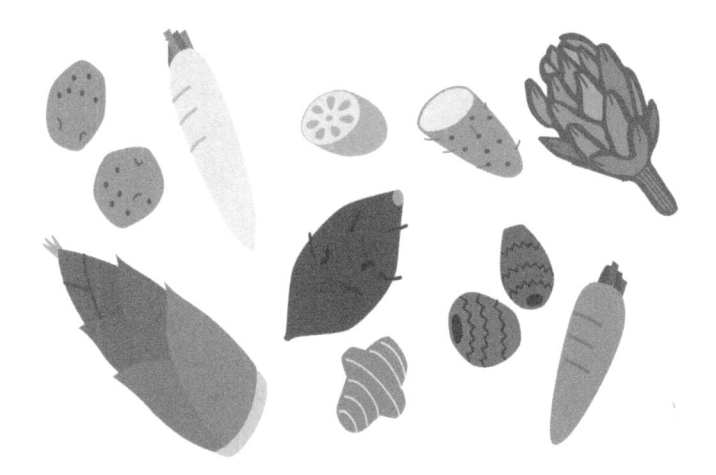

Roots like parsnip, potato and swede should all be cooked before eating, ideally steamed to retain nutrients. Carrots offer up different benefits when raw or cooked.[8] Heat makes beta-carotene, a precursor to vitamin A, more available than raw, and their antioxidant levels double when carrots are cooked with their skins on. The same applies to beetroot too.

If you are near a farmers' market or farm shop, see you if can find colourful versions of roots and tubers, like rainbow carrots, yellow beetroots or intensely flavoured purple sweet potatoes and keep experimenting with ones you don't normally eat. Shred celeriac and eat it raw in salads rather than cooked, or add radishes to curry. Remember, variety is the spice of life, particularly when it comes to beneficial nutrients for your body, and microbiome. Try not to overdo it though - even the most innocuous vegetable can cause a digestive upset if eaten in large quantities.

Aim to eat one or two portions from this group every day, mixing them up from day to day as much as you can.

Bulbs and stems

This flavoursome group is dominated by the *Alliaceae* family – onions, shallots, leeks, chives, and the foe to vampires, garlic. Other tasty stems include asparagus, celery, bamboo shoots and rhubarb. All contain prebiotic fibre that the microbiome loves to eat, particularly onions and garlic, alongside pungent sulphur-containing compounds and a host of antioxidants, including quercetin and allicin. Unfortunately, many people with digestive issues struggle to tolerate some or all the Allium family and so tend to avoid them. 'Bad' bacteria in the microbiome or even higher up in the small intestine overreact to these compounds, creating excess gas, bloating and flatulence. Gradually improving microbiome diversity by slowly increasing the variety of plant foods eaten can help improve the situation and even make onions and garlic tolerable again. Heat also reduces sulphur levels, making them less irritating, and marinating raw onion in lemon or vinegar also helps by softening the cell walls and releasing the sulphur compounds. If you struggle with the most pungent offenders – onions and garlic – you may be fine with leeks and chives, so do give them a try.

> **Asparagus wee?** These delightful stems are a seasonal favourite of mine, but they do come with an aromatic after-effect. The sulphur compounds in asparagus are so pungent, the aroma hangs around when you next have a wee. Not for everyone though; some people can't smell it – lucky them! For a few unlucky people, the smell is so overwhelming they choose not to eat asparagus at all – a shame because, alongside their delicious flavour, asparagus contains vitamins A, C, E and K as well as a heap of antioxidants like flavonoids and polyphenols. If you manage to find purple asparagus, you'll gain brain-loving anthocyanins too.

Try to eat at least one portion from this group every day. If you find them hard to tolerate, eat a small, cooked amount a few days a week to start with and gradually build up depending on how you respond. If it's too uncomfortable, avoid for a couple of weeks, then try again. It can change; I couldn't eat garlic for two years. It has improved, but still only when cooked.

'Fruit' vegetables

A surprising number of vegetables commonly eaten are actually fruit. Tomatoes, aubergine, courgettes and peas all fall into this group. Botanically, a fruit is a seed-bearing structure that develops from the ovary of a plant. For culinary purposes, it doesn't really matter as they're all amazingly tasty and packed full of powerful nutrients, antioxidants and fibre.

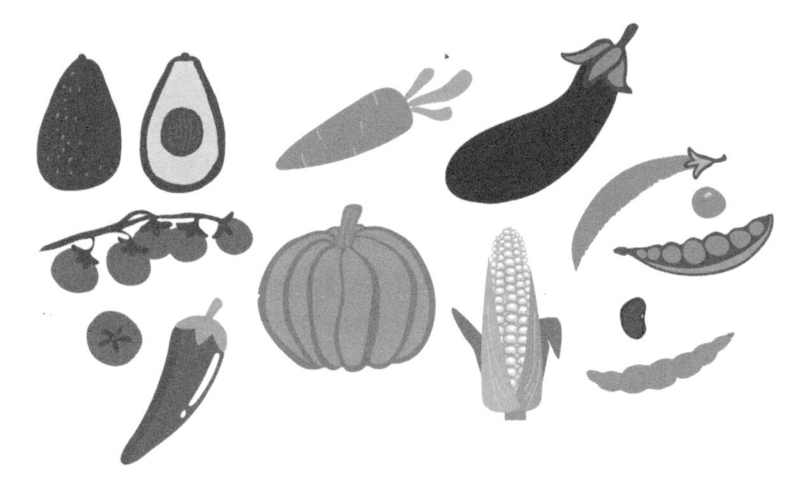

All the beautiful rainbow colours are found in this group, which means they're packed with antioxidants and other phytonutrients, particularly polyphenols. Some antioxidants, like lycopene in tomatoes, protective against prostate cancer, are only released when cooked. Many in this group feature in the healthful Mediterranean diet pattern, the world's most researched, health-promoting dietary pattern, full of anti-inflammatory compounds.

You may have noticed that many of the nightshade family are in this group which, as I covered in Chapter 6, might not be an issue for you. If you do react to one, see how you are with the others before banishing the whole group from your diet.

Try to eat one or two from this group every day, mixing it up to include all the colours during the week.

Fungi, algae and sea vegetables

Whilst fungi, algae and sea vegetables are not officially 'plants', they tend to be included in the 'vegetable' category. 'The food of the Gods' in Roman times, mushrooms and other fungi are a group of non-animal organisms that humans have consumed for thousands of years as food or medicine. Medicinal mushrooms have featured in Chinese medicine for over 2000 years and Hippocrates used them for their anti-inflammatory properties in 450 BCE. There's even evidence of use by our Neolithic ancestors over 5000 years ago. Not all mushrooms are good to eat though, which is why I've never been foraging for mushrooms in case I find the wrong type!

Although there are around 700 different types of edible mushroom and fungi around the world, it can be hard to find more than two or three in a standard UK supermarket. Some upmarket ones may stock oyster, shiitake, or a mix of 'woodland' mushrooms, but often you need to visit an Asian supermarket or large city market to discover exciting alternatives.

Mushrooms and other fungi contain a wealth of healthful nutrients like B vitamins, selenium, potassium and zinc. If left gill side up, mushrooms will also manufacture vitamin D; this makes them the only non-animal organism to contain a naturally made form of this vitamin and shows that fungi love to sunbathe as much as we do. They also contain a heap of antioxidants like polyphenols and a type of fibre called beta-glucan. In general health, beta-glucan is thought to help lower cholesterol and fats by binding to them in the gut as well as to help manage blood sugar levels.

Mushrooms also have an immunomodulatory effect,[9] which means they directly impact our innate and adaptive immune response. Research into inflammatory bowel disease (IBD) and rheumatoid arthritis (RA) shows that mushrooms and other fungi have a positive effect, but for lupus it's mixed.[10, 11] However, these are lab studies using extracts rather than studies of humans eating whole foods. Some have concerns that the 'immune boosting' effects may be too strong for people with autoimmune disease, especially for people on immune-suppression medications. Other research however, suggests that fungi can support T helper cells, dampening down autoimmune reactions and support healing.[12]

One other potential issue is gut health. Dysbiosis can create an overgrowth of moulds and yeasts perpetuated by eating mushrooms, especially in people with thrush or the herpes virus. Interestingly, research suggests that reishi mushrooms can help with this.[13] If you think mushrooms are a problem for you, leave them out of your diet for a couple of weeks and observe how you feel, then reintroduce them in small amounts and see if anything changes. Hopefully, you will be fine as mushrooms add flavour and texture to lots of recipes in addition to their beneficial nutrients.

Unless you enjoy sushi, sea vegetables might not feature much in your daily diet. In the past, though, coast-dwellers would have regularly eaten dulse and samphire, dubbed 'sea asparagus' due to their tasty, if rather salty, tender stems. Algae like spirulina are often added to smoothies for their strong nutritional properties, including an array of B vitamins, omega 3, protein, iron, magnesium, potassium and zinc plus phytonutrients like phycocyanin that provides its blue/green colour. It's not for everyone though as, to my taste-buds anyway, it also tastes of pond.

Sea vegetables are a good non-animal source of iodine, important for thyroid function and often lacking in plant-based diets. If you have thyroid issues, take care with foods like kombu which can carry excessive amounts; nori and wakame have more moderate amounts and are less likely to cause problems.

Nori is a useful ingredient to keep in the store cupboard, especially if you want to recreate a 'fishy' kind of flavour. I regularly make no-fish pie or no-fish cakes using nori – it adds an extra flavour as well as the nutrients. Edible seaweed can also be bought as flakes and used instead of salt, adding flavour and iodine in one go.

Beans and lentils (legumes)

One of the oldest cultivated plants, legumes have been eaten since prehistoric times and remain key foods for a huge swathe of the world's population. Often looked down upon as the poor man's meat, legumes are a great source of plant protein along with fibre, minerals and even polyphenols in colourful skins. Beans and legumes are so healthy they support longevity. Studies have found a dose-dependent link between legumes and a reduction in all-cause mortality[14]: every 2 tablespoons of beans reduces the risk of death by 8%. That's impressive! No wonder some have suggested legumes should be renamed 'healthy people's meat'.

The downside of beans and lentils is they can create a lot of flatulence, especially in anyone with dysbiosis. As covered in Chapter 4, legumes are high in FODMAPs and can cause painful bloating and noxious wind. A low-FODMAP diet in the short run can help, but avoiding them completely won't improve the situation in the long run as you'll miss out on the benefits they offer for healing the microbiome and the body.

It does take time to shift, though. How do I know? I had severe dysbiosis before starting my plant-based journey. Years of living with an undiagnosed dairy intolerance and a love for all things sweet, I had a reputation for being super-windy in my family. Odorous wafts could erupt for hours. Eliminating dairy made a huge difference but I could still go through phases of explosive wind after eating high-fibrous foods, including some beans. Once fully plant-based and as my gut started to heal, I found legumes had fewer and fewer after-effects, which was a great relief to everyone.

Some beans with a tough outer layer, like soya or fava beans, may cause a bigger reaction than smaller beans or split lentils. The skin is highly fermentable; removing it when soaking dried beans can make a big difference. Haricot and butter (lima) beans are high in oligosaccharides and are notorious for their fart factor too. You might want to limit your intake of these to start with, focusing on black or aduki beans and lentils at first, introducing the others in small amounts. Everyone's microbiome reacts differently, which is why there are no set rules to the timing of moving to a whole-food plant-based diet. Some people can change overnight without malodorous after-effects (or ones they confess to!). Others with a more delicate gut composition will take time. But every change pushes you in a positive direction, so don't delay too long or you might just be prolonging the problem unnecessarily.

As discussed in Chapter 6, beans and lentils must be cooked before eating. Tins and packets of ready-to-eat legumes are cheap and easy to find. A cheaper option still is to buy dried goods to cook at home. This can take some forward planning, but cooking at home with a little bicarbonate of soda in the water can help reduce the oligosaccharide issue, although it can make them rather mushy if cooked for too long.

> **Tricia's story:** Tinned baked beans were the first type of beans Tricia could tolerate after her Crohn's flare up. After that, she gradually introduced more tinned beans and lentils, making sure she still cooked them for some time to make them more digestible.

If you're not sure how to prepare and cook dried beans and lentils, check out my website https://thesensitivefoodiekitchen.com/a-quick-guide-to-preparing-beans-and-lentils/ for my in-depth guide.

> **Sprouting:** Legumes are seeds, ready to spring into life when conditions are right with warmth, light and water. Soaking and sprouting beans and lentils can start this process off, making the nutrients within more available and digestible – a double bonus. Health food stores often sell ready-sprouted legume sprouts, but they are easy to do at home as well. All you need is a large jar to soak the beans or lentils in plus something to drain the water through – a cover made of muslin works well. Alternatively, you can buy specially designed jars for sprouting.
> - Rinse the legumes then pop in the jar, cover with water and leave to soak for 24 hours.
> - Drain out the water, rinse and drain again, then leave somewhere light but not in direct sunlight.
> - After 12 hours, rinse, drain and leave again.
> - Depending on the type of legume, sprouting should start after 48 hours. Once tiny white strands appear, you can eat them. Or leave them to grow a bit more, rinsing and draining every 12 hours.
> - When they're ready, store the sprouted legumes in the fridge in an air-tight container for up to three days. Don't let them go manky, though.
>
> See *The Sprout Book* by Doug Evans (page 321) for everything you need to know and more.

I can't leave a section on beans and lentils without mentioning the elephant in the room – soya beans. These small beans, vibrant green, yellow or even black when fresh, dull and wrinkled when dry, have carried the heavy weight of controversy for decades. From environmental destruction and man-boobs to cancer and 'Frankenstein food', soya has more bad press than any other plant food.

Yes, soya farming is contributing to the destruction of the Amazon rainforest. It is also grown as a mono crop in some areas, is often genetically modified and carries high levels of pesticides and other chemicals. The vegan movement is not behind these issues, though, but animal agriculture and the rising demand for meat.

Globally, only 7% of soya is eaten directly by humans.[15] That includes China and Japan where it's a daily staple. Over 70% is used to feed animals farmed for meat and dairy, even though soya is not ideal for many animals, particularly cows. It makes them fart too and contributes to increasing methane levels in the atmosphere, causing global warming. A lot of the negativity about soya as a food sources comes out of the US. Previously the largest grower of soya beans (it's now second to Brazil – rainforest destruction in action), 94% are genetically modified – the 'Frankenstein food'. This has caused alarm in health communities, with fears about knock on effects in humans from environmental contamination and residue in meat products.

As a plant-based food source for humans, the humble soya bean comes with a plethora of benefits, including high levels of plant protein, excellent amounts of essential fatty acids and a range of beneficial plant compounds, including phytosterols that help lower blood cholesterol levels and isoflavones or phytoestrogen. These last compounds underlie media scare stories claiming soya gives men man-boobs even though a high dairy and fat intake is much more likely to do that. Phytoestrogens do have a similar effect to mammal oestrogen, attaching to oestrogen receptors without disrupting normal hormonal processes. Indeed, soya is thought to help balance fluctuating oestrogen levels during perimenopause and can provide some of the protective elements provided by oestrogen, including supporting the immune system.[16] And counter to another common internet rumour about soya and increased cancer risk, research also shows these natural compounds have an anti-cancer effect instead. For autoimmune disease, oestrogen appears to have varied impacts in different conditions.[17] In MS, for example, it has a protective effect, but the opposite is true in lupus. These are animal experiments using oestrogen rather than phytoestrogens. Studies using phytoestrogens show a positive effect for RA,[18] which is good news.

Whole, or minimally-processed, soya products, like edamame beans, tofu, tempeh, soya milk and yoghurt, are best; avoid ultra-processed meat-replacement products that contain altered and concentrated soya protein. Fermentation can help break down FODMAPs and increase digestibility; tempeh is made from fermented whole beans packed together into a firm 'cake'. It has a slightly odd taste but, like tofu, absorbs other flavours well and can be used in a range of savoury dishes. If you are unsure about how to cook with soya products, have a look at my guide in the bonus book features on my website: https://thesensitivefoodiekitchen.com/cooking-with-soya-products/.

Soya is often flagged up as a food to avoid with autoimmune disease, which is a shame as it contains so many healthful properties. If it's not something you react to then try to include two portions a day.

> **My top tips** for buying soya products are:
> - Buy organic
> - Buy calcium-set tofu to increase your calcium intake
> - Check for hidden added sugars and emulsifiers in soya milk
> - Buy unsweetened, plain soya yoghurt and add fruit at home
> - Check the ingredients list and avoid 'hydrolysed' soya protein.

Grains

Back in Chapter 6 we explored the issue around gluten and autoimmune disease (page 117). Whole grains remain a key part of a whole-food plant-based diet as they provide a good number of calories, essential vitamins, minerals and, of course, fibre. Fortunately, if you do need to avoid gluten, there is still a great selection of whole grains to choose from, including oats, buckwheat and millet as long as you don't have coeliac disease (CD), non-coeliac gluten intolerance (NCGI), or a gluten allergy. Be aware there is a risk of cross-contamination in factories processing gluten-containing grains. If gluten is a big issue for you, always check the label.

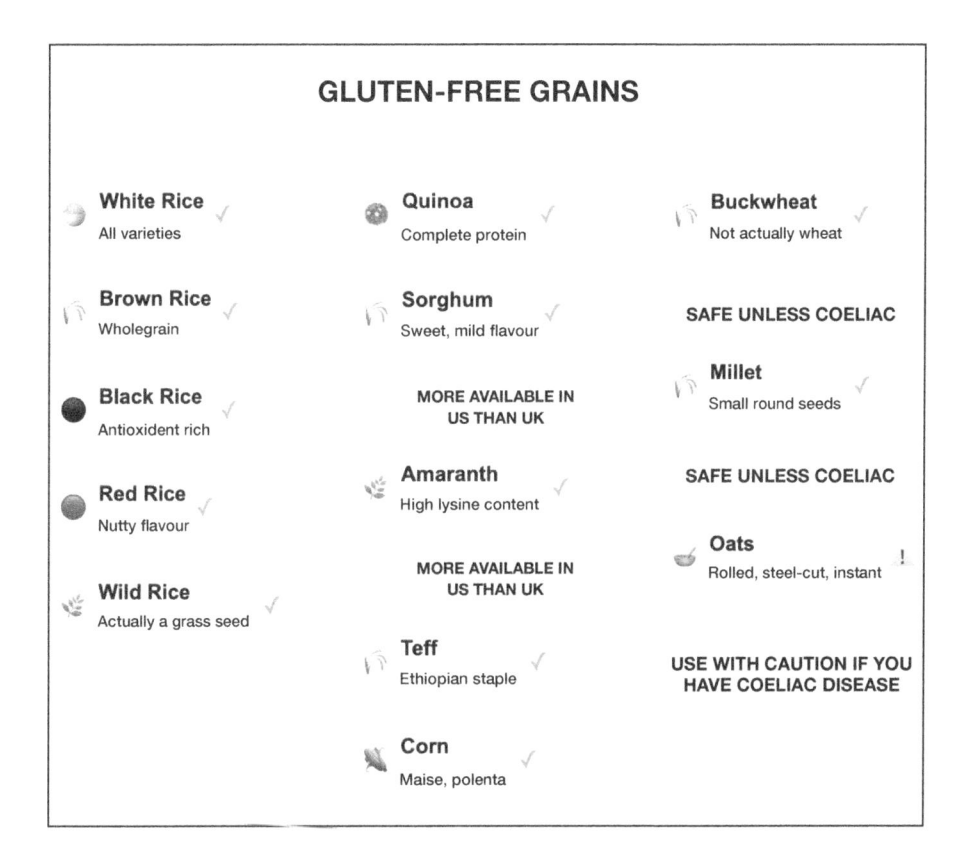

GLUTEN-FREE GRAINS

White Rice ✓ — All varieties	**Quinoa** ✓ — Complete protein	**Buckwheat** ✓ — Not actually wheat
Brown Rice ✓ — Wholegrain	**Sorghum** ✓ — Sweet, mild flavour	**SAFE UNLESS COELIAC**
Black Rice ✓ — Antioxident rich	MORE AVAILABLE IN US THAN UK	**Millet** ✓ — Small round seeds
Red Rice ✓ — Nutty flavour	**Amaranth** ✓ — High lysine content	**SAFE UNLESS COELIAC**
Wild Rice ✓ — Actually a grass seed	MORE AVAILABLE IN US THAN UK	**Oats** ! — Rolled, steel-cut, instant
	Teff ✓ — Ethiopian staple	**USE WITH CAUTION IF YOU HAVE COELIAC DISEASE**
	Corn ✓ — Maise, polenta	

Many of these are seeds rather than grains that contain a wealth of nutrients like plant protein, iron, calcium, essential fatty acids, B vitamins and vitamin E with its strong antioxidant capacity and, of course, fibre. Some of these pseudo-grains are mass-produced using pesticides and herbicides, so buy organic products wherever possible and affordable.

Variety is the key once again, so take time to explore and experiment with different products. Whilst oats for breakfast are great, eating them every day won't ensure your microbiome gets everything it needs to thrive. If you have a leaky gut, eating the same item every day can increase the risk of intolerance, so try mixing it up and experiment with new things. For example, quinoa or millet porridge makes a delicious change to oat-based. As for rice, there are so many different types and colours to try that plain white rice will soon become a thing of the past. Whilst it does take longer to cook, soaking in water for a few hours beforehand cuts the time dramatically.

Nuts and seeds

During my 'dieting years', I spent a long time on a very low-fat diet, avoiding all nuts apart from chestnuts. Seeds were not a big thing in the 1980s so I didn't eat these either. That's a big regret now I know more about nutrition. Nuts and seeds are a nutrient powerhouse packed with healthy fats, minerals, fat-soluble vitamins, antioxidants and fibre, all connected with reducing chronic inflammation. A 2022 meta-analysis found a daily intake of around 30 g of nuts or seeds led to a 21% reduction in heart disease, 11% reduction in cancer and a 22% reduction in death from all causes.[19]

What about autoimmune conditions? We've already explored concerns regarding phytates in Chapter 6 and we know that our early ancestors ate them, even though the paleo approach excludes them. Plus, soaking and sprouting can make nuts and seeds more digestible, even with conditions like coeliac disease where nutrient absorption is an issue. As a group of conditions, the research is scant, however. There is more on specific conditions like RA where studies show the essential fatty acid and antioxidant profile has a positive effect on inflammatory markers.[20] Or lupus, where a recent study suggests that eating nuts and seeds reduces the risk of developing lupus by 41%.[21] In MS, nuts and seeds can help reduce the risk of developing it and also help reduce symptoms.[22]

Regular nut consumption leads to lower levels of inflammatory biomarkers, which is good news and is part of the Mediterranean way of eating, known for longevity and healthy outcomes. Most nuts are a good source of calcium, great for bone health, but should be eaten away from medications like thyroxine as calcium interferes with its absorption. Nuts also contain zinc, magnesium and iron as well as the lesser-known trace minerals like manganese, selenium, silicon and chromium. Just three medium Brazil nuts provide enough selenium for the day as well as good amounts of other minerals plus plant protein, healthy fats and of course fibre. Not that I'm suggesting you just eat three Brazil nuts; all nuts contain these essential minerals in varying amounts, so eating different types during the week not only gives you a good range of nutrients but variety and tasty recipes too.

Seeds, especially flax and chia seeds, contain high levels of omega 3 fatty acids; this helps reduce inflammation and is particularly beneficial for autoimmune disease. They also contain isoflavones/phytoestrogens that can support hormonal health. Cold-pressed flaxseed oil is a powerful way of consuming higher amounts of these anti-inflammatory compounds, but beware of where you buy it as it rapidly goes off if not stored correctly. When rancid, it's foul! Flaxseeds themselves must be ground before eating as the tough outer layer is indigestible, keeping the healthy nutrients and fibre locked up. Grind them in a high-speed blender and store in the fridge to keep those volatile oils stable. Be careful how much you eat in one go as flaxseed can stimulate gut motility more readily than you might wish if you're not used to it. Start with 1 teaspoon and increase gradually; 1-2 tablespoons a day is plenty. Hemp seeds are also a good source of omega 3 fatty acids, plant protein and minerals like magnesium, calcium and iron. Hemp hearts are easier to use and can be sprinkled on food or blended to make tasty dressings and garnishes that liven up the dullest of dishes.

Herbs and spices

Used for thousands of years as the only medicine available, 80% of the world's population still use or rely on herbs and spices in traditional medicines for their healthcare needs. They can play a powerful role in the anti-inflammatory kitchen too.

Herbs like boswellia, ashwagandha, *Ginkgo biloba* and St John's wort are often taken as supplements by people with autoimmune disease. I'm not going to focus on these, though, as I'm not a herbalist; instead, let's have a look at how herbs and spices can be used in everyday cooking.

I can't think of a recipe that doesn't benefit from a scattering of herbs or pinch of spice. It's not just flavour they add but powerful phytonutrients and antioxidants as well as antibacterial properties. Some, like black pepper, also stimulate the release of stomach acid to aid digestion. Along with other spices like cumin and ginger, black pepper calms digestive issues, helps break down fat and aids the absorption of some vitamins and minerals. Black pepper also works in partnership with other phytonutrients – for example, an active compound called piperine, enables the absorption of the curcuminoids in turmeric. That's a lot for one small peppercorn that's just treated as a flavouring.

Turmeric has been extensively studied, and benefits have been found for almost every chronic inflammatory condition. Used for joint pain and inflammation for thousands of years, turmeric has antimicrobial, antiviral, and anti-inflammatory properties; adding it to food on a regular basis has positive side benefits rather than the side effects associated with many pain medications. Just remember to add the black pepper.

> **The healing power of turmeric:** I first began to understand its power when living in India. Being a key component of Indian cuisine, it was of course everywhere, displayed in alluring, glowing piles in the markets. One day when I met a local Indian friend, I noticed she had a thick coating of turmeric on the back of her forearm. She explained she'd burnt herself and applied a turmeric poultice which soothed the pain and would help it heal. I was rather sceptical but when I saw her the following week, there was almost no sign of the burn; it had all healed beautifully.

Ginger is another powerful root that can help reduce pain and inflammation, as well as support gut health. Fresh, dried or pickled, there are hundreds of different types of ginger, but generally it's just common ginger available in UK supermarkets, and sometimes galangal in the Japanese food section. Used for thousands of years to relieve nausea, the volatile compounds in ginger have a calming effect on the gut, especially when paired with other spices like cinnamon and cardamom. Dried ginger powder can be used as a painkiller; studies have shown that ground ginger is as effective as other painkillers for period pain.[23] Compounds called gingerols prevent the formation of inflammatory chemical messengers that cause joint pain; a tasty way to reduce inflammation, that's for sure.

It's not just herbs and spices from the East that provide these wonderful properties. Traditional herbs like rosemary (a strong antibacterial that is also good for the brain), thyme (anti-spasmodic and antibacterial) and parsley (anti-cancer and overall anti-inflammatory effects) are just as effective and can be easily grown in the garden or in pots on balconies or kitchen windowsills. There's something rather wonderful about going out and harvesting fresh herbs. I find their strong aromas elicit comforting and familiar memories which make me feel good, even before I've eaten them.

There's not enough space here to cover every spice and herb – if you want to know more, check out a couple of book recommendations in the Resources section (page 321). For now, though, just remember that every time you add a pinch of cinnamon, a sprinkle of rosemary or a scattering of basil, you are adding a little bit of medicinal plant magic along with the beautiful flavours and aromas.

Although it's not a herb or spice, I want to include green tea here with its many marvellous anti-inflammatory phytonutrients that are known to be good for both gut health and autoimmune disease. Green tea contains lots of polyphenols including catechins, which calm the innate and adaptive immune responses.[24] Research has focused on green tea extracts, but including it as part of your daily intake is still helpful and, with so many types on the market, like 'standard' green tea, floral jasmine, powerful gunpowder tea and musty maccha, there's plenty to choose from to suit your taste. I drink at least two cups a day, often more – I do love my tea!

Fermented foods

Fermentation has been used to preserve food for thousands of years. In recent times, as the importance of gut health has been recognised, fermented foods have been increasingly researched. Studies indicate that the bacteria and other microbes produced through fermentation can support the immune system as well as the microbiome and help reduce systemic inflammation and the effects of autoimmune disease.[25] These beneficial microbes, known as probiotics, populate the microbiome and help to overcome the less beneficial, inflammatory microbes creating havoc in the gut. The extra SCFAs produced by a happy, well-fed and balanced microbiome support anti-inflammatory signalling and reduce the creation of inflammatory cytokines and oxidative stress at cellular level.

Vegetables, soya beans and dairy products are the main fermented foods used functionally today, with sauerkraut, kimchi and yoghurt being amongst the most eaten in the West. Fermented soya products like tempeh, natto and miso are becoming more popular, particularly miso which adds a deep umami flavour to many plant-based recipes. Sourdough bread using a fermented wheat starter is making a comeback now the downsides of industrially made, ultra-processed bread are being recognised. Home-baked sourdough became a craze during the Covid-19 lockdowns, and a homemade starter collects the microbes in your own home, making it personalised to your surroundings. Fermentation can make wheat products more digestible, including gluten, especially in ancient wheats like spelt, rye and emmer, although these remain off the menu for people who must avoid it. Unfortunately, I have had no luck in creating gluten free sourdough bread despite reading up on it. I'm sure there's a way!

Home-made benefits apply to all fermented foods. Sauerkraut is super-easy to make and again carries a bacterial signature of your own home. Tasty and crunchy, it takes just a few days to ferment and can be kept in the fridge for weeks as you work your way through the batch. If you like a bit of spice, kimchi is also easy to make with the spice mix readily available in online stores. Kombucha can be made at home too. A 'mother' starter is needed. It's possible to make these from scratch yourself (it takes time, but I have done it), although it's easier to find someone local who can spare some of their productive 'mother'. Only buy chilled fermented products in the shops; anything on the shelves will be pasteurised, killing off the beneficial bacteria.

> **Kate's story:** Kate recommends making kimchi at home. Now she's mastered the technique, it's easy and cheap, plus it uses bacteria found in their environment. Don't worry if it doesn't work out right the first few times; Kate recommends you keep experimenting – success will be achieved in the end.

Much of the research conducted on autoimmune disease and fermented foods has been done in labs or on animals. The main benefits found have included modulation of inflammatory signalling in the gut and an increase in SCFAs. Fermented turmeric enhanced the availability of its curcumin content; sauerkraut and kimchi improved inflammatory bowel disease symptoms; and fermented soya helped reduce neuroinflammation.[26]

Probiotic supplementation is currently a huge area of research and potentially a highly lucrative market. However, supplementation alone will not have the same benefits if dietary changes are not made and may not be necessary as eating a whole-food plant-based diet packed with fibre and polyphenols supports gut health. Adding fermented foods can boost and support beneficial bacteria that will then flourish in a nutrient-dense environment.

A word of caution, though: fermented foods are not for everyone, particularly those who cannot tolerate yeast or histamine. Personally, I only eat them occasionally as I struggle to digest them, even when made at home. I also suggest you don't rush out and buy five different types of fermented foods to eat all at the same time. Someone I know did this and felt terrible after three days. It took a while for him to understand that his body just wasn't ready for an intense bombardment of multiple microbes. Less is better than more. Fermented foods like miso, sauerkraut and kimchi are also very high in salt. In Chapter 3, we explored the connection between salt and autoimmunity, so it's best to eat these only occasionally, especially if you suffer from high blood pressure or kidney issues. Finally, some of the bioactive compounds can interfere with certain medications for depression or anxiety, so please check with your doctor or pharmacist before adding fermented foods to your daily diet.

What about drinks?

Having mentioned the benefits of drinking green tea and kombucha, this seems a good point to quickly explore what else is good to drink during the day and what to avoid.

As boring as it may seem, good old plain water is always the number one fluid of choice. Humans are around 66% water, so it makes sense that we need to drink a good amount to maintain a healthy balance. Many people are permanently dehydrated or consume lots of dehydrating drinks like coffee or sugar-sweetened fizzy drinks. Dehydration can cause constipation, lack of energy, reduced brain function and make the body work harder, increasing the release of inflammatory free radicals. It also contributes to heart conditions, dizziness and recurrent urine infections (UTIs). People with autoimmune disease have a higher incidence of UTIs, and these can trigger symptoms and potentially a relapse.[27] 'Have you got a UTI?' is certainly the first question I get asked by my MS team if I'm not feeling quite right.

The ideal fluid intake varies from person to person and is influenced by size, level of physical activity and often personal preference. I know people who seem to drink twice as much as I do during the day. They also tend to get over-heated more easily and have a different metabolic rate. The standard recommendation is between six and eight glasses of water a day, which works out to around 2 litres. That's just water – other drinks are added on top of that. Interestingly, a whole-food plant-based diet has a high-water content, so you gain extra fluids through eating this way and may feel that six glasses a day is just fine for you.

Too much water can be just as bad as not enough. Drinking a high volume of water in a relatively short period of time, especially when it's not needed, dilutes the blood and lowers sodium levels. Low levels can lead to neurological dysfunction, even loss of consciousness and, on occasion, death. I know many people who have found themselves in dire straits due to excess water consumption, including my own mum. Once she recovered, she got a right ticking off!

Water doesn't have to be boring. I enjoy carbonated water infused with lemon or lime. Cucumber water is refreshing, especially in summer, and water infused with berries is a tasty treat. Hot infusions are lovely too, either with herbal teabags or fresh spices like ginger, cinnamon and cardamom, lemon and ginger, or fresh mint tea.

And what about alcohol? For most chronic health conditions, it's been found to promote systemic inflammation. Studies on autoimmune disease are not so clear, however. Some research suggests a light or moderate intake may have a protective effect for a range of conditions due to its immunomodulatory role.[28] Whilst I'm not suggesting you knock back a bottle of wine or gin a night, it's good to know that the odd drink not only won't do any harm but maybe some good. Do remember that some medications interact with alcohol, though, and this might not be good if you have other health conditions.

Summary

Much has been covered in this chapter. Hopefully you are now feeling confident that you have a vast array of foods to choose from and won't go hungry. Eating a rainbow mix of fruit, vegetables, whole grains, nuts, seeds and legumes provides a wonderful array of flavours, textures and nutrients that you and your microbiome will love. Every meal is a chance to reduce inflammation and help your body heal.

Chapter 8

Final things to consider

Introduction

Much has been covered in the last seven chapters. Hopefully you are now feeling confident about the nourishing benefits of a whole-food plant-based diet that can push you towards a less inflammatory, more healing state, and that you are excited about the abundance, flexibility and choice that comes with this way of eating.

Autoimmunity is for life; a whole-food plant-based diet is not a quick fix or a temporary discomfort. Eating nourishing and enjoyable foods can become part of normal life; different and often challenging to start with, but once you've adapted and start experiencing how it feels to be 'well', your old way of eating won't be so tempting. That's certainly how I feel. Adopting a whole-food plant-based diet was definitely one of my better life choices. If I was suddenly told 'you don't have MS', I wouldn't change the way I eat, that's for sure. I'm not the only one who feels like that, and it's not just people using food as medicine either! Eating this way fills you with an energy and vitality you don't realise is possible.

> Rosa's parents have benefited from moving to a whole-food plant-based diet, as has Kate's husband. The powerful anti-inflammatory, body-loving nutrients can help everyone live better for longer.

In this chapter, I'm going to share a few more tips and things to consider, including cooking techniques, potential medication issues, how fasting may help and, most importantly, the fundamental importance of kindness, to yourself and others.

Go at your own pace

Back in Chapter 5, I gave you my Seven Steps to wellness, with the proviso that you go at your own pace. I really cannot emphasise that enough. Changes need to work for you. When you remove certain foods, like dairy, sugar or gluten, from your diet, you can feel worse in the short term. Supported by the bad bacteria that thrive on these foods, the brain fires off craving messages that affect your mood, cause headaches or worsen fatigue, especially if you do it all at once without adding in anti-inflammatory foods. Some people push through, but if you can't, don't completely give up. Try again, but this time do one thing at a time whilst being more mindful about what you're doing.

Dairy can be particularly hard, especially cheese as it's super-addictive. What are you replacing it with? Most vegan cheeses are made with coconut oil and need to be avoided due to the high levels of saturated fat, plus they don't contain the compounds that your cheese addiction will be craving. Nuts, seeds, nutritional yeast and garlic powder can create tasty cheese alternatives, supported by lots of nutrient-dense vegetables. Adding different foods can make a big difference; you don't want to feel deprived. Of course, these alternatives are not the same as cheese, but the cravings will pass eventually. As a reformed cheese addict, I can't even bear the smell of it now.

> **Rosa's story:** Rosa didn't find it hard to move to a plant-based diet and her taste-buds changed pretty quickly. Cheese was the hardest food to let go of, although she now enjoys the increasing selection of plant-based cheese alternatives.

There's no prescribed right way to make change, no 'failure' if you make a less healthful choice. On the other hand, doing nothing is not an option if you want your body to start healing. Disease-modifying medications can help manage your symptoms and possibly slow disease progression, but they won't help your body to heal or thrive as a stand-alone. Indeed, research is now suggesting these therapies are more effective when coupled with diet and lifestyle changes. If you're tempted not to bother or feel overwhelmed, just remember the food you eat is a disease-modifying apparatus you can wield three times a day.

Learn new ways of cooking

A whole-food plant-based diet uses different cooking techniques to avoid the use of highly refined oils or saturated fats and to maximise nutrient loss. Taste-buds love the texture and flavour of fried food, but taste-buds have a high turnover. Once you've stopped eating them for a few weeks, these foods won't be so appealing, instead leaving an unpleasant after-taste and coating on your tongue if you eat them. Your microbiome won't enjoy it either as it struggles to cope with these toxic oils. There are three main ways to consider – 'frying' in water or stock, baking, or using an air fryer, instead of deep frying, and steaming to retain nutrients.

Frying without oil

Chefs around the world advocate for frying food in some form of fat at a high temperature, whether for speed or flavour. It was one of the first things I was taught in school home economics lessons, and you see it on every cooking show on TV. Cooking in water or stock is anathema to them. However, it works just as well and produces tasty dishes without the addition of adulterated oils. I have even managed to win over the chef who attended my Eat Well Live Well course with this technique, a great relief as I failed cookery at school and have no formal chef training! It's exciting to see many chefs now discovering how delicious oil-free, whole plant foods can be, creating wonderful flavour combinations and dishes.

Frying with water or stock may take a few attempts to get right, but the key essentials are a good pan, a medium heat and paying attention. Water can only reach 100°C before evaporating, unlike oil or butter which can go up to 190°C. High temperatures change the structure of oils and proteins, releasing toxins like acrylamide and advanced glycation end products (AGEs) that stimulate cell degeneration – literally ageing you. The risk is higher when cooking with animal products; frying in water or stock at lower temperatures minimises it. Food can be prevented from sticking to the pan with the addition of a little extra stock or water, but take care not to add too much or you move from 'frying' to poaching which provides a very different flavour. It's best to use good quality stainless steel pans that emit an equal heat, and adding a tiny pinch of salt helps draw out natural fluids to reduce the 'sticking risk'. Using a lid to cover the pan stops the fluid evaporating so quickly and can enhance the flavour too.

Oils like extra-virgin olive oil, walnut or sesame that enhance the overall flavour of the dish can still be used but as a garnish at the end of cooking, not during these first stages. This is particularly important for cold-pressed flaxseed oil; this should never be exposed to high heats but added to food once it's served. If the heat is tolerable for your mouth, it's okay for the oil too.

Bake or air fry

Air fryers have become an essential kitchen item since the cost-of-living crisis as they use less power than conventional ovens. Like a fan oven, air fryers circulate hot air at high temperatures, resulting in a crispy, tasty texture.

Whether you bake in an oven or use an air fryer, the benefits when it comes to health are similar – no heated refined, toxic oils. The temperature settings may be similar to a traditional fryer but it's a circulating heat that doesn't have direct contact with the food being cooked. Try to keep the settings at 180°C or below though to be on the safe side. Low and slow may take more time but it's the flavours that will be developing, not toxic compounds. To prevent food sticking to trays or dishes, invest in a reusable silicon baking mat or non-stick baking paper.

Steam

The UK still has a bad reputation for stinky cabbage aromas, mushy cauliflower and carrots boiled to death – there's nothing enticing, or healthy about those. British cuisine has certainly moved on from that, though some people still boil most or all of their vegetables, which can destroy their nutrients as well as texture and flavour. Steaming is a much better option that retains colour, vitality and beneficial compounds and many vegetables only need a few minutes in the steamer before they are perfectly *al dente*.

A great kitchen gadget is a rice cooker that can also be used to steam vegetables in the top tray. As it's programmable, the timer can be set earlier in the day so you can return with dinner ready and waiting. Any nutrients lost in the veg can drip down and be absorbed by the rice below – an added bonus. Rice cookers aside, small steamer saucepans are easy to find and cheap to buy. You can even buy a steamer 'flower' to pop in the base of a normal pan – just remember to add water! Once the veggies are cooked, use the nutrient-rich steamer water in soups and stews.

You'll find all these cooking methods in the recipes section. It may take a little while to perfect them, but keep exploring and experimenting and soon you won't even have to think about it.

Give your gut a break

Most of us have access to food 24 hours a day from well-stocked fridges and cupboards, nearby takeaways or home delivery services. Just a few taps on your phone and almost any cuisine can be delivered in minutes, even when you live in the middle of the countryside like I do. Snacks are everywhere, from the bakery to the fuel station and beyond. Clever marketing tells us they're essential, but do we really need them? Maybe if we're not satiated with processed food, probably not if we're eating satisfying and filling whole foods.

Despite what the media and food companies may tell us, humans are not designed to eat all day long. Our bodies need a break from digesting and assimilating nutrients to repair, clean up and rest. The best time for this is during sleep, but many people with chronic health conditions, particularly autoimmune disease, don't sleep well, sometimes only a few hours. Being awake or up and about during the night breaks the body's natural sleep-and-restore cycle. Many people have a snack before bed and another as soon as they wake, no matter how much sleep they've had. Fatigue from poor sleep makes you feel exhausted and run down and it's easy to turn to high sugar and fat snacks for an energy boost, grazing throughout the day even though they rarely help.

Nightshift workers know how that feels. I worked a mix of night and day shifts for many years; nights always made me feel exhausted and swapping between day and night was even worse. It took days for me to feel back to normal. Night shifts mess with the body's circadian rhythm; night is the time for detoxification and repair.[1] Instead, the body is forced to function and respond normally, putting it under great strain. I used to graze on biscuits or sweets and drink as much tea as possible whenever there was time; 4:00 am was always the worst, the lowest point in the body's energy cycle and often the quietest time on the ward, so more time to snack. Once I changed to eating whole plant foods, I snacked less but still needed something to keep me going until the day shift arrived. People who work night shifts have higher rates of chronic health problems including autoimmune disease and cancer[2]; the body just doesn't like it.

Cleaning up with autophagy

Research over the last few years has highlighted how taking a break from eating is important for health. It forces the body to use energy stores in the liver and adipose tissue and clears out old and damaged cells, a process called autophagy.[3] Greek for 'self-devouring', autophagy is the body's internal recycling system, reusing useful elements and eliminating the rest as waste. Autophagy should occur when cells are damaged and there's a lack of incoming nutrients. When food is constantly eaten, the body must prioritise its processing rather than cleaning. Plus, when stressed or inflamed, the body becomes overburdened with damaged cells, making healthy cells work even harder. Eventually, the body becomes exhausted and moves into self-protection mode – maybe this is why fatigue is so common in people with autoimmune disease?

Autophagy is promoted by exercise and taking a breaking in eating, otherwise known as fasting. This could be time-restricted eating, intermittent fasting, low-calorie intake or patterns like the 5:2 plan where you have a very low-calorie intake for two days a week. The keto diet has also been included in this, where a low-carb and high-fat diet pushes the body into ketosis, creating ketone bodies for energy. I am not a keto fan as it's hard to do properly and to maintain. I felt terrible when I tried it and I have met many people who have experienced negative outcomes or severe dysbiosis, although some people thrive on it. Water fasts are another approach but should not be done for more than 24 hours without clinical supervision and never by anyone with type 1 diabetes or blood sugar issues.*

Fasting as a religious practice is common. During Ramadan, Muslims avoid consuming food during daylight hours and eat after dark for a month. Lent, a period of 40 days leading up to Easter in Christianity, could be seen as another type of fasting, although many people just avoid one type of food (often chocolate) rather than restricting their eating overall.

Time restriction or fasting?

Time-restricted eating and intermittent fasting are often used interchangeably although they are different. Time-restricted eating limits the number of hours in which you eat. The 8:16 pattern is popular, with an 8-hour window for food and 16 hours rest or 10:14, with a 10-hour eating window which can be easier for many people to follow. Research suggests both are effective. Even a 12:12 pattern can make a difference, particularly in areas with high cell turnover like the gut.

---

*NB: If you have type 1 diabetes and don't have a constant insulin infusion or monitoring system, please first discuss trying a time-restricted eating pattern with your diabetic nurse or health professional to ensure that it is right for you, to avoid hypoglycaemic or ketoacidosis events.

TYPES OF FASTING

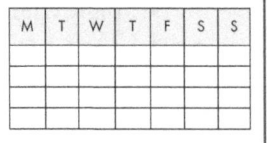

5:2 Diet
Eat low calorie, 2 days a week

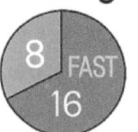

Time-Restricted Eating
Eat normally in a restricted time

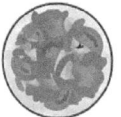

Very Low Calorie
800 calories a day (not long term)

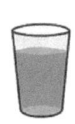

Water Fasts
A few days only (medical supervision advised)

Intermittent fasting refers more to extended periods of limited or no-calorie intake. This could be fasting every other day, for a couple of days a week, or having a very low-calorie intake for a few days at a time. All methods seem to be effective when researched but daily life is different, so finding a method that works for you is key. This is particularly important if you are physically active or participating in high-energy sports, when a low-calorie intake is not advisable. Autophagy is only effective for a short time. Once the recycled materials have been used up, supplies of fresh raw materials are needed to support bodily processes. If they're not, starvation mode will kick in and resources will be scavenged from organs you don't want broken down, like heart muscle. Getting the right balance is important.

Research suggests that autophagy through time-restricted eating can break down and expel damaged immune cells and reduce systemic inflammation and the symptoms of autoimmune disease. Valter Longo is an expert in this field – you can find his book in the Resources section (page 321). Time-restricted eating is a lifestyle modification most of us can do, although an 8:16 ratio may be too much to start with, especially if your current pattern is the exact opposite – 16 hours of eating and only 8 hours of rest. If that is the case, start by aiming for a 12:12 pattern and go from there. It's a new habit that will develop over time. Or if work makes it hard to be so structured, restricted calories two days a week might be easier for you.

Understand medications

Many people with autoimmune disease take prescribed medications. These could be disease-modifying therapies, painkillers or treatments for depression or anxiety. Or they could be medications for other chronic health conditions like hypertension or heart disease.

When changing to a whole-food plant-based diet, it's worth exploring whether there are any contraindications with your prescribed medications. Your pharmacist should be able to help you, but if you are still unsure, please consult your specialist or a plant-based dietitian or nutritionist.

Issues around calcium and thyroxine apply to all dietary patterns, so you should already know when to time taking them. There are a few other common interactions that are worth knowing – Table 8.1 lists the main ones. It's not an exhaustive list, so please do check if you are concerned about potential issues.

This list highlights just how powerful whole plant foods can be – they can have whole-body benefits rather than side effects. If eating a banana or avocado can help reduce blood pressure, surely that's better than taking medication with potential side effects? You do need to take care if you are taking blood pressure or diabetic medications, as changing to a whole-food plant-based diet can have positive effects in just a couple of days. Please monitor yourself and liaise with your doctor or health practitioner; as your body heals, you may well be able to reduce and even stop these medications, but do not stop taking prescribed meds without medical support. Some painkillers or antidepressants cannot be stopped immediately but reduced slowly. It's important to have the right guidance.

Table 8.1: Common interactions between foods and medications

Grapefruit	Avoid if you're taking statins for high cholesterol as it can prevent its metabolism and increase side effects. Can reduce the effectiveness of some anti-hypertensives and anxiety drugs
Green leafy and cruciferous vegetables	Contain high levels of vitamin K that can interfere with blood thinners if eaten in large quantities, particularly warfarin. Eat a regular amount and ask your GP to amend the dose to keep levels stable. High calcium levels can interfere with absorption of thyroxine, digoxin and even antibiotics. Avoid eating 2 hours before or after these medications
Bananas and avocados	Their higher potassium content can interfere with ACE inhibitors for high blood pressure
Liquorice	Can interact with ACE inhibitors and anti-coagulants
High-fibre, low-sugar diet	Be careful with diabetic medications that lower blood sugar levels – monitor carefully.

Some disease-modifying therapies for autoimmune conditions need to be taken around or with food. For example, Tecfidera, taken by many people with MS, is best taken alongside higher-in-fat food like nuts, tofu or avocado to help reduce side effects. Steroids, commonly used as a first line treatment for many autoimmune conditions, should always be taken with food as they can irritate the gut lining. Again, if you are not sure, always check with your pharmacist or healthcare specialist.

Find your tribe (carefully)

Humans are social beings. Most of us enjoy being part of a group, whether it is based on family, friends, workplace, hobby or religion. Belonging is important; loneliness is known to contribute to chronic health conditions and early death. An autoimmune diagnosis can be isolating, especially if you don't know anyone with the same condition or how to explain invisible symptoms like fatigue and pain. No one really gets it unless they're going through the same thing.

Finding a community that understands is so important. Most autoimmune conditions have organisations that offer support, and social media has enabled people all around the world to connect. It can be such a relief to finally find your tribe, somewhere you don't have to explain yourself.

A word of warning though. Online groups aren't always the answer. It can become a toxic environment full of negativity and criticism, or so much woe and desperation it can impact your mental health. It's easy to feel guilty if you're 'not that bad' or offer solutions that are dismissed or attacked by others, especially if it's about diet or exercise. When people are in a low place, positive ideas can be taken as personal criticism or an unobtainable goal. It's easy to get pulled into the same pool of negativity when your energy is low and your body aches from head to toe.

> **Rosa's story:** Rosa and her mum joined a sarcoidosis Facebook group but found the negativity too overwhelming. As an unregulated forum for people to share their symptoms and struggles, the stories were too hard for them to deal with, and both decided to leave the group. When you are trying to come to terms with the trauma of your own diagnosis, those of other people may be overwhelming; you are often not in the right place to deal with other people's difficulties. Walking away is a healthy choice.

Fortunately, not all groups are like that. A well-moderated online group of like-minded people can be a wonderful place to find inspiration and encouragement. It may take a while to find, or you could start your own if you have the inclination and energy to do so. Organisations and charities that run lifestyle medicine programmes offering positive solutions and strong community support, like Overcoming MS or the Plants for Joints programme (see Resources on page 321) are great examples of this. Local plant-based groups that meet up in person can also be a positive environment if the aim is focused on health rather than vegan activism. Not that I have anything against such activism; it's just not the same purpose.

Many cities and large towns have community kitchens that focus on encouraging whole-food plant-based eating for health – these can be a great place to connect with like-minded people and learn more about eating this way. I've added the details of some in the Resources section (page 321).

If the thought of putting yourself out there is exhausting, you're not alone. It can take time and energy to feel comfortable with any group. In the short term, your tribe might be supportive family and friends. Changing to a whole-food plant-based diet might be seen as a bit radical, so talking to them about what you want to do and why is important. This is imperative if you're not the main cook in the home as you will need them to get on board and learn new skills. Ideally, your partner or family will join you on the adventure, but most people start on their own. However, once they see the positive effects that you gain and start to try the delicious food, they will hopefully join you on the adventure. It certainly makes it easier.

Friends can be more challenging than family, and changing to a whole-food plant-based diet can affect what's left of your social life. Fortunately, plant-based options at restaurants and cafes are becoming much easier, especially in larger towns and cities – even rural spots like mine in Devon. Alternatively, invite friends to yours for dinner – it doesn't have to be flash, just tasty. Some friends may fall out of your life, unwilling to understand or adapt whereas others may surprise you with their support.

Finally, medical professionals can be an ally or a challenge. Until recently, the impacts of diet and other lifestyle changes have been dismissed due to lack of evidence. This is changing rapidly, and you may be more up-to-date than them! If your consultant is dismissive about your changes, you are at liberty to find a new one. Fortunately, there are an increasing number of informed and forward-thinking health professionals who either practise lifestyle medicine or are interested in the positive effects lifestyle has on long-term chronic health conditions. Working in partnership with your health professional not only supports you, but them as well. You can inform and inspire them and demonstrate the effectiveness of these changes, which in turn will equip them with knowledge and examples so they can support other patients in a similar situation. A win for everyone.

Make a start – today!

There's never a best time to make changes, so why not do it today? An easy place to start is to revisit Chapter 5, the Seven Steps, to start healing from the inside out – simple changes with a positive bias that focus on what you can add rather than take-away. Then explore the recipes in the second half of this book, starting on page 169. All tasty, filling and packed with whole plant nutrients and fibre, there are options to suit everyone's taste. If you're not used to cooking and eating this way, don't worry. My recipes are simple to make, using ingredients available in supermarkets and health food shops. Once you've tried them a couple of times, you should be able to create tasty nutrient-packed meals in 30 minutes or less.

You don't have to stick with the recipes here; there are lots of great books with tasty whole plant recipes out there. My first book, *Eat Well Live Well with The Sensitive Foodie* has over 100 recipes to keep you going and there are a few other recommendations in the Resources section (page 321). Once you feel confident, start experimenting and creating dishes with your own twist. My recipes are a guide; feel free to make changes. You'll soon have a selection of tasty meals you'll look forward to eating.

PORTIONS OF WHOLE PLANT FOODS PER DAY

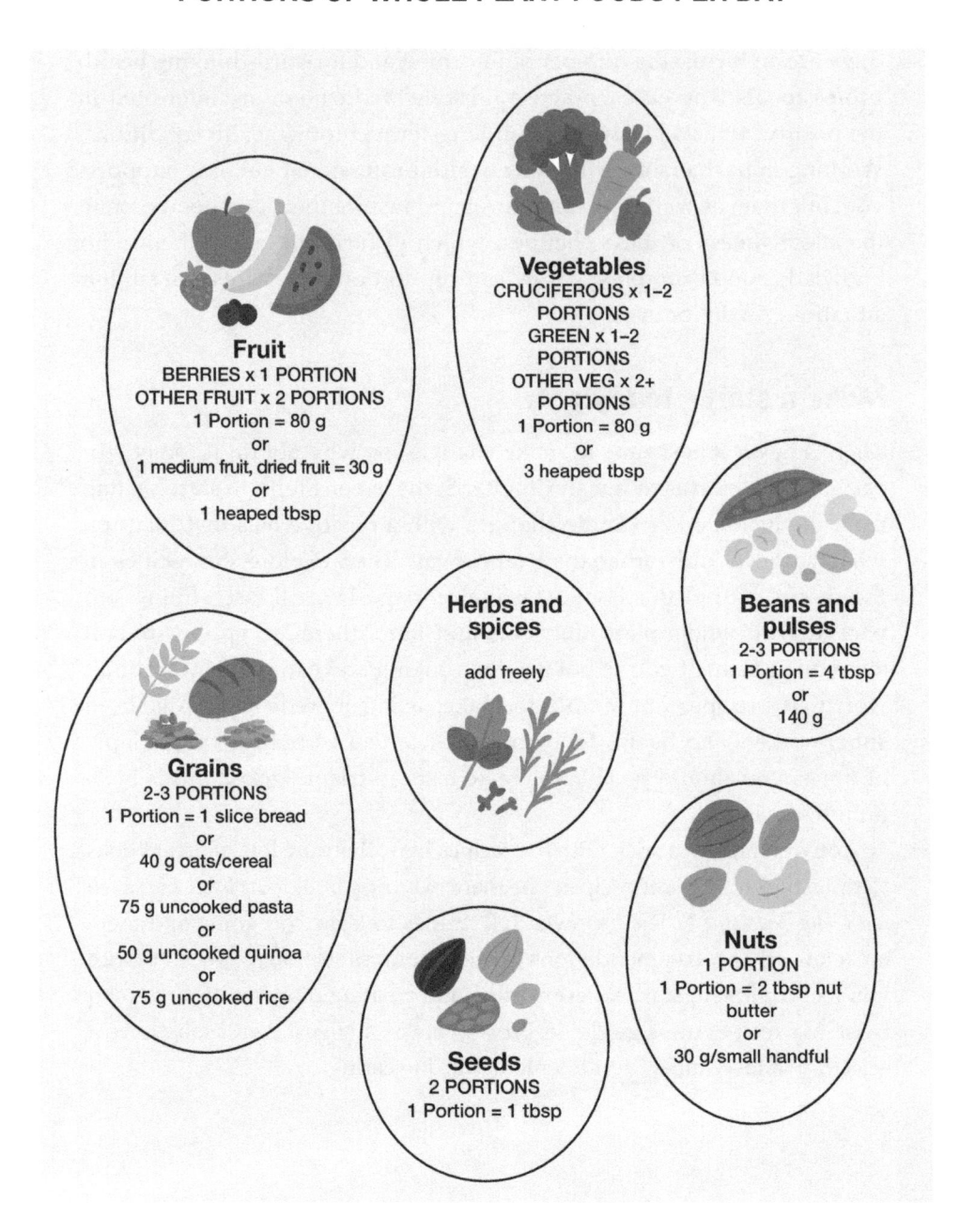

Fruit
BERRIES x 1 PORTION
OTHER FRUIT x 2 PORTIONS
1 Portion = 80 g
or
1 medium fruit, dried fruit = 30 g
or
1 heaped tbsp

Vegetables
CRUCIFEROUS x 1–2 PORTIONS
GREEN x 1–2 PORTIONS
OTHER VEG x 2+ PORTIONS
1 Portion = 80 g
or
3 heaped tbsp

Herbs and spices
add freely

Beans and pulses
2-3 PORTIONS
1 Portion = 4 tbsp
or
140 g

Grains
2-3 PORTIONS
1 Portion = 1 slice bread
or
40 g oats/cereal
or
75 g uncooked pasta
or
50 g uncooked quinoa
or
75 g uncooked rice

Seeds
2 PORTIONS
1 Portion = 1 tbsp

Nuts
1 PORTION
1 Portion = 2 tbsp nut butter
or
30 g/small handful

> **Favourite meals:** Rosa loves marinated tofu and vegetables with hoisin sauce, Iricla's favourite is a nut roast, cauliflower 'cheese' and roast potatoes, whereas Kate has found it hard to decide as there are so many delicious foods to choose from. She narrowed it down to chickpea and vegetable curry with lots of fresh herbs and spices. Yum!

There are a few guidelines to follow though. Make sure you eat enough. This is not a restrictive approach, although generally lower in calories than the standard Western diet. Also, eat a variety of foods throughout the day to ensure you consume enough protein, healthy fat, fibre, minerals, vitamins and phytonutrients. Exactly how that looks is up to you, but the infographic opposite provides a guide to help you make sure you get everything you need without having to calculate grams, micrograms or calories. If you want to do that, there are plenty of apps to help you.

Summary

That's it! You're now fully equipped to start your own tasty, healing journey. My final words are 'be kind', to yourself and others around you, as you start to make changes. Ideally it will be plain sailing, but if not, just go with it in your own time and way. Let it be an adventure of discovery and, most importantly, be patient. It generally takes years to tip over into autoimmunity, so an overnight miracle is not on the cards. Hopefully, though, you will quickly start to feel the benefits like me and the other people featured in this book and wonder why you ever ate any other way.

Now it's over to you. Enjoy!

THE PLANT-BASED WHOLE-FOOD RECIPES

Introduction to the recipes	173
Three-day sample menu:	175
Breakfast	**176**
Black forest fruit smoothie	176
Green smoothie bowl	177
Crunchy fruit yoghurt pot	178
Almond and apricot chia breakfast pot	179
Gluten-free pancakes	180
Vegan Spanish omelette/tortilla	181
Morning veggie scramble	182
Beans, greens and mushrooms	184
Tempeh 'bacon'	185
Banana breakfast bars	186
Soups	**188**
'Moroccan' soup	189
Broccoli and almond soup	190
Creamy celeriac soup with spicy chickpea croutons	191
Split green pea soup	193
Spinach, squash and coriander soup	194
Golden soup	195
Spinach and rosemary soup	197
Italian bean soup	198
Sweet potato and red lentil soup	199
Black bean soup	200
Salads	**202**
Warm broad bean, mangetout and new potato salad with crispy smoked tofu	202
Two-bean salad	204
Roasted sweet potato and kale salad	205
Sprouted mung bean salad	206
Lentil salad	208
Rainbow carrot and thyme salad	209

Red kale and pear salad	210	Mushroom, squash and kale root vegetable pie	241
Herby millet tabbouleh	211	**Magnificent mains**	**243**
Beetroot and watercress salad	212	Vegetable curry with chickpea dumplings	243
Asparagus, pea and rocket salad	213	Walnut and white bean bake	245
Lunch or light meals	**215**	Tempeh, hazelnut and apricot bake	247
Smashed chickpeas	215	Moussaka	248
Crunchy cauliflower bites	216	Comforting root vegetable stew and herby dumplings	250
Tempeh onion bhajis	217		
Chickpeas and chard	219		
Amaranth and millet pancakes	220	Shiitake mushrooms and smoked tofu noodle bowl	252
Quinoa and vegetable patties	221	Broccoli and kale tart	254
Smoky beans	223	Cumin and turmeric traybake	256
Baked bubble and squeak	224	Sesame-baked butternut squash rings with smoky chickpeas	258
Aloo tikki balls	225		
Carrot flapjacks	226		
Easy recipes	**228**	Roasted cabbage slices, aromatic millet and tahini dressing	260
Tempeh and vegetable skewers	228		
Creamy cauliflower curry	229	**Baking**	**262**
Ethiopian split pea stew	231	Apple, apricot and oat bars	262
Quick Jambalaya	233	Black bean chocolate brownies	264
Baked mini Romanesco cauliflower	234	Pear and ginger muffins	266
Stuffed sweet potatoes	235	Sticky date and ginger cake	267
Green kitcheri	237	Cherry Bakewell flapjacks	268
Asparagus and broccoli pasta with white bean sauce	238	Spiced cookies	269
		Sweet carrot scones	271
Quick broccoli and smoked tofu rice	239		

The plant-based whole-food recipes

Plum and cardamom cake	273	Tamarind stir-fry sauce	297
Carrot and maple muffins	274	Lemon and herb dressing	298
Almond and cardamom balls	276	Turmeric ginger tahini dressing	298
Desserts	**278**	Leafy green sauce	299
Rhubarb and strawberry crumble	278	Elderflower dressing	300
Raspberry mousse	280	Simple cashew cream	301
Chia chocolate pudding	281	Raw chocolate sauce	301
Raw blueberry lemon tarts	282	Raspberry sauce	302
Raspberry Bakewell tart	284	**Spreads and breads**	**304**
Blackberry and apple tray bake	286	Turmeric hummus	304
Baked crunchy nectarines	287	White bean, thyme and roasted garlic dip	305
Baked 'cheesecake'	288	Smoky red lentil dip	306
Ginger and pear rice pudding	291	Green pea dip	307
Apple and salted caramel slice	292	Melty vegan 'cheese'	308
Sauces and dressings	**295**	'Ricotta' two ways	309
White bean sauce	295	Mushroom paté	310
Sweet and sour sauce	296	Sweet potato flatbread	311
		Buckwheat bread	313
		Red lentil bread	314

Notes on the recipes

Check the recipe you've chosen for serving size as these range from one to six. Most are easily increased or halved. Some specific ingredients are seasonal; I try to offer up tasty alternatives to make the recipes usable all year round.

All recipe measurements are in grams – apologies to readers in the US, Australia and elsewhere who use cup measurements. I recommend buying a small set of scales that you can balance different-sized bowls and jugs on to weigh directly into, or download an app like Cooking Units Converter from Infinite Fork SL.

In this book I use these abbreviations:

g = grams
ml = millilitre
tbsp = tablespoon
dsp = dessertspoon
tsp = teaspoon

Oven temperatures are based on an electric fan oven measured in Centigrade. Please note the following conversions for Fahrenheit or gas ovens. Refer to your manufacturer's handbook for full confirmation as every oven is slightly different.

Centigrade	Fahrenheit	Gas
150	300	2
165	325	3
180	350	4
190	375	5
200	400	6

Introduction to the recipes

Welcome to the tasty part of the book, the recipes. There are 100 different ones to try, covering all meals and times of the day. All are gluten free and use a selection of whole plant foods, so each one is nutrient packed. Feel free to use them however you like, but try not to eat the same meal every day. Remember, variety is key to gut health and overall health; we need exposure to a full range of vitamins, minerals, healthy fats, amino acids, polyphenols and, of course, fibre.

Whilst I prefer not to be prescriptive, I'm aware if you're new to this it might all seem overwhelming, so I have included a suggested three-day menu plan to give you an idea of how you might like to mix them up. Don't look for perfection from day one or try to do all of this overnight; just start trying a few recipes and gradually build up your repertoire. Refer to the end of the last chapter (page 166) for guidelines on portions to include every day if you want to make sure you're including everything you need.

If you are an 'all or nothing' person then a complete overnight change might well be what you prefer. This, of course, is fine but be warned – your body may well feel worse before it starts to feel better if you do it this way. Think of it like training for a marathon. If you never or rarely run, it's highly unlikely you will be able to run 26 miles in one go, and if you did you'd feel wrecked afterwards, maybe even cause some damage. You need to train your body, which takes time and concerted effort, expecting it to hurt from time to time.

The same principle applies to changing to a whole-food plant-based diet, especially if you've been eating high amounts of animal products and not much fibre. Time after time I've heard people say, 'I gave up dairy and/or gluten and/or meat for two weeks and felt terrible, so that doesn't work for me'. I'm not surprised! That's a lot for the body to deal with in one go. If they had focused on one at a time, reduced the food group they were giving up gradually before omitting it completely, whilst replacing it with a suitable alternative, their bodies would have reacted in a much less dramatic way. It's much kinder to train your body this way, but if you just have to go all in, then relax and enjoy the (bumpy) ride!

If you need to increase your vegetable intake, focus on eating a soup, a salad and a portion of cooked vegetables every day. The soup and salad recipes often include some form of legume, so you'll be increasing those too without any extra effort. As you increase your fibre intake, don't forget to drink more water to help it move along in your gut.

One important thing to remember when you start cooking plant-based meals is that fresh produce has a high water content that gets released into the pan as it's heated. For soups and stews in particular, I usually recommend using less stock or water than stated in the ingredients list in the first instance, then adding more as needed to get the consistency you enjoy. My mantra is 'you can always add but you can't take away' when it comes to fluids, spices and seasoning. Checking the flavours as you go is really important to ensure you end up with a delicious tasty meal that your taste-buds will love just as much as your body!

Here are a few more tips to help to get a routine established:
- Have a set day to plan the week ahead and put aside an hour to do meal prep if you have a busy week ahead.
- In your plan, identify any meals that could be batch cooked so you have extra for another day or to keep in the freezer.
- Plan simple, easy meals for busy days. The same goes if you are struggling with energy – don't add more pressure on yourself. Simple foods are often just what you need.
- Think about variety and eating the rainbow every day. What can you add to gain those extra colourful benefits? Things like a handful of blueberries on a salad or extra greens in a curry count.
- Make sure you're eating enough calories, especially on days you want to exercise.
- Keep bags of frozen chopped vegetables in the freezer so you always have something to hand.
- Bulk-buy nuts, seeds and pulses to make them cheaper – if you have somewhere to store them. Tinned beans and lentils are very useful for quick meals.
- If you react to a certain food, avoid it for a few days and then try it

again. If it's still an issue, you may need to omit it for longer
- Keep an open mind and keep experimenting. Remember, you're training your gut and, like all training programmes, it might not be a smooth journey.

Ultimately, though, my main piece of advice it to have fun and enjoy what you're eating. I believe making lasting changes that support the body and promote healing must be enjoyable, otherwise they just won't work. Be kind to yourself with an open mind and before you know it, you'll wonder why you ate any other way.

Three-day sample menu

I included a sample menu in my first book, and it's had more positive comments than anything else I wrote, so I'm including another one. Hopefully it will be as helpful as the last.

Day	Breakfast	Lunch	Dinner
Day 1 (weekend)	Beans and greens with tempeh bacon	Sweet potato and red lentil soup Warm broad bean and mangetout salad	Walnut and white bean bake with a selection of seasonal veg steamed or roasted Strawberry and rhubarb crumble with cashew cream or dairy-free yoghurt
Day 2	Apricot and almond chia pot	Spinach and rosemary soup Smokey beans on toasted buckwheat bread, watercress and beetroot salad	Tempeh vegetable skewers with sweet potato and kale salad Raspberry mousse
Day 3	Green smoothie	Italian bean soup Red kale and pear salad with turmeric hummus and red lentil bread	Shiitake mushroom and smoked tofu noodle bowl Fruity rice pudding

Breakfast

I'm a big fan of breakfast so I've included a range of options for you to try, from super-simple to larger, brunch ideas. There's more in my first book too as I like to show people that there's more to breakfast than processed cereal or toast. Having said that, whole-grain muesli and granola are tasty, simple breakfasts, as is porridge, which can be made with more than just oats. Quinoa, amaranth and millet are all delicious options, as is rice. Yes, I don't see anything wrong with having rice 'pudding' for breakfast, especially if it's loaded with seasonal fruit. I've not included recipes for these options here as there are so many ideas to share – don't rule them out though as additional awesome options.

Breakfast is a good time to get your fruit fix for the day, especially if you struggle with an overactive microbiome. Eating fruit on an empty stomach allows it to have free passage through the digestive tract, unhindered by complex fibres and proteins that take longer to break down. Remember that frozen fruit retains a lot of nutrients and polyphenols and can be a more affordable option, especially when they're out of season. Mix up the colours and types of fruit you eat every day and you'll naturally gain their wonderful rainbow properties with minimal effort and maximum taste.

Black Forest fruit smoothie

Serves 1

There's a whole glassful of powerful anti-inflammatory nutrients in this smoothie along with plant protein and healthy fats from the hemp and flaxseeds. Black Forest fruit mixes include sweet and sour cherries; both contain anthocyanins, and sour cherries can aid muscle recovery after exercise. Bags are available in the freezer section making this a year-round option. The squeeze of lime is super-important; not only will it help you absorb nutrients in the greens, but it gives it a lovely zing that brings the whole smoothie alive. Sub the Swiss chard with any greens you prefer or have in the fridge.

Ingredients

100 g frozen Black Forest fruit mix (defrosted if preferred)
1 tbsp shelled hemp seeds
1 tbsp ground flaxseed
30 g Swiss chard (or greens of choice)
50 g banana (optional but good)
100 ml dairy-free milk of choice
½ lime, juice only

Method

1. Pop all the ingredients into a blender/high-speed blender jug and blend until smooth.
2. Add more dairy-free milk or lime juice if needed and blend again.
3. Drink straight away.

Green smoothie bowl

Serves 1

I enjoy my smoothies thick and creamy – somehow, they feel more satisfying. Using frozen ingredients means you can have your smoothie super-thick in a bowl and take your time eating it. Of course, if you're in a hurry, just add more fluid, drink the smoothie and eat the fruit, nuts and seeds separately.

Frozen spinach is cheap and easy to find in supermarkets. It often contains a higher level of nutrients than fresh spinach as it's harvested and frozen within a few hours. Feel free to add fresh or other greens or even a green powder like spirulina if you prefer. Don't skip the lemon juice – it helps you to absorb all those awesome ingredients and enhances the flavour too.

Ingredients

1 medium banana, sliced and frozen
80 g frozen spinach (defrosted for 5 minutes so it's not solid)
1 tbsp ground flaxseed or chia seeds

¼ ripe avocado (optional)
1 tsp lemon juice
130 ml dairy-free milk of choice

To top:
1 tbsp pumpkin seeds
2 tbsp fresh berries of choice
1 tbsp chopped walnuts

Method
1. Place the smoothie ingredients into a blender jug and blend until smooth.
2. Pour the green smoothie into a bowl and top with the fruit, nuts and seeds.
3. Eat immediately whilst the smoothie is firm.

Crunchy fruit yoghurt pot
Serves 1

Fruit, yoghurt and granola are the perfect breakfast combo. It's also surprisingly filling and will keep you going until lunchtime. Use whatever fruit is in season or go for frozen. Remember to defrost it in the fridge overnight so it's ready for you in the morning. Use unsweetened dairy-free yoghurt – almond and soya are the main two options in the shops. It is possible to make your own at home with other plant milks but, with a zero-success rate, I can't give you a recipe! Look out for low added sugar and oil granola or make some yourself and store it in an air-tight container. I have a simple but tasty recipe in my first book if you want to check it out.

The instructions guide you to create a pretty arrangement of fruit, yoghurt and granola. If you're short on time, just pop it all in a bowl and eat it – not as pretty but it tastes just the same!

Ingredients
4 tbsp dairy-free yoghurt of choice
1 handful raspberries or strawberries

1 handful blueberries
½ nectarine or peach or any combination of fresh/frozen fruit you like
2 tbsp granola

Method
1. Wash the fruit and chop it into small pieces where needed.
2. Place ½ of the granola in the base of a bowl/large glass. Cover with ⅓ of the prepared fruit then, add ½ the yoghurt.
3. Add another ⅓ of the fruit, top with the remaining yoghurt, the remaining granola and finish with the last of the fruit.
4. Eat straight away.

Almond and apricot chia breakfast pot
Serves 1

Almond and apricot are a magical combo; the almond butter in this chia pot adds flavour and creaminess to the texture along with extra protein that makes it very satisfying. Use soft dried apricots rather than really tough ones, sulphite free if you can find them. They're darker in colour but taste great.

Ingredients
130 ml almond milk (or dairy-free milk of choice)
1 tbsp maple syrup
1 tbsp almond butter
2 tbsp chia seeds
3 dried apricots

Method
1. Prepare the night before. Pour the milk into a bowl or jug. Add the almond butter and maple syrup. Stir well to combine.
2. Add the chia seeds and stir again.
3. Chop the apricots into small pieces. Place in the bottom of a breakfast bowl. Pour the almond milk mix over the top.
4. Place in the fridge overnight – it will be thick and ready to eat in the morning.

Gluten-free pancakes
Serves 4

Successful plant-based gluten-free pancakes can be a challenge as gluten and egg normally bind pancakes together. After many attempts, I've found success with this combination of flours and a lot of patience. A good non-stick crêpe or frying pan is essential as just a light wipe of olive oil is added to the pan. Once the mix is in the pan, ensure the heat is medium-low and wait until the bubbles stop appearing on the surface before attempting to turn the pancake over. As always, the first one will undoubtedly fail, but don't give up as the next will be better, I promise.

Make a batch and store them in the fridge, separated by non-stick baking paper. Gently re-heat in the pan when you're ready to finish them off.

Ingredients
40 g gluten-free flour mix
60 g chickpea/gram flour
25 g cornflour or tapioca flour
1 pinch salt
1 tbsp brown sugar or maple syrup (optional)
250 ml soya milk or dairy-free milk of choice

Method
1. Place the flours, salt, and sugar if using, into a medium-sized bowl and mix well. Add the soya milk and whisk with a balloon whisk until you get a batter with no lumps (you might want to use a blender if your flour is a bit lumpy).
2. Leave to rest for 15 minutes.
3. Add a few drops of extra-virgin olive oil to the pan and wipe it around with some kitchen roll. Pre-heat the pan for 3 minutes on a medium-low heat.
4. Pour half a ladleful of mix into the middle of the pan. Spread it out gently with the back of the ladle.
5. Cook for 2-3 minutes. Bubbles will form on the top.
6. When the bubbles have finished appearing, gently loosen the edges of the pancake with a fish slice and flip over.

7. Cook for another minute until that side is lightly browned.
8. Transfer to a warm plate and repeat until all the mix is used up.
9. Serve with toppings as desired.

Vegan Spanish omelette/tortilla

Serves 4-6

Sometimes, there are recipes that look complicated or too much like hard work. You might feel this is one of them, but don't dismiss it until you've tried it. Once you've mastered the cooking of this gorgeous plant-based tortilla, it will become a firm favourite.

Perfect for a weekend brunch, it tastes even better cold or re-heated a day or so later, making it a tasty on-the-go breakfast, packed lunch or quick evening meal. Cook the potatoes the day before and keep in the fridge until you're ready to make the full recipe to save time. Kala namuk (Indian black salt) is a great ingredient to have on hand as it provides the sulphur-like aroma and flavour you get from eggs. You can find it in Asian stores – a small amount goes a long way, so it lasts for ages.

Ingredients

500 g potatoes
1 large onion diced or one large leek, rinsed and sliced
4 medium mushrooms, sliced (optional)
pinch salt
60 ml soya milk
300 g silken tofu, drained
1 tsp Dijon mustard
45 g gram (chickpea) flour
2 tbsp nutritional yeast flakes
2 tbsp cornflour
¼ tsp ground turmeric
¼ tsp black salt (optional – adds an 'eggy' flavour)
olive oil for greasing the pan

Method
1. If the potatoes haven't been cooked yet, wash them and peel if necessary. Cut into 2½-cm slices and place in a steamer basket. Steam for 10-15 minutes until just cooked – don't let them overcook or they'll collapse. Turn off the heat and leave to cool for a few minutes.
2. Heat 2 tbsp water in a large non-stick frying pan on a medium-low heat and cook the onion or leek with a pinch of salt, stirring now and then. If it starts to stick, add a little more water.
3. Make the batter by placing the milk, silken tofu, mustard, gram flour, nutritional yeast, cornflour, turmeric and black salt (if using) in a blender jug and blend to smooth. Pour into a bowl.
4. When the onions are soft, add the mushrooms to the pan if using and cook for 3 minutes. Tip the potatoes into the pan and continue cooking for 2-3 minutes on medium heat. Stir regularly until the potatoes are slightly browned. Tip the veggies into the bowl with the tofu mix and stir well to combine.
5. Pre-heat the grill to high.
6. Carefully tip the mix back into the pan. Cook on a low heat for 8-10 minutes until the base is lightly browned and the centre is firm. Pop the pan under the grill (keeping the handle away from the heat) and cook for another 5 minutes until golden and the centre is set.
7. Carefully remove from under the grill. Leave to settle for a couple of minutes then loosen the sides with a spatula and slide the tortilla out onto a plate.
8. Cut into 4 slices and eat straight away or leave to cool and wrap it up for work or school. This can also be gently re-heated before eating if desired.

Morning veggie scramble
Serves 2

Scrambled tofu is my usual go-to weekend breakfast dish. However, not everyone likes or can tolerate tofu, so this veggie scramble mix is a fantastic alternative. Use whatever vegetables you like or have to hand and the chickpea flour mix adds some plant protein and really fills you up. The end result looks a little gloopy but tastes amazing.

Serve on toast, with extra veggies on the side, or with tempeh 'bacon' or beans and greens for the perfect filling brunch.

Ingredients

Veggies – my suggestions but choose what you prefer:
¼ medium red or white onion, finely chopped
3 medium mushrooms, washed and finely chopped
½ small courgette, finely chopped
3 handfuls spinach, rinsed and roughly chopped

Scramble mix:
50 g gram (chickpea) flour
1 tbsp ground flaxseed
½ tsp baking powder
¼ ground turmeric
1 pinch kala namuk (Indian black salt) or table salt
black pepper to taste
1 tbsp nutritional yeast (optional)
180 ml water

Method

1. Add 2-3 tbsp of water to the base of your frying pan. Pop in the chopped onion and sauté over a medium heat for 5 minutes until it starts to soften. Stir from time to time and add more water if needed.
2. Add the mushrooms and/or courgettes (if using) and cook for another 2-3 minutes. Finally add the spinach and continue to cook, allowing the water in the veg to come out.
3. Whilst the veggies are cooking, pop all the scramble ingredients in the blender jug and whiz for 30 seconds to make sure everything is combined and there are no flour lumps.
4. Once the veg are soft and ready to eat, carefully tip them into the blender jug and mix with a fork (don't whiz again or you'll lose the texture). Pop the pan back over the heat and pour the mix into the pan.
5. Stir with a flat-ended wooden spatula. As the mix cooks on the base of the pan,

scrape it up and mix it into the wet mixture. Continue doing this until the mix is super thick.
6. Continue cooking on a medium heat – stop stirring for 2 minutes then give the base of the pan a good scrape. The mix will have stuck, but the browned bits add flavour and texture to the scramble.
7. Once the mix is dry, it's ready to serve. Make sure you soak your pan after serving!

Beans, greens and mushrooms
Serves 2 big portions

This improved version of baked beans is easy to make and provides you with a nutrient-packed start to the day. I love this with small black beans that give extra polyphenols, but feel free to use whatever you enjoy or have in the cupboard.

If you avoid tomatoes, just add the water instead. It won't look quite as attractive, but it will taste great – just remember to add the lemon juice at the end to help you absorb all the lovely nutrients.

Ingredients
2 handfuls kale, chard or spinach
4-6 medium mushrooms of choice
2 tbsp tomato purée
1 x 400-g tin cooked beans
1 pinch garlic powder (optional)
flavouring of choice – tamari/coconut amines/chilli sauce/miso paste etc
salt and pepper to taste

Method
1. Wash and roughly chop the greens. Wash the mushrooms and chop.
2. Pop the tomato purée into a small pan and add 4 tbsp water. Stir to combine. Turn on a low heat.
3. Add the shredded greens and mushrooms to the pan and cook for 2-3 minutes

until the leaves wilt and the mushrooms soften.
4. Drain and rinse the beans then add to the pan along with your flavourings. Stir to combine and cook on a low heat for another 2-3 minutes until everything is hot.
5. Serve on toast or with scrambled tofu or chickpeas and/or tempeh bacon.

Tempeh 'bacon'
Serves 2

If you enjoy the salty, smoky flavour of bacon, then this high-protein plant-based version is for you. Slice the tempeh super-thin and ideally marinade it for a few hours – overnight is even better if you want it for breakfast the next day. Alternatively, dice the tempeh before popping it into the marinade to use in pasta, quiche or salads.

Ingredients
100 g tempeh
1 tbsp tamari/soya sauce/coconut amines
1 tsp smoked paprika
1 tbsp maple syrup
½ tsp liquid smoke (if you have it)
chilli flakes/powder (optional if you like it spicy)

Method
1. Slice the tempeh as thinly as you can.
2. Mix the marinade ingredients in a lidded container.
3. Place the tempeh slices into the marinade, pop on the lid, turn it a few times to make sure everything is coated, then leave to marinate for at least 1 hour.
4. Pre-heat the oven to 180°C. Place the marinated tempeh on a baking tray lined with non-stick baking paper and bake in the oven for 10 minutes, then turn over and bake for another 10. Alternatively, place in an air fryer for 6-8 minutes at 180ºC.
5. Serve whilst hot or store in the fridge for up to 4 days and re-heat when required.

Banana breakfast bars

Makes 9 bars

Sometimes you need breakfast on the go or something convenient to take to work; these bars hit the spot. Packed full of fibre, protein, healthy fats and sugars, they will keep you going for hours. If you must avoid ripe bananas, use unsweetened apple sauce instead. Feel free to sub the seeds with chopped nuts or add in sesame or chia seeds instead, and also extra spices like ground ginger or a pinch of nutmeg.

These bars are also great for lunchboxes, on-the-go snacks or just to enjoy at home when you fancy an energy boost during the day. They also freeze well, so you don't have to eat them all at once.

Ingredients
2 medium soft or mushy bananas
2 tbsp ground flaxseed
3 tbsp water
50 ml extra-virgin olive oil
75 ml maple syrup or date syrup
200 g oats
50 g pumpkin seeds
30 g sunflower seeds
20 g hempseeds
60 g sultanas or raisins or dried cranberries
2 tsp ground cinnamon
1 pinch salt

Method
1. Pre-heat the oven to 180°C. Line a baking tray with non-stick baking paper.
2. Peel the ripe bananas and drop them into a large bowl. Mash with a fork or potato masher until smooth.
3. Add the ground flaxseed, water, olive oil and maple syrup. Stir well to combine.
4. Add the remaining ingredients to the banana mix and stir well, making sure everything is well combined. It will be very thick.

5. Transfer the mix to the prepared baking tin. Spread it out, pressing it into the corners and flattening the top.
6. Place in the oven and bake for 15 minutes then turn the tin around in the oven and bake for another 5 minutes or until the top is starting to brown.
7. Remove from the oven and leave for 5 minutes before lifting the bake out of the tin with the baking paper. Place on a cooling rack and mark out 9 squares with a sharp knife.
8. Once completely cooled, fully cut into squares. Store in an air-tight container in a cool place for up to 4 days.

Soups

I am a big fan of soup and make it at home all year round. There are so many combinations to choose from, it's hard to get bored. Plus, it's a great way to use up the odds and ends floundering in the bottom of the fridge.

Cooking vegetables breaks down tough cell wall, releasing their nutrients and making them more readily available for absorption in the gut, which is great for those with delicate digestion and for those of us in need of healing nutrients. Heat does destroy some of these healthful compounds but many leach out into the cooking fluid, which of course is a key part of the soup itself.

Most of the recipes call for vegetable stock. However, shop-bought stock cubes often contain less than ideal ingredients, including emulsifiers, palm oil and gluten. Bouillion is slightly better; gluten- and yeast-free versions are available. Vegetable stock is sometimes available in sachets but is expensive and again, often contains additives. If you have the time, home-made vegetable stock is great. However, most of us don't have the time or energy to do that, so, what's the answer?

One option is to use cooking water from steamed or boiled vegetables; this retains nutrients and some flavour. The other is just to add boiling water and enhance the flavour of the soup with lots of herbs, seasoning and a simple but not often mentioned ingredient, celery salt. Most stocks contain concentrated celery for the savoury element. Using celery salt instead provides that savoury flavour without all the other additives. A pinch is enough. It's usually found in the spices section in larger supermarkets, health food shops or online.

All these soups can be frozen. If you want to batch cook, double the amounts then freeze in individual containers. Perfect to take to work or use on those days when you are lacking time or energy to cook something fresh. Just remember to label the pots, unless you like a surprise!

'Moroccan' soup
Serves 4

This is a satisfying soup packed full of colourful veggies, healing spices and lots of fibre. If your gut is a little tender or sensitive, leave out the chilli. You might also want to wait to add the extra chickpeas until serving if you find them a little gassy. Dish them out to the others or keep in the fridge for another recipe.

Ingredients
1 medium onion (white or red)
1 large stick celery, washed and trimmed
1 large or 2 medium carrots
1 red bell pepper
1 fat clove garlic
1 x 400-g tin chickpeas, drained
1 x 400-g tin chopped tomatoes
½ tsp red chilli powder (optional)
1 tsp ground cumin
1 tsp ground coriander
¼-½ tsp ground cinnamon
500 ml vegetable stock (or hot water)
salt and pepper
2 tbsp fresh coriander – to garnish

Method
1. Finely chop the onion, celery, carrots and red pepper.
2. Heat 2-3 tbsp water in the base of a large pan. Add the prepared veggies and sauté on a medium heat for 5 minutes until the veg start to soften. Add a little more water if they start to stick.
3. Whilst the veg are cooking, peel and grate the garlic. Drain and rinse the chickpeas.
4. Add the garlic to the pan and cook for another 2 minutes.
5. Pour in the chopped tomatoes and add the spices. Stir well and simmer for

a couple of minutes before adding **half** the chickpeas and enough stock to cover everything.
6. Bring to the boil, then cover with the pan lid and simmer for 20 minutes or so until all the veggies are cooked.
7. Turn off the heat and blend with a stick blender until the mix is broken down but still a little chunky.
8. Add the remaining chickpeas to the pan and season with salt and pepper as desired. Re-heat gently until piping hot, then serve with a garnish of fresh coriander.
9. Store leftovers in the fridge for up to 3 days or freeze for use another day.

Broccoli and almond soup
Makes 4 moderate portions

Broccoli and almonds are the perfect combo when it comes to nurturing nutrients. Being a member of the cruciferous family, broccoli rocks when it comes to anti-inflammatory phytonutrients. And almonds carry good amounts of minerals like magnesium, calcium and potassium, and lots of fibre. Great for heart health – and gut health too.

If you must avoid almonds, sub with sunflower seeds or potato instead.

Ingredients
1 small white onion – or ½ medium
2 fat cloves garlic
1 full head calabrese broccoli
75 g chard or spinach
1 bay leaf
3 tbsp ground almonds
600 ml vegetable stock
salt and pepper to taste
a few flaked almonds to garnish

Method
1. Peel and finely chop the onion. Peel and grate the garlic.
2. Wash the broccoli under a running tap. Separate the florets from the stem and put to one side. Trim any tough outer layers off the broccoli stem then finely chop any remaining stem.
3. Wash the chard then separate the stems from the leaves. Chop both, putting the stem with the broccoli stem.
4. Heat 2-3 tbsp water in the base of a large pan. Add the onion, chopped broccoli stems, chard stems and bay leaf. Sauté for 5 minutes until the onion starts to soften. Add more water to the pan as necessary, so it doesn't stick.
5. Add the grated garlic, stir well and cook for another 2 minutes.
6. Stir in the ground almonds then add 400 ml of the stock. Bring to a gentle boil then reduce the heat, pop on the pan lid and simmer for 10 minutes.
7. Chop the broccoli florets into small pieces. Add to the pan – add a bit more stock if needed to ensure everything is just covered. Simmer for 5 minutes.
8. Finally, add the chopped chard leaves to the pan and cook for another 5 minutes.
9. Turn off the heat and remove the bay leaf.
10. Blend to smooth, adding more stock if needed to get the thickness you desire.
11. Season with salt and pepper and serve with a few flaked almonds on top.
12. Store leftovers in the fridge and use within 3 days.

Creamy celeriac soup with spicy chickpea croutons
Serves 4 portions

Celeriac is one of the odder-looking root vegetables, but looks can be deceiving; this knobbly ball is full of fabulous flavour when both raw and cooked. It's also packed full of antioxidants, vitamin C and fibre.

When cooked in soups, celeriac provides a rich, creamy texture, perfect for a luxuriant consistency. Do try to add the celery salt; it turns a lovely flavour into an awesome one with just a pinch. It's magic. Top with roasted spiced chickpeas or mixed seeds if desired.

Ingredients

½ medium white onion
2 medium sticks celery
1 medium celeriac
2 fat cloves garlic
1 tbsp dried thyme
1 pinch celery salt
500 ml vegetable stock or hot water
200 ml soya or almond milk
salt and pepper

For the chickpea croutons:
100 g chickpeas
½ tsp smoked paprika
½ tsp chilli powder
1 pinch salt

Method

1. Peel and finely dice the onion. Wash and trim the celery but keep any leaves. Finely chop. Peel and chop the celeriac – there's usually quite a bit of waste to remove the woody knobbly bits. Chop into small pieces as it reduces the cooking time.
2. Heat 2-3 tbsp water in the base of a large pan. Add the onion, celery and celeriac with a pinch of salt. Sauté on a medium heat for 5 minutes until the veggies start to soften – add more water to prevent sticking if needed.
3. Grate the garlic and add it to the pan. Cook for another 2 minutes.
4. Pour in the vegetable stock or hot water. Add the thyme and celery salt. Bring to the boil then reduce the heat, pop on the lid and simmer for 25 minutes until the celeriac is soft. You'll need longer if your chunks were large.
5. Whilst the soup is simmering, make the chickpea croutons. Heat the oven to 180°C or use an air fryer. Rinse the chickpeas and mix the spices together in a bowl. Tip in the damp chickpeas and toss to coat them. Tip them into a baking tin or air fryer drawer and roast for 10 minutes, turning once. Put to one side until the soup is ready.

6. Once the celeriac is soft, turn off the heat and leave to cool for 2-3 minutes. Pour half the soya or almond milk into the pan and blend with a stick blender until smooth, thick and creamy. Add more 'milk' if needed.
7. Re-heat the soup and serve once it's piping hot with a glug of flaxseed oil and scattering of the chickpea croutons. Keep leftovers in the fridge for up to 3 days.

Split green pea soup
Serves 4

Split green peas are a veritable powerhouse of nutrients, and super-cheap too. Packed with fibre, plant protein and an array of minerals, they are a great addition to all sorts of recipes and make a great soup too.

Cooking times depend on where you buy your peas. Packs in supermarkets tend to be quick cook, whereas if sourced from a whole-food shop or online store, they can take ages to soften. If the pack doesn't say 'quick cook', then it's a good idea to soak them beforehand. Overnight is hassle free as long as you remember.

Ingredients
100 g dried split green peas
1 medium white onion
2 medium carrots
2 medium sticks celery
1 bay leaf
1 fat clove garlic (or more if you love it)
700 ml vegetable stock
1 tbsp mixed dried herbs and/or thyme
salt and pepper
1 tbsp lemon juice

Method
1. Weigh out the peas, pop in a sieve and wash under a running tap. If needed,

soak in a bowl of water for 5 hours or overnight.
2. Peel the onion and finely dice. Peel and dice the carrots. Wash the celery sticks and trim before finely dicing.
3. Heat 2 tbsp water in the base of a large saucepan. Add the onion, carrots, celery and bay leaf. Sauté for 5 minutes over a medium heat until the veggies start to soften.
4. Grate the garlic and add to the pan. Sauté for another 2 minutes with a bit of vegetable stock if needed to stop it sticking.
5. Pour the vegetable stock into the pan and add the herbs. Drain the peas (if soaking) and add to the pan. Bring to the boil then reduce the heat, pop on the lid and simmer for 30 minutes or until the peas are soft and mushy.
6. Turn off the heat then blend with a stick blender. Season with salt and pepper as desired and add the lemon juice. Serve with chunks of fresh, warm bread or flatbread (see page 311).

Spinach, squash and coriander soup
Serves 4

This tasty soup combines the sweetness of squash with the warmth of ginger and garlic, with a good helping of greens added in – perfect for lunches on chilly autumn days, but it can also be enjoyed all year round with whatever squash is in season.

Squash and spinach have a high water content, so care needs to be taken when adding fluid; less is more until they're both fully cooked. Extra stock or water can be added then to get the consistency you desire, although you can always serve it in a mug if you accidently put too much in. It will taste just as awesome either way.

Ingredients
1 medium white or red onion
2-cm piece fresh ginger
2 cloves garlic
1 small squash
500 ml vegetable stock or hot water

150 g spinach
20 g fresh coriander (or parsley)
salt and pepper to taste
glug extra-virgin olive oil or cold-pressed flaxseed oil to garnish

Method
1. Peel and finely dice the onion. Peel the ginger and garlic and grate. Cut the squash into manageable pieces, peel and then dice finely. The smaller the pieces, the quicker they cook.
2. Wash the spinach and coriander. Separate the stems and the leaves for both. Keep a few coriander leaves for garnish. Chop the stems and put to one side. Roughly chop the spinach and coriander leaves.
3. Heat 2 tbsp water in the base of a large pan. Add the onion and a pinch of salt. Sauté for 5 minutes until the onion has softened – add more water if needed.
4. Add the grated ginger and garlic to the pan. Sauté for another 2 minutes then add the chopped spinach and coriander **stems**. Cook for 2 more minutes.
5. Tip the chopped squash into the pan and stir well. Pour in enough stock or hot water to just cover the veggies. Bring to the boil then reduce the heat, pop on the lid and simmer for 20 minutes or until the squash is lovely and squashy. Turn off the heat.
6. Blend to smooth with a stick blender then pop back on the heat.
7. Add the chopped spinach and coriander leaves to the pan, stir well and simmer for 2 minutes until the leaves have wilted into the soup.
8. If your soup is too thick, now add extra stock or hot water to get the consistency you want.
9. Season with salt and pepper and serve with a glug of oil and scattering of reserved coriander leaves.

Golden soup
Serves 4

This soup is so vibrantly yellow, it must be good for you! Turmeric provides the golden glow, a spice that's packed full of anti-inflammatory phytonutrients.

This healthful root needs to be served with fat and piperine, a compound in black pepper, so the active compounds can be absorbed in the gut. The cashew nuts add the fat plus a lovely creamy texture. Just remember to add lashings of black pepper to season at the end and you'll end up glowing as bright as the soup.

Ingredients

1 small onion
1 medium carrot
1 fat clove garlic
1 small cauliflower
½–1 tsp ground turmeric
75 g cashew nuts
500 ml vegetable stock or hot water
salt and pepper to taste

Method

1. Peel and finely chop the onion. Peel and dice the carrot. Peel and grate the garlic.
2. Remove any tough outer cauliflower leaves but keep small, tender ones. Cut out the hard core then chop the florets and softer stems plus small leaves.
3. Place the cashew nuts into a bowl of hot water to soak.
4. Heat 2 tbsp water in the base of a large pan. Add the onion and carrot. Sauté on a medium heat for 5 minutes until the veggies start to soften.
5. Add the garlic and cook for another 2 minutes.
6. Pop in the chopped cauliflower and ground turmeric and stir well. Drain the cashews and add them to the pan. Pour in the vegetable stock, bring to the boil then pop on the lid and reduce the heat. Simmer for 20 minutes until the veggies are soft.
7. Turn off the heat then blend to smooth with a stick blender.
8. Season well with black pepper and a little salt if desired.
9. Serve piping hot with a swirl of dairy-free yoghurt and extra black pepper if desired.

Spinach and rosemary soup
Serves 4

This soup is very green and pungent. It's also utterly delicious, especially if you remember to add the lemon juice at the end. This rather magically lifts the flavours. It will also help you absorb more of the iron from the green leaves – more plant magic!

Rosemary and spinach complement each other rather beautifully. If you're not a fan, add thyme or even fresh oregano for a more Mediterranean feel.

Ingredients
1 white onion
1 stick celery
1 medium potato
350 g spinach or Swiss chard (or a mix of both)
1 tbsp fresh rosemary leaves
450 ml vegetable stock
200 ml dairy-free milk of choice
salt and pepper
soya yoghurt, lemon juice and extra rosemary leaves to serve

Method
1. Peel and finely chop the onion. Rinse and trim the celery then finely dice. Peel and finely dice the potato.
2. Heat 2-3 tbsp water in the base of a large pan. Add the onion, celery and potato plus a pinch of salt. Pop the pan lid on and sweat the veggies on a medium heat for 10 minutes – stir from time to time to make sure they don't stick to the pan. Add a little extra water if needed.
3. Whilst the veg are cooking, wash and roughly chop the spinach and/or chard leaves. Pick the rosemary leaves off the tough stalk and finely chop.
4. Pour over the vegetable stock and add the rosemary. Bring to the boil then reduce the heat and simmer for another 10 minutes with the lid on.
5. Add the spinach or chard leaves and cook for another 2-3 minutes until fully

wilted, then turn off the heat.

6. Pour the mix into a blender jug and add a little dairy-free milk. Blend to smooth, adding more milk to get the consistency you like.
7. Season with salt and pepper and gently re-heat until piping hot. Serve with a swirl of dairy-free yoghurt, a squeeze of lemon and the remaining rosemary leaves.

Italian bean soup

Serves 4

This is a tasty, filling soup full of fresh Italian flavours. Packed with vegetables, the beans add extra plant protein, fibre and texture. Upgrade the soup to almost a meal by adding small gluten-free pasta, orzo or rice. You'll also need a bit of extra stock, or the soup might get so thick you'll be able to stand your spoon up in it.

Use whichever Italian herbs you like or have. I always have a jar of dried Italian herbs which is the perfect mix – if you use them, you don't need to add any of the ones I've specified, unless you want to, of course.

Ingredients
1 red or white onion
1 medium leek
2 medium carrots
2 sticks celery
1 red bell pepper
2 cloves garlic
100 ml passata
1 heaped tsp dried oregano
1 tsp dried thyme
½ tsp dried basil
3 medium fresh tomatoes
700 ml vegetable stock or hot water
1 x 400-g tin cannellini beans or aduki beans
salt and pepper
glug extra-virgin olive oil or cold-pressed flaxseed oil to serve

Method

1. Peel the onion and finely chop. Trim and rinse the leek, then shred into small pieces. Peel and dice the carrots. Wash and trim the celery then finely chop. Wash and de-seed the pepper and cut into small pieces.
2. Heat 2-3 tbsp water in the base of a large pan. Add the prepared veggies and sauté on a medium heat for 5-7 minutes. Add more water if needed to prevent any sticking on the pan base.
3. Peel the garlic cloves and grate. Add to the pan and cook for 2 more minutes.
4. Pour in the passata, herbs, chopped fresh tomatoes and vegetable stock. (If you are adding small pasta, orzo or rice, add this now too.) Bring to the boil then reduce the heat and simmer with the lid on for 15 minutes.
5. Rinse and drain the tinned beans. Add to the pan and simmer for another 5 minutes.
6. Turn off the heat and season with salt and pepper to taste.
7. Serve with a drizzle of oil and a few fresh chopped herbs if you have them.

Sweet potato and red lentil soup

Serves 4

Red lentils are a super-cheap way to add plant protein and fibre to your diet. They also cook quickly, which is great when time is short. Sweet potato is a veritable powerhouse of nutrients, including beta-carotene and polyphenols, great for the microbiome and you too. They also taste gorgeous. Orange and purple ones are the best for nutrients; choose orange for this soup.

I've used a selection of lovely anti-inflammatory spices in this soup. Make sure you add a good amount of black pepper to make the turmeric bioavailable.

Ingredients

1 red onion
2 celery sticks
½ red bell pepper
1 medium sweet potato

2 cloves garlic
120 g red lentils
½ tsp ground turmeric
1 tsp smoked paprika
1 tsp ground cumin
1 x 400-g tin chopped tomatoes
800 ml vegetable stock
salt and black pepper

Method

1. Peel and chop the onion. Rinse the celery sticks and finely chop. Dice the red pepper. Peel and dice the sweet potato.
2. Heat 2-3 tbsp water in the base of a large pan. Add the onion, celery, pepper and sweet potato. Sauté over a medium heat for 5 minutes.
3. Peel the garlic and grate into the pan. Stir to combine and sauté for another 2 minutes, adding extra water if needed to prevent it sticking to the pan.
4. Rinse the lentils in a sieve under a running tap then tip into the pan. Stir well.
5. Add the spices, tinned tomatoes and vegetable stock. Bring to the boil then reduce the heat and simmer for 25 minutes with the lid on.
6. Turn off the heat and leave to stand for 2-3 minutes. Pour 2 ladles' worth of soup into a large bowl and blend the remaining soup with a stick blender.
7. Return the reserved soup into the pan – this gives a bit of texture overall. Season with salt and pepper and serve piping hot.
8. Keep leftovers in the fridge for up to 3 day or freeze portions for use later.

Black bean soup

Serves 4

This is another chunky, nutrient-packed soup that can work as a meal. Black beans contain powerful, purple-coloured anthocyanins in the skin, the most anti-inflammatory phytonutrients. They're also packed with plant protein and fibre and work well in all sorts of Tex-Mex-inspired dishes.

Ingredients

1 red onion
½ red bell pepper
1 fat garlic clove
2 medium fresh tomatoes
500 ml vegetable stock
2 tbsp tomato purée
140 g frozen or fresh sweetcorn kernels
350 g cooked black beans
2 tsp ground cumin
¼ cayenne pepper
salt and pepper
fresh coriander, chopped avocado, dairy-free yoghurt to serve

Method

1. Peel and finely chop the onion. Finely chop the pepper. Peel and grate the garlic. Chop the fresh tomatoes.
2. Heat 2 tbsp water in the base of a large pan. Add the onion and red pepper. Sauté over a medium heat for 5 minutes. Add the grated garlic and chopped tomatoes and cook for another 2 minutes, stirring well.
3. Pour the vegetable stock into the pan. Add the tomato purée, sweetcorn, black beans, cumin and cayenne. Bring to the boil then reduce the heat and simmer with the lid on for 15 minutes.
4. Turn off the heat and season with salt and pepper.
5. Serve in bowls topped with fresh coriander, avocado and dairy-free yoghurt as desired.

Salads

Salad has come a long way since I was a child – and thank goodness for that. Limp lettuce, flavourless tomatoes and super-soggy cucumber should now be a distant, disappointing memory, replaced by vibrant, tasty bowls as a feast for the eyes as much as for your taste-buds, and of course, body.

A beautiful accompaniment or star of the show, salads enable you to eat a fabulous variety of vegetables, pulses, grains, nuts and seeds as well as some sneaky fruit if you so wish. The combinations are endless, easily adaptable to suit the season and can include a combination of raw and cooked ingredients if you so desire.

Desire is what I want to inspire in you, maybe even cravings! Once you begin to enjoy a nutrient-packed salad every day, don't be surprised if you start looking forward to them. Skip them for a few days, then tune into your body and see what it really wants – I bet it will be a salad.

Eating a salad every day is a super-simple way of increasing your fruit and vegetable intake. Whether it's a main component for lunch, a starter or side for dinner, or even a crunchy start to the day at breakfast, you'll gain amazing nutritional benefits as well as a huge repertoire of go-to dishes.

Here are 10 options to get you started, but don't stop there. There are plenty more combinations to explore. I have lots on my website and in my first book as well, or you can just explore what's in season and create your own favourite combinations. Don't forget to add a bit of citrus or vinegar to boost the nutrient intake though.

Warm broad bean, mangetout and new potato salad with crispy smoked tofu

Serves 2 as a main, 4 as a side

This is a hearty late Spring/early Summer salad that is full of great sources of plant protein in the broad beans and tofu as well as nutrient-packed veggies. Mangetout are deliciously sweet and have a delightful crunch that brings this salad to life. Enjoy them at their best in May and June (in the UK) and substitute with green beans through the summer and broccoli later in the year. Broad beans can be found in the freezer section when they're not in season. It may seem like a faff to remove the outer skin but don't miss this step as your taste-buds and digestion will thank you.

Ingredients

200 g new potatoes, scrubbed with skins on
100 g mangetout/sugar snap peas
100 g podded broad beans, fresh or frozen (defrosted)
2 big handfuls mixed salad leaves, washed and roughly torn
6 baby tomatoes, washed and cut into quarters
2 portions lemon and mixed herb dressing

For the tofu:
150 g smoked tofu, chopped into small pieces but not dried
1 tsp cornflour or gram (chickpea) flour
1 pinch paprika
1 tsp mixed dried herbs
salt and pepper

Method
1. Cut the new potatoes into halves or quarters depending on size. Steam for 15 minutes or so, until soft when pierced with a knife.
2. Whilst the potatoes are cooking, blanche the broad beans by popping them into the same pan for 1-2 minutes (depending on size). Remove with a slotted spoon, then peel off the bitter outer skin to reveal the tasty, vibrant green inner pod. Discard the skins and leave the beans to cool.
3. Steam the mangetout or sugar snap peas for 3 minutes. Remove from the heat whilst they're still *al dente* (you can eat them raw if super-fresh).
4. Cook the tofu: measure the cornflour, mixed herbs and paprika into a bowl. Add salt and pepper and mix well to combine. Drop in the smoked tofu pieces and lightly coat with the mixture.
5. Pop the tofu in an air fryer and 'fry' for 10 minutes until crispy on the outside and soft in the middle. Start cooking this just as the potatoes are ready.

6. Drain the potatoes and leave to cool slightly in the sieve then cut into bite-sized chunks.
7. Chop the mangetout roughly.
8. Grab two bowls or one large bowl if serving as a side salad. Drop the salad leaves in the bottom. Scatter potato, mangetout, broad beans and tomatoes over the leaves. Once the tofu is crispy, pop on top then pour over the lemon and herb dressing.
9. Serve immediately.

Two-bean salad
Serves 1

A super-tasty, hearty lunchtime dish, this salad features one fresh bean and one tinned. I love fresh green beans and grow a variety of colours in my veg patch. They are gorgeous picked fresh and rarely need any cooking when small and tender.

Use whatever fresh and tinned beans you have to hand. If green beans are not in season, substitute with another type of tinned bean or fresh greens, like long-stemmed broccoli or kale – much better than buying produce that has been flown halfway across the world.

If you find red onion difficult to digest, leave it to soak in the dressing for a good 30 minutes before you want to eat. The acids soften the onion and make it more digestible. However, if onion is not for you, leave it out. The salad will still taste gorgeous.

Ingredients
20 g red onion
2 handfuls mixed salad leaves
4 tbsp tinned flageolet beans
60 g fresh green beans of choice
6 almonds, roughly chopped or sliced

For the dressing:
1 tbsp lemon juice
2 tbsp cold-pressed flaxseed oil or extra-virgin olive oil
½ tsp mustard
1 tbsp fresh herbs such as oregano, thyme, parsley
salt and pepper to taste

Method
1. Slice the red onion. Wash the salad leaves. Drain and rinse the tinned flageolet beans.
2. Wash and finely chop the fresh herbs. Place the dressing ingredients in a small bowl and whisk to combine. Add the red onion and leave it to soak for 30 minutes or so if desired.
3. Wash and trim the green beans. Steam for 2-3 minutes if needed and leave to cool.
4. Scatter the mixed leaves in the base of a shallow bowl. Scatter one third of the red onion dressing over the top followed by half of both types of bean. Add another third of the onion dressing and the remaining beans.
5. Add the remaining dressing and garnish with almonds and a few extra fresh herbs.

Roasted sweet potato and kale salad
Serves 2 hearty portions

This winter salad is packed full of rainbow nutrients that will brighten the dullest of winter days. Roast the sweet potato in advance to save time on the day, but don't skip the time between prepping the kale and eating it. Chopping the kale activates enzymes that promote the bioavailability of fabulous nutrients contained within. Massaging with the lemon juice supports this process as well as making the leaves easier to chew.

Pomegranate seeds are lovely additions and contain fabulous antioxidants and vitamin C, essential to support health in the cold winter months, but do mind your teeth!

Ingredients

1 large sweet potato
¼ medium red onion
100 g kale of choice
2 tbsp lemon juice
50 g peppery salad leaves
100 g cooked chickpeas
2 tbsp pomegranate seeds
1-2 tbsp balsamic vinegar
salt and pepper to taste

Method

1. Peel the sweet potato and cut into chunks. Pop in a baking tin with a little olive oil (optional) and roast for 20 minutes or so until lightly brown and just soft. Leave to cool.
2. Wash the kale well and chop into small pieces.
3. Place the lemon juice in the bottom of a bowl. Add the kale and sliced onion. Mix with your hands and leave to soften for 30 minutes or so.
4. Once the sweet potato has cooled and the kale and onion have softened, construct the salad. Pop the sweet potato chunks in with the kale and onion. Add the peppery leaves, chickpeas, balsamic vinegar and salt and pepper. Toss the mix to ensure the flavours are distributed.
5. Decorate with the pomegranate seeds on top and serve straight away.

Sprouted mung bean salad

Serves 1

Mung beans are super-easy to sprout at home, and cheap too. As we saw in Chapter 7, sprouting beans, seeds and grains can make them easier to digest and increases nutrient bioavailability.

This crunchy salad is full of fresh flavours with an Asian slant. If your digestion is a bit delicate, omit the chilli and be cautious with the spring onions if necessary. This recipe serves one but can easily double or quadruple if you have more mouths to feed.

You can use shop-bought bean sprouts if you don't sprout at home. Make sure they are well in date and rinse them well under running water and prepare according to the packaging before eating.

Ingredients
½ tsp cumin seeds
½ tsp black mustard seeds
2 spring onions
5-cm chunk cucumber
4 cherry tomatoes
100 g sprouted mung beans
¼ red chilli
1 tbsp fresh coriander or parsley leaves
½ lime, juice only
salt and pepper to taste

Method
1. Place the cumin and mustard seeds in a small pan and toast over a medium heat for 2 minutes until the seeds start to pop. Turn off the heat and put to one side to cool.
2. Wash the spring onions and trim before slicing into small pieces. Chop the cucumber and cherry tomatoes. Slice the red chilli if using.
3. Place the sprouted mung beans in a bowl with the spring onions, cucumber, tomatoes, chilli and coriander or parsley leaves. Add the toasted seeds, lime juice, salt and pepper. Toss to combine all the ingredients and serve immediately.

Lentil salad
Serves 2

Lentils are a great source of fibre and plant protein; they can, however, be a bit windy for some. Sprouted lentils work well in this salad, reducing the gas factor whilst making the nutrients more bioavailable.

If you don't have sprouted to hand, don't worry as any type of whole green, brown or puy lentil will do nicely. You can cook your lentils in advance or use one of the many types of ready-cooked lentils available in the supermarket. I particularly like sachets of puy lentils as they keep their texture and have a deep, earthy flavour.

Ingredients
¼ green cucumber
6 cherry tomatoes
¼ red pepper
¼ red onion or 2 spring onions (optional)
1 handful fresh parsley, chives or coriander
125 g cooked or sprouted lentils
1 tbsp toasted sesame seeds

For the dressing:
½ tsp Dijon mustard
1 lemon, juice only
2 tbsp extra-virgin olive
salt and pepper

Method
1. Wash and finely chop the cucumber, cherry tomatoes and pepper. Finely dice the onion if using. Wash and finely chop the herbs.
2. Place all the dressing ingredients into a small jar, pop on the lid and shake to combine. Check the flavour and add more mustard, lemon juice or seasoning as desired.
3. Mix the lentils, vegetables and most of the herbs together in a bowl. Add the

dressing and stir well to combine.
4. Garnish with sesame seeds and the remaining chopped herbs before serving.

Rainbow carrot and thyme salad
Serves 4

When it comes to carrots, orange is not the only colour in town – they come in shades of yellow, red and purple too. Found more often in farm shops or veg box schemes, each colour provides a different selection of polyphenols which, as we have seen in Chapter 4, support both the microbiome and our cellular processes.

Carrots are one of those vegetables that release different nutrients when cooked or raw. Here, they are lightly roasted. You could steam them or cook half and have half raw. Or even cut the carrots into thin sticks and eat fully raw. It's up to you.

If you can only find orange carrots, don't worry. This salad still tastes as good. It just won't have the same rainbow hues when served.

Ingredients
4-6 medium-sized carrots of different colours
1 tbsp fresh thyme or lemon thyme leaves
150 g spinach
juice ½ lemon
salt and pepper to taste
2 tbsp balsamic vinegar

Method
1. Pre-heat the oven to 180°C. Line a baking tray with non-stick baking paper.
2. Scrub the carrots, trim the ends and peel if necessary.
3. Cut into small lengths and pop into a colander. Rinse under a running tap.
4. Tip the carrots onto the baking sheet and scatter half the thyme leaves over the top.
5. Pop the tray in the oven and roast for 15 minutes or until the carrots start to soften

and are lightly browned.
6. Wash the spinach leaves and dry. Scatter them over a serving dish and drizzle the lemon juice over the top.
7. When the carrots are ready, remove the tray from the oven. Carefully add them on top of the spinach which will wilt slightly from the heat.
8. Season with salt and pepper. Scatter the remaining thyme leaves over the top then drizzle on the balsamic vinegar.
9. This salad can be served immediately whilst still warm or once it has cooled.

Red kale and pear salad
Serves 2

If you find raw kale a bit too difficult to eat, it might be that you need to give it a bit of TLC before you pop it in your mouth. Chopping kale leaves releases enzymes that help release all the wonderful nutrients within. Massaging the leaves with an acid, like lemon juice, tenderises them, making them easier to chew, digest and gain all the loveliness within.

The key is remembering to do it. When you make this simple salad, start it an hour before you want to eat it. It will be much more enjoyable, and nutritious too.

Ingredients
90 g red or green kale or cavolo nero
½ small white or red onion or 3 spring onions
½ lemon, juice only
1 large ripe pear
2 tbsp fresh parsley leaves
1 tbsp lightly toasted sesame seeds or seeds/nuts of choice
salt and pepper to taste
1 tbsp flaxseed oil or extra-virgin olive oil to garnish (optional)

Method
1. Wash the kale and cut out the tough central spine. Chop the leaves into bite-sized pieces and tip into a bowl. Slice the onion.
2. Add the lemon juice and massage into the leaves with your fingertips for about 5 minutes. Add the sliced onion and put to one side to rest, for about an hour if you can.
3. When it's time to build the salad, core and slice the pear. Chop the parsley leaves.
4. Add the sliced pear, parsley, sesame seeds, salt and pepper and mix well. Drizzle the flaxseed or extra-virgin olive oil over the top and it's ready to serve.

Herby millet tabbouleh
Serves 2-4 people

Tabbouleh is a Middle Eastern grain-based dish, traditionally made with cracked wheat. My gluten-free option uses millet instead. With its slightly nutty flavour and firm texture, it's an ideal replacement. It's also packed with fibre and plant protein. This recipe provides two good-sized portions; double the ingredients if you are cooking for more. It stores well in the fridge for up to 3 days, so prepare ahead if you have a busy week.

Ingredients
100 g millet
300 ml vegetable stock
½ small bunch parsley
few handfuls of other fresh herbs – oregano, tarragon, chives etc
1 lemon, juice only
salt and pepper to taste
2 tbsp pistachio nuts or nuts of choice, chopped and/or
2 tbsp mixed seeds or seeds of choice
1 glug cold-pressed flaxseed oil or extra-virgin olive oil to garnish (optional)

Method
1. Rinse the millet under a running tap and leave to drain.
2. Bring the stock to the boil in a small pan and carefully pour in the millet. Reduce the heat and simmer with the lid on for 15 minutes or so until the stock has been absorbed, and the millet is soft but not stodgy. Drain off any excess fluid and tip into a large bowl or plate. Spread the millet out so it cools and stops cooking.
3. Whilst the millet is cooking, finely chop the herbs and roughly chop the nuts.
4. Once fully cooled, transfer the millet to a serving bowl and add the remaining ingredients. Mix well, taste and adjust the seasoning as needed.

Beetroot and watercress salad
Serves 2

The simplest ingredients often create the most delicious combination of flavours. This tasty salad is one of them, with sweet beetroot, peppery watercress and crunchy, rich walnuts offering a wonderful collection of nutrients too.

The elderflower dressing finishes this simple salad off beautifully but if you're in a hurry, a drizzle of extra-virgin olive oil and squeeze of lemon will do nicely.

Ingredients
2 smallish, cooked beetroot
45 g watercress, around half a bunch
50 g walnuts
10 g fresh parsley
1 portion of elderflower dressing (see page 300)

Method
1. Peel the cooked beetroot if it's a bit rough and cut into bite-sized chunks.
2. Wash the watercress and dry well before breaking it up slightly with your hands.
3. Scatter the watercress in the bottom of a bowl. Add the beetroot and walnuts.
4. Roughly chop the parsley and scatter over the top.
5. Pour the dressing over the top and serve immediately.

Asparagus, pea and rocket salad
Serves 2

In the UK, the asparagus season is short so I try to make the most of it by eating it as often as I can when available. These tasty spears have strong anti-inflammatory phytonutrients including lots of vitamin C as well as soluble and insoluble fibre, including inulin. This is a particular favourite of the microbiome and has been connected to longevity in various research studies.

Asparagus are usually served cooked, but I love this vegetable raw. Thin, tender stems are best for this, otherwise they can be a bit woody. If raw is too much for you, then lightly steam the spears for 2-3 minutes and cool under running water straight away to retain as many nutrients as possible. If you grow your own peas or sugar snap peas, then pick the pods when small and tender and add these to the salad as well. Otherwise, frozen peas are great.

This salad is light and tasty. Eat as a side dish or add a rice or gluten-free grain salad to make a more filling meal.

Ingredients
20 g pine nuts
6-8 slender asparagus spears
50 g peas in their pods or frozen, defrosted
6 radishes
2-3 handfuls rocket or other salad leaf

For the dressing:
1 lemon, juiced
1 tbsp extra-virgin olive oil or cold-pressed flaxseed oil
1 small clove garlic, grated (optional)
salt and pepper to taste

Method

1. Pop the pine nuts in a small pan and lightly toast over a medium-low heat. Watch carefully as they can easily burn. Leave to cool.
2. Wash the asparagus and trim off the woody ends. Thinly slice with a sharp knife or vegetable peeler (mind your fingertips!).
3. Wash and trim the pea pods if using, splitting them open to reveal the peas. Alternatively, make sure frozen peas are fully defrosted.
4. Slice the radishes thinly.
5. Mix the dressing ingredients together in a small jar and shake to combine.
6. Pop the asparagus, peas, radishes and rocket or other leaves into a bowl. Pour over the dressing and toss the salad before scattering the pine nuts over the top.

Lunch or light meals

In the past, my lunch was always some type of sandwich, usually cheese – functional but uninspiring and not nutrient-packed. Discovering I had an intolerance to yeast meant bread was no longer an option; moving to a whole-food plant-based diet required some imagination when it came to lunchtime. There's always soup and salad, but sometimes you need a bit more.

The following selection of recipes are a mix to make and eat at home or suitable to pop in a lunch box. They can also be eaten at any time of the day; many make great snacks for hungry tummies or light evening meals. Most can be made in bulk and frozen for when you need to grab and go, and some are great as a sandwich or wrap filling, so there are plenty of options. If you were looking for hummus or dip ideas, then go straight to the last section 'spreads and breads' (page 304); they all make marvellous lunch options too.

Smashed chickpeas
Serves 2

This first recipe is a simple filling for wraps or baked potatoes, or a topping for toast. It's particularly good on toasted slices of the lentil bread you'll find in the last section (page 314). The mustard, lemon and capers make this tangy and sharp which complements the mellow chickpeas. You can substitute chickpeas with other beans if preferred.

Ingredients
1 lemon
1 medium spring onion (optional but good)
1 tbsp fresh parsley and chives
4 heaped tbsp cooked chickpeas
1 tsp Dijon mustard

salt and pepper to taste

1 tsp capers (optional)

Method
1. Juice the lemon and grate the rind (optional). Trim and finely chop the spring onion, using the green leaves as well as the bulb. Wash and finely chop the herbs and capers.
2. Place the chickpeas in a bowl with the lemon juice and Dijon mustard. Mash with a fork, adding a little water if it's too dry. You want soft, mushed chickpeas with a little texture and a thick sauce.
3. Stir in the spring onion, herbs, seasoning and capers. Mix well and check the flavour; add more seasoning, lemon or Dijon mustard as required.
4. Keeps in the fridge for 2 days.

Crunchy cauliflower bites
Serves 2

Cauliflower tastes gorgeous when it's cooked in the oven or air fryer, creating a lovely savoury flavour when lightly browned. Coat the cauliflower pieces with a slightly spicy sauce, sprinkle some sesame seeds on top and they're even better.

These cauliflower bites make a lovely snack or lunch treat. Add them to a wrap with salad, top a hot bowl of soup with them or just eat them as they are, dipped in a tasty sauce (see the sauces section for ideas – page 295); they're crunchy and full of flavour and nutrients without a drop of oil in sight.

Feel free to play around with the spices, increasing or omitting the cayenne pepper, adding some chilli flakes or ground cumin if you wish. Once they're hot and crispy, they must be eaten straight away or they lose their crunch, so they are best eaten at home rather than added to a lunch box.

Ingredients
200 g cauliflower

4 tbsp gram (chickpea) flour or green pea flour

1 tbsp cornflour

¼-½ tsp cayenne pepper (optional)

¼ tsp turmeric

¼ tsp garlic powder

salt and black pepper to taste

4 tbsp water

3 tbsp sesame seeds

Method
1. Pre-heat the oven to 180°C and line a baking tray with non-stick baking paper. If you are using an air fryer, pre-heat if required to 180°C.
2. Cut the cauliflower into bite-sized pieces, pop in a colander and wash under a running tap.
3. Add the gram flour, cornflour, spices and seasoning to a large bowl and mix well to combine. Add 3 tbsp water and stir well with a whisk to create a thick, smooth batter. If it's too thick, add more water a little at a time until it's the consistency of double cream.
4. Add the cauliflower to the bowl and stir well, making sure every floret is covered in batter. Transfer each floret onto the baking sheet or air fryer drawer/bowl with a spoon then sprinkle the sesame seeds over the top.
5. In the oven, bake for 10 minutes then turn the bites over and bake for another 5 minutes or so until lightly brown and crispy. In the air fryer, 'fry' for 10 minutes then shake the basket and bake for another 5 minutes. Eat immediately.

Tempeh onion bhajis
Serves 4

My first taste of Indian food was 'going out for a curry' to celebrate a boyfriend's 17th birthday. I had never had spicy food before and the korma I ordered seemed super-hot (it wasn't!) so I wasn't that keen. The onion bhaji, however, was gorgeous. A ball of crispy, crunchy onions dripping with oil was a taste sensation and I've loved them ever since; fortunately, I found a way to make them without the lashings of oil. Onions are delicious when baked and whilst they might not get quite as crispy, they're still one of my favourite snacks or starters.

I've added some grated tempeh into this recipe partly to add a little plant protein, but also to make them more substantial so they can be eaten as a light lunch if desired. Feel free to leave it out if you're not a fan. Like the cauliflower bites on page 216, use the oven or air fryer to get these little lovelies nice and crispy. Dipping these tasty bhajis into dairy-free yoghurt and mango chutney creates a taste sensation in one mouthful.

Ingredients
1 large or 2 medium onions, red or white
½ tsp salt
4 tbsp gram (chickpea) or green pea flour
black pepper
1 pinch turmeric
1 tsp ground cumin or ½ tsp garum masala
1 pinch chilli flakes
50 g tempeh, grated

To serve:
fresh coriander, dairy-free yoghurt, mango chutney (optional)

Method
1. Slice the onions, pop into a bowl and sprinkle the salt over the top. Leave to rest for a few minutes whilst you get the other ingredients ready. The salt will draw water out of them.
2. Pre-heat the oven to 180°C and line a baking tray with non-stick baking paper. Or pre-heat the air fryer if required.
3. Place the gram or green pea flour, spices and black pepper in a small bowl and mix together. Add the tempeh if using and stir again.
4. Once the onion has released some fluid, tip the flour mix into the onion and stir well. The mix will be super-thick, and the onion pieces will clump together.
5. Place a large spoonful of mix onto the baking tray/air fryer basket, pushing it

together to form a ball/patty if needed. Repeat until the mix is used up.
6. Bake or air fry for 15 minutes then turn and bake for another 5 minutes or so until the bhajis are crispy. Serve immediately whilst piping hot.

Chickpeas and chard
Serves 4

This is a super-tasty little dish that can be made with any greens you have to hand. I grow rainbow chard in my veg patch at home, so I always seem to have some to hand. If you're looking to up your intake of greens for the calcium, then kale or seasonal greens are a better option. Don't forget to add the squeeze of lemon just before you eat – the flavour lifts and it help you absorb more of those cell-loving nutrients.

You can eat this on its own as a light lunch or with rice, quinoa or flatbread on the side.

Ingredients
1 small onion
2 cloves garlic
2-cm piece ginger
1 green chilli (optional)
200 g fresh Swiss chard
1 x 400-g tin chickpeas, drained
salt and pepper to taste
1 tbsp toasted sesame seeds (optional) and fresh coriander to serve
1 lemon, cut into chunks

Method
1. Roughly chop the onion, garlic, ginger and chilli if using. Separate the chard stems and leaves and roughly chop both.
2. Pop the onion, garlic, ginger and chilli into a small blender pot with a little water. Blitz for 20 seconds or so until it forms a thick paste.

3. Pour the paste into a non-stick pan with the chopped chard stems. Cook over a medium heat for 5 minutes or so until the onion is soft and the flavours released.
4. Add the chopped leaves to the pan. Cook for another few minutes until it starts to wilt then add the drained chickpeas, salt and pepper.
5. Simmer for a few more minutes until everything is piping hot.
6. Scatter sesame seeds and fresh coriander on top and serve with a chunk of lemon on the side.

Amaranth and millet pancakes
Makes 4

I've called these 'pancakes' but they're more a type of hot flatbread that can be added as a side to dishes like the chickpeas and chard above or as the star of the meal, loaded with roasted veggies, chilli, curry or anything you like. The millet will need blitzing in a high-speed blender to make a flour, although you can use ragi if you have it (Indian millet flour).

As with all these recipes, you can add whatever flavouring you like and enjoy. I like the flavour of cumin and it's a great digestive aid, as are nigella seeds. If you enjoy some spice, add chilli flakes or even cayenne pepper. These pancakes can be eaten straight away or left to cool and kept in the fridge until you want them. Use non-stick baking paper to separate them, though, as they do have a habit of sticking together.

Ingredients
75 g millet (or ragi flour if you have it)
75 g amaranth flour
1 tsp baking powder
½ tsp salt
2 tbsp ground flaxseed
¼ tsp turmeric powder
black pepper
1 tsp each cumin and nigella seeds
chilli flakes, cayenne pepper (optional if you like heat)
350 ml dairy-free milk of choice

Method
1. Grind the millet into flour by blitzing in a high-speed blender for a few seconds.
2. Tip the millet flour into a bowl and add the amaranth, baking powder, salt, ground flaxseed, turmeric, black pepper, seeds and any other flavourings. Stir well to combine.
3. Add the dairy-free milk and whisk well to combine, making sure there are no lumps hiding at the bottom of the bowl.
4. Place a good non-stick frying or crêpe pan over a medium heat. Wipe a tiny amount of extra-virgin olive oil over the pan and leave to pre-heat for a minute or so.
5. Pour a ladle's worth of batter into the centre of the pan and swirl it from side to side to spread out evenly. Leave it to cook on a medium heat for 2-3 minutes without touching it whilst the bubbles appear on the top.
6. Once the bubbles stop, gently loosen the base of the pancake with a spatula. Once it moves freely, carefully turn it over and cook the other side for another 2-3 minutes until firm and lightly browned.
7. Transfer the pancake to a plate and keep warm until you have made the remaining three pancakes then serve as desired.

Quinoa and vegetable patties
Makes 12

Despite my best efforts, I always seem to overestimate the amount of grains or pasta we need for one meal. It's probably a hangover from having two very hungry teens at home in need of constant feeding; even though they have both left home, my portion measurement is stuck in the past. Fortunately, having leftovers means I have lots of opportunity for creating new recipes, so nothing is wasted.

These lovely patties are a great way to use leftover quinoa and any bits and bobs of vegetables floundering in the bottom of the fridge. If you have a different leftover whole grain, like rice or millet, then use that instead. A sachet of ready-cooked quinoa is also a great option to save time. These patties store in the fridge for a couple of days and freeze well, so why not double the amounts and make a batch for use on a busy or low-energy day? Serve with one of the savoury sauces in the sauce section and a side salad for a lovely lunch or light evening meal.

Ingredients

½ medium red onion
¼ head broccoli, stems and florets separated
1 medium carrot
70 g sweetcorn
2 tbsp ground flaxseed
250 g **cooked** quinoa
½ tsp garlic powder
1 tsp dried oregano
1 pinch chilli flakes (optional) or fresh chives
salt and pepper to taste

Method

1. Finely chop the onion, broccoli stems and florets. Peel and grate the carrot. Defrost the sweetcorn if using frozen or remove nibs from the corn cob if using fresh.
2. Pop the ground flaxseed into a small bowl and add 4 tbsp water to create a thick flax 'egg'. Stir and leave it to thicken.
3. Heat 2-3 tbsp water in the base of a pan and sauté the onion, broccoli stems and grated carrot over a medium heat for 5 minutes. Add the broccoli florets and sweetcorn and sauté for another 2-3 minutes until the veg are softened. Turn off the heat.
4. Line a baking tray with non-stick baking paper.
5. Tip the cooked veg into a food processor along with the cooked quinoa, herbs, spices, flax 'egg' and seasoning. Pulse a few times to break everything down but keep some texture. After a few good pulses the mix should start sticking together.
6. Remove a large spoonful of the mix and form it into a patty with your hands. Place on the prepared baking sheet and repeat until all the mix is used up. There should be enough for 12 patties.

7. Pop the baking sheet in the fridge for 10 minutes and pre-heat the oven to 180°C.
8. Place the patties in the oven and bake for 30 minutes, turning once, until they are golden brown. Serve hot.

Smoky beans
Serves 2

I have always been a big fan of baked beans. Sadly, the tinned version I grew up on contains a lot of added sugar and salt and just doesn't taste as good as it used to. This version might take a little longer to prepare than opening a tin and re-heating, but it's worth the effort. Serve on a baked potato, toast or an amaranth and millet pancake topped with fresh green herbs and a glug of cold-pressed flaxseed oil or extra-virgin olive oil and you have yourself a nourishing, tasty meal.

Ingredients
1 small onion, white or red
200 ml passata or sieved tinned tomatoes
100 ml water
1 tsp garlic powder
1 tsp smoked paprika
1 tsp maple syrup
1 x 400-g tin white beans of choice (e.g. butterbeans, cannellini, flageolet)
1 tbsp lemon juice
black pepper (optional)

Method
1. Finely chop the onion and pop it in a small pan with a little water. Sauté on a medium heat for 5 minutes until it's soft.
2. Add the passata, water, garlic powder, smoked paprika and maple syrup to the pan and simmer for 5 minutes.
3. Add the beans and lemon juice and simmer for another 5 minutes.
4. Season with black pepper if desired and serve hot. Store any leftovers in the fridge for up to 3 days.

Baked bubble and squeak
Serves 4

Another great recipe for using up leftovers, bubble and squeak will always remind me of Christmas and my dad. He was rarely found in the kitchen, but making bubble and squeak with the leftover vegetables from Christmas dinner became an annual tradition for him. He fried his in lots of butter, so I'm not sure what he'd make of my baked version. To me they're just as tasty and of course can be eaten any time of the year, not just for Christmas.

Serve with pickles, chutney or sauerkraut or something from the sauce section (page 295).

Ingredients
350 g cold, cooked vegetables that ideally include potato and cabbage plus whatever else you have. Brussels sprouts are particularly good
2 tbsp dairy-free milk of choice
salt and pepper

Method
1. Pre-heat the oven to 180°C and line a baking tray with non-stick baking paper.
2. Chop the cold, cooked vegetables into small pieces and place in a bowl. Add 1 tbsp of dairy-free milk and the seasoning.
3. Mash together until everything starts to stick. Add more milk if needed.
4. Separate the mix into 4 portions. Using a burger mould or free hand, press out 4 separate patties onto the lined baking sheet.
5. Bake in the oven for 20 minutes then carefully turn over and bake for another 10 minutes until firm and brown. Serve immediately.

Aloo tikki balls
Makes 14

Aloo tikki is a super-tasty Indian snack traditionally made with potato and spices rolled into a ball or patty and deep fried. My recipe uses sweet potato and is baked rather than fried. The combination of fresh and dried spices is great for gut health and every ball is packed with a delicious range of anti-inflammatory polyphenols.

I utilise the freezer for this recipe – for the ingredients rather than storing the finished product. Bags of prepared sweet potato, onion, garlic and ginger are readily available and save time and energy. Keeping a stash of these in the freezer means you always have raw ingredients to hand even when the fridge is empty.

Rice flour is integral to this recipe as it provides a little texture as well as helping to bind the balls together. You could substitute with gram flour, but I don't think it works quite as well. These tikki balls are lovely piping hot straight out of the oven but also make a great lunch box addition. Serve with mango chutney, sweet chilli or tamarind sauce.

Ingredients
300 g sweet potato
4 tbsp finely chopped onion
1 heaped tbsp frozen chopped ginger or grated fresh
1 tbsp frozen garlic or grated fresh
2 tbsp fresh coriander
40 g cashew nuts (or sunflower seeds if nut free)
4 tbsp rice flour
1 lime, juice only (optional)
1 tsp ground cumin
½ tsp ground cinnamon
1 pinch cloves
1 pinch chilli flakes (optional)
salt and pepper to taste

Method
1. Peel and dice a large sweet potato and steam until soft. Alternatively, pop frozen sweet potato into the steamer and cook until soft. Leave to cool slightly.
2. Heat 2 tbsp water in the base of a small pan and add the diced onion. Sauté for 5 minutes on a medium heat then add the ginger and garlic. Separate the coriander leaves and stems, finely chop the stems and add to the pan. Cook for 2-3 minutes until everything is soft then turn off the heat.
3. Pop the cashews or seeds into a small blender pot and whizz a few times to break them down – keep some texture. Add the cooked vegetables, rice flour, coriander leaves, spices and seasoning. Blend to bring everything together – the mix should be soft but not sticky, with a little texture.
4. Pre-heat the oven to 180°C and line a baking tray with non-stick baking paper.
5. Take a spoonful of mix and gently roll it into a ball with your fingers. Place on the baking tray and repeat until all the mix is used up.
6. Place the tray in the middle of the oven and bake for 10 minutes. Turn the tray and bake for another 10 until the outside is firm and lightly crisped.
7. Serve immediately if eating hot.

Carrot flapjacks
Makes 8

Having always been a big fan of flapjacks, I started to wonder about why they were always sweet and not savoury. Oats are so adaptable and so good for gut health (as long as you can tolerate them) with all its soluble fibre, I decided there must be a way to create a savoury snack option. After some experimentation, the carrot flapjack was born.

Oats are paired with different types of seeds that provide healthy fats, protein and minerals as well as fibre, and carrots, that gloriously orange source of beta-carotene, the precursor to vitamin A and strong antioxidant. Mix in some herbs and flavourings and *voila*, a delicious savoury flapjack, perfect for lunch boxes, picnics or post work-out snack.

Ingredients

1 ½ tbsp ground flaxseed

5 tbsp water

1 tsp Dijon mustard (optional)

200 g carrot

175 g oats

1 tsp mixed herbs

½ tsp garlic powder (optional but good)

2 tbsp mixed seeds

2 tbsp nutritional yeast (optional)

salt and pepper to taste

For the topping:

1 tbsp hemp seeds

1 tbsp nutritional yeast (optional)

Method

1. Pre-heat the oven to 180°C and line a 20-cm square baking tin with non-stick baking paper.
2. Place the ground flaxseeds in a small bowl and add the water and mustard (if using). Stir well to combine and leave to thicken for a few minutes.
3. Peel and finely grate the carrots into a large bowl. Add the oats, herbs, garlic powder, seeds, nutritional yeast, salt and pepper. Stir well to combine.
4. Pour the ground flaxseed mix into the oat mix and stir well. The mix should stick when pressed together with your fingers. If not, add a little more water but be very careful not to add much or it will be too soggy.
5. Spoon the mix into the prepared baking tin, pressing it into the corners. Smooth the top and sprinkle the hemp seeds and extra nutritional yeast over the top.
6. Bake for 20 minutes or until the top is lightly browned. Remove from the oven and leave to cool in the tin.
7. Cut into 8 equal slices and store in an air-tight container in the fridge for up to 4 days.

Easy recipes

As much as I enjoy cooking, there are days when I'm low on 'can be bothered'. Busy days can leave anyone jaded and lacking in the enthusiasm required to create a marvellous feast, especially if you have an autoimmune disease where energy is at a premium and fatigue hovers at all times, waiting to strike. Quick and simple recipes can be tasty and nutritious and can help you save whatever energy you have for the rest of the day.

None of the following recipes should take more than half an hour to make and all use ingredients readily available in the supermarket. Many can be frozen, so double up the ingredients to stock up the freezer for use on those really challenging days. Simply defrost, re-heat and *voila*, you're done. That really is an easy recipe.

Tempeh and vegetable skewers
Makes 2-4 skewers (depending on their length)

This is a super-tasty and filling meal that looks like a bit of hassle but doesn't take too long. Prepare the ingredients a few hours before you want to eat to let them soak up the tasty marinade. Tempeh gives you a good amount of plant protein and lots of fibre. As it's fermented, many people find it easy to digest, and it will give your gut bugs a little boost too. If you don't have tempeh to hand, use extra firm tofu instead.

Ingredients
For the marinade:
2 tbsp tamari or coconut amines
2 tbsp maple syrup
2 tbsp white wine, apple cider or malt vinegar,
    or lemon juice if you can't have vinegar
1 tsp smoked paprika
½ tsp garlic powder

½ tsp dried thyme
black pepper

For the skewers:
150 g tempeh
½ medium red bell pepper
½ medium courgette
¼ medium red onion

Method
1. Mix the marinade ingredients together in a container with an air-tight lid.
2. Cut the tempeh into 3-cm squares. Slice the pepper and red onion into thin wedges and cut the courgette into thickish slices.
3. Place the tempeh and veggies into the container, pop on the lid and gently shake to make sure everything is covered.
4. Leave to marinade for 1-2 hours if possible, turning the container from time to time to distribute the marinade.
5. When you are ready to cook, slide a slice of the onion, courgette, pepper and a cube of tempeh onto a metal skewer and repeat until the ingredients are equally divided and arranged onto the skewers.
6. Cook under a pre-heated grill or on a pre-heated BBQ for 10 minutes, turning regularly – don't put it right by a flame. Baste with leftover marinade once or twice to make sure it doesn't burn.
7. Pour the leftover marinade into a small non-stick pan. Bring to the boil then simmer for 10 minutes or so until reduced and thick.
8. Once the skewers are cooked, transfer to a plate and drizzle the reduced marinade over the top. Serve with salad and wraps.

Creamy cauliflower curry
Serves 4

We do love a good curry in our house. Living in India opened our eyes to much more than the standard dishes you find in the UK. Regional variations of style, ingredients and flavour meant there was always something new to discover. Some of the best dishes I ate were served in friends' homes, not in fancy restaurants. They always apologised for the food being simple, but it was the simplicity that allowed the vegetables and spices to shine.

Cauliflower makes a wonderful base to curries, although it's important not to overcook it otherwise it turns to mush. Traditionally partnered with potato, I've used sweet potato in this recipe, although feel free to revert to white potato if you like. Tomato is usually a main ingredient in Indian sauces; here, tofu forms the creamy sauce, avoiding the need for juicy tomatoes, good news for those of you who need to avoid them.

Flavour is key in this recipe, not heat from chilli peppers. Feel free to add them if you like, but I prefer the combination of turmeric and garum masala for tastiness without a burn.

Ingredients

1 tsp each of cumin and black mustard seeds
1 onion
2 medium sweet potatoes or white potatoes
1 fat clove garlic
2-cm piece fresh ginger
1 medium cauliflower
75 g spinach or kale
300 g silken tofu
¼ tsp ground turmeric
1 tsp garum masala
1 tsp ground cumin
½ tsp chilli flakes (optional)
salt and black pepper
fresh chopped coriander to garnish

Method

1. Finely chop the onion. Trim or peel the potatoes and dice small. Peel the garlic

and ginger and grate. Remove the hard outer leaves of the cauliflower (you can use the small, inner ones) and chop into small florets. Wash under running water. Wash and shred the spinach or kale.
2. Place a medium-sized pan over a medium heat and add the cumin and mustard seeds. Dry fry for a minute or so until they start to pop.
3. Take the pan off the heat for a moment and carefully add 2-3 tbsp water (it will sizzle and spit). Pop the pan back on the heat and add the onion. Sauté over a medium heat for 5 minutes, adding more water if needed to stop it sticking.
4. Add the potato and grated garlic and ginger. Sauté for a few more minutes, again adding extra water if needed.
5. Add the spices to the pan along with 200 ml water. Stir well and bring to the boil. Reduce the heat and simmer with the lid on for 10 minutes.
6. Next, add the cauliflower and kale to the pan (if using spinach, it can be added later). Simmer for another 10 minutes until the veggies are just soft.
7. Whilst the cauliflower is cooking, pop the silken tofu into a small blender pot and blend to smooth.
8. Add the tofu and spinach (if using) to the pan and stir well to combine. Simmer for another 2-3 minutes, then turn off the heat and season with salt and pepper.
9. Serve garnished with fresh coriander and rice or flatbread.

Ethiopian split pea stew
Serves 4

Berbere is a traditional Ethiopian spice blend containing a wide range of whole spices including cardamom, coriander seeds, fenugreek, clove and nigella seeds. You can make your own, but I feel it's a bit of a compromise. Berbere spice mix can be found online or in larger ethnic stores. It's worth the effort in finding it as it adds a beautifully rich and warming flavour to a very simple dish.

Yellow split peas are super-cheap and easy to find in supermarkets. You could try alternative ones like split Flamingo peas from Hodmedod's (see Resources section, page 321), split fava beans or even split green peas. The peas are cooked separately then added to the veg near the end, so you could prepare them in advance and re-heat them whilst sautéing the veg for a super-quick but tasty mid-week dinner. Serve with the amaranth and millet pancake (page 220) or plain steamed wholegrain or red rice.

Ingredients
250 g yellow spilt peas
2 onions
3 cloves garlic
2-cm knob fresh ginger
100 g spinach or seasonal greens
1 tsp ground turmeric
1-2 tsp berbere spice mix
salt and black pepper
lemon or lime wedges to serve

Method
1. Rinse the yellow split peas in a sieve under running water. Pour 750 ml water into a pan and bring to the boil. Add the peas, reduce the heat and leave to simmer for 30-45 minutes until they're soft and most of the water has been absorbed. Drain using a sieve. Soaking the peas for a few hours beforehand will reduce the cooking time.
2. Once you are ready to make the stew, finely chop the onion, peel and grate the garlic and ginger, wash and shred the spinach or greens.
3. Heat 2-3 tbsp water in the base of a medium-sized pan and add the onion with a pinch of salt. Sauté for 10 minutes until it is soft, adding more water as needed.
4. Add the grated garlic and ginger to the pan and sauté for another few minutes – make sure they don't burn by adding a little more water as necessary.
5. Turn off the heat and stir in the ground turmeric and berbere spice mix before adding the cooked yellow peas to the pan. Stir well to combine.
6. Turn the heat back on and carefully bring the stew to just bubbling. Add the chopped spinach or greens to the pan and simmer for another 5 minutes until they are fully wilted.
7. Season with salt and black pepper. Serve in bowls with flatbread and a wedge of lemon or lime on the side.

Quick Jambalaya
Serves 2

Finding the energy to prepare and cook delicious, nutritious meals can be hard. This tasty recipe uses ingredients where the hard work has been done for you; all you need is a few minutes to bring it all together.

Frozen vegetables retain a good proportion of their healthful nutrients, often more than their 'fresh' counterparts. They're cost-effective and great for portion control, which helps reduce food waste too. I've used mixed peppers in this recipe, but choose an alternative veg if you avoid them and adjust the spice level to suit your taste-buds.

Ingredients
2 tbsp frozen chopped onions
100 g frozen sliced mixed peppers
150 g frozen diced sweet potato
2 tomatoes, diced (omit if not tolerated)
200 g frozen peas
½ tsp garlic powder
1 tbsp Cajun spice mix or fajita mix
1 x 250-g sachet cooked whole-grain rice
1 x 400-g tin butterbeans or black beans
salt and pepper to taste
1 handful rocket or spinach to serve

Method
1. Heat 2 tbsp water in the base of a pan and add the onion and peppers. Sauté for 5 minutes.
2. Add the sweet potato and chopped tomato, if using, to the pan. Continue cooking for another 5 minutes with the lid on over a medium/low heat.
3. Pour hot water over the peas whilst the other veggies are cooking to defrost them.
4. Add the garlic powder, spice mix and rice to the pan with another 2-3 tbsp

water and stir well to combine. Simmer for 2 minutes.
5. Drain and rinse the tinned beans. Drain the defrosted peas. Add both to the pan and stir well.
6. Simmer for another few minutes until everything is piping hot. Season with salt and pepper as needed.
7. Serve in bowls with the green leaves scattered on top.

Baked mini Romanesco cauliflower
Serves 2

I'm fascinated by romanesco. Somewhere between a cauliflower and broccoli, this quirky member of the cruciferous family looks like a group of pale green tiny Christmas trees. Packed full of healthful nutrients, they also taste delicious when roasted. Being small, they can be kept whole and served with a sauce – I've given you two options here to try, smoky tomato or cashew 'cheese', both delicious. If you can't find romanesco, use small cauliflowers or heads of broccoli instead.

Ingredients
2 mini romanescos or cauliflowers

For the smoky tomato sauce:
200 g chopped tomatoes
1 tsp smoked paprika
½ tsp garlic powder
½ lemon, juice and rind
1 tbsp tamari or coconut amines
1 tsp balsamic vinegar (optional)
1 tsp dried thyme

For the cashew cheese sauce:
70 g cashews
3-4 tbsp nutritional yeast
1 tsp Dijon mustard (optional)

½ tsp garlic powder
salt and pepper to taste

To serve:
1 tbsp toasted pumpkin or sesame seeds
1 tbsp chopped parsley

Method
1. Pre-heat the oven to 180°C. Wash and trim the romanesco, cutting a cross into the solid core underneath. Rub a little extra-virgin olive oil over each one and pop them in a baking tray and into the oven to roast for 20-25 minutes until they are easily pierced with a knife. Keep an eye on them and cover with foil to prevent them burning.
2. In the meantime, make your sauce of choice.
3. *For the smoky tomato sauce,* pour the chopped tomatoes into a small pan and add the other ingredients. Gently heat and simmer for 5-10 minutes to allow the flavours to develop.
4. *For the cashew cheese sauce,* pour boiling water over the cashews and leave to soak for 10 minutes. Drain then pop the cashews into a high-speed blender jug and just cover with fresh water. Blend to smooth then add the remaining ingredients and blend again. Check the flavour and add more seasoning if required.
5. Place the roasted romanesco in serving bowls and pour your sauce over the top. Serve with a mixed green salad and flatbread (page 311) or amaranth and millet pancake (page 220).

Stuffed sweet potatoes
Serves 2

I'm a big fan of baked potatoes, especially sweet potatoes. Their nutrient-rich flesh goes all soft and gooey in the oven and they match perfectly with so many different toppings. I'm particularly fond of this tasty black bean mix, which can also be served with rice or other whole grains if baked potatoes aren't your thing. Orange sweet potatoes are readily available in supermarkets; if you find purple ones, do try them. They're intense but somehow magical.

You can add an extra dimension by topping these stuffed potatoes with cashew cheese sauce (see above) or even a drizzle of tahini and lemon. Both are delicious additions. These stuffed sweet potatoes can be made in advance and re-heated as needed (without the sauce) or frozen so increase the amounts and make a batch to use on busy or low-energy days.

Ingredients
2 medium, sweet potatoes
1 small onion
½ red pepper
1 small courgette
1 clove garlic
200 g chopped tomatoes or passata
1 tsp smoked paprika
1 tsp ground cumin
240 g cooked black beans

Optional:
1 portion cashew cheese sauce (see recipe on page 235) or
1 tbsp tahini mixed with lemon juice, salt and pepper

Method
1. Wash and trim the sweet potatoes. Prick them a few times with a sharp knife and place them on a baking tray in the oven at 180°C.
2. Whilst the potatoes are baking, finely chop the onion, pepper and courgette. Grate the garlic.
3. Heat 2-3 tbsp water in the base of a small pan. Add the onion, pepper and courgette and sauté on a medium heat for 7 minutes. Add the garlic and continue cooking for another 2-3 minutes.
4. Pour in the tomato, spices and beans and simmer for 5 more minutes, then turn off the heat.
5. Once the sweet potatoes are baked, take the tray out of the oven and leave them to cool for a few minutes. Once you can handle them, cut in half and carefully scoop out the flesh, leaving a thin layer next to the skin so it doesn't

break. Leave the skins on the baking tray.
6. Add the sweet potato insides to the beans and stir well to combine. Spoon the mix back into the sweet potato skins – they will be bulging with filling! If you are topping with cashew cheese sauce, pour 2-3 spoonsful over each potato and return them to the oven.
7. Bake for 5-10 minutes until everything is piping hot and the sauce lightly browned (if using).
8. Remove from the oven and serve immediately with wilted greens on the side. Add the tahini sauce at this point if that's your sauce of choice.

Green kitcheri
Serves 4

Kitcheri is a traditional Indian dish valued for its high nutrition and easy digestibility, often used in Ayurvedic practice and a renowned comfort food dish. Usually made with mung beans, rice and spices, I've added in some leafy greens for extra goodness and the option of lentils in case mung beans are hard to find. If, however, you have a packet in the cupboard, try sprouting them for a few days then use them to make this dish. Sprouting releases even more nutrients and gives a lovely crunchy texture.

Ingredients
1 onion
2-cm piece fresh ginger
2 cloves garlic
1 tsp cumin seeds
1 tsp black mustard seeds
160 g mung beans or green lentils
270 g wholegrain basmati rice
1 tsp ground coriander
¼ tsp turmeric
1 pinch salt and black pepper
1 litre water

100 g leafy greens of choice
1 lemon, juice only
2 handfuls fresh coriander

Method
1. Peel and finely chop the onion and garlic. Peel and grate the ginger.
2. Add the cumin and black mustard seeds to a large pan over a medium heat. Lightly toast until they start to pop and release their aromas.
3. Carefully add 2-3 tbsp water to the pan (it will spit so stand back) along with the onion and ginger. Sauté for 5 minutes, adding more water to prevent sticking.
4. Place the lentils or mung beans and rice in a sieve and rinse well under a running tap.
5. Add the garlic to the pan and cook for another 2-3 minutes.
6. Tip the lentils or beans and rice into the pan with the spices and a pinch of salt. Mix well and cook for 1 minute before adding the water.
7. Bring to the boil then reduce the heat and simmer with the lid on for 30 minutes or so until the water has been absorbed.
8. Wash and shred the greens then add them to the pan. Stir well and leave them to wilt into the kitchiri for a few minutes.
9. Turn off the heat, season with salt, pepper and lemon juice. Scatter the fresh coriander on the top.
10. Serve with a simple cucumber salad if desired and dairy-free yoghurt.

Asparagus and broccoli pasta with white bean sauce
Serves 2

I love asparagus and broccoli and add them into dishes wherever I can. You can, however, use the veggies you enjoy or are in season. Gluten-free pasta is widely available now with more options than the standard, rather boring corn option. I love brown rice or red lentil pasta as they provide more nutrients and fibre than corn. I also eat less of it as they are both super-filling.

The white bean sauce is super-simple to make, which means this is a quick evening meal to enjoy when time is short.

Ingredients
100-120 g dried pasta (depending on appetite size)
6-8 spears asparagus
½ head broccoli or 6-8 spears long-stem broccoli
1 handful fresh herbs like oregano, chives or parsley
1 portion white bean sauce (see sauce section, page 295)
Drizzle of cold-pressed flaxseed oil to garnish (optional)

Method
1. Bring a large pan of water to the boil and cook the pasta according to packet instructions.
2. Wash and trim the asparagus, then chop into pieces. Wash and trim the broccoli and cut into small pieces. Wash and finely chop the herbs.
3. Make the white bean sauce as per recipe.
4. Heat 2-3 tbsp water in the base of a small frying pan and sauté the asparagus stems for 2-3 minutes. Add the tips and cook for another minute or so then turn off the heat.
5. Just before the pasta is cooked, add the broccoli to the pan and simmer for a few minutes until *al dente*. Drain the pasta and broccoli and return to the pan.
6. Add the just-cooked asparagus and white bean sauce to the pasta and broccoli. Stir well to combine and warm through on a very low heat for 2-3 minutes.
7. Serve with a drizzle of flaxseed oil and a sprinkle of fresh herbs on top.

Quick broccoli and smoked tofu rice
Serves 2-3

One pot meals are the best when it comes to time, energy – and space. I first made this tasty rice dish when we were travelling in our campervan, and I only had a tiny space to cook in and 1½ rings to cook on. There were a few tantrums, but it taught me to appreciate the joys of simple, space-efficient cooking.

Packs of pre-cooked rice are readily available in the shops and can come in handy when time and energy are low. You can also cook rice specifically for this dish or use any left over from a previous meal – just make sure it's properly re-heated. I've used an array of rainbow veg, but feel free to use what you have to hand – the freezer can come in handy here again. Smoked tofu provides a good amount of plant protein and matches with lovely smoked paprika.

Ingredients
½ red onion
½ head broccoli
½ red pepper
½ large courgette
2 medium tomatoes (optional)
1 large clove garlic
1 tsp smoked paprika
1 pinch chilli flakes (optional)
200 g smoked tofu
1 pack cooked whole-grain rice or mixed whole-grain and wild rice or
    250 g cooked rice
salt and pepper
1 tbsp fresh parsley (optional)
2 tbsp dairy-free yoghurt (optional)

Method
1. Peel and finely chop the onion. Separate the broccoli florets from the stem – trim woody bits off the stem but keep the inner bits and finely chop. Chop the florets but keep them separate. Finely chop the red pepper and courgette. Chop the tomatoes and grate the garlic.
2. Place 2 tbsp of water in the base of a pan and add the onion and broccoli stem. Sauté for 5 minutes then add the pepper and courgette. Continue to cook for another 5 minutes, adding more water if needed.

3. Add the broccoli florets, chopped tomatoes and garlic and cook for another 3 minutes.
4. Crumble the smoked tofu and add it to the pan with the cooked rice, smoked paprika, salt and pepper. Add a little water if the mix is too dry. Cover and simmer on a low heat for 3-4 minutes or until the rice is piping hot.
5. Serve in bowls with chopped parsley and dairy-free yoghurt if using.

Mushroom, squash and kale root vegetable pie
Serves 2

Autumn brings a wonderful collection of wild mushrooms and squashes packed full of beta-carotene and polyphenols, preparing us for the colder weather and comfort food of winter. This tasty pie might look out-of-place in the 'easy' section, but it doesn't take too long to prepare and cook. If you can't be doing with the faff of peeling and chopping squash, grab a bag of ready-prepared frozen squash from the supermarket instead.

You can use good old white potatoes for the mash, but I've gone for a mix of celeriac and carrot. Any root vegetable works though, so feel free to mix it up and find a combo you love. The same goes for the mushrooms. Woodland mixes provide a lovely variety of flavours and textures, but white or chestnut mushrooms will work just as well. Double the ingredients to serve 4 and make one large pie, or freeze the extra for another day.

Ingredients
½ medium celeriac
2 carrots
1 small leek
100 g squash
1 clove garlic
200 g woodland mushrooms
100 g kale or cavolo nero
200 ml dairy-free cream

2 tbsp fresh tarragon or 1 tbsp dried
salt and pepper to taste

Method
1. Peel the celeriac and carrots and dice small. Pop into a pan of boiling water and cook until soft and mashable.
2. Wash and trim the leek before shredding. Peel the squash and chop into bite-sized pieces. Grate the garlic. Wipe the mushrooms clean and roughly chop. Wash the kale and shred.
3. Heat 2-3 tbsp water in a medium-sized pan and add the leek and squash. Simmer for 10 minutes until the squash starts to soften, adding more water as needed to prevent it sticking to the pan.
4. Add the garlic and cook for 2-3 minutes before adding the mushrooms and chopped kale. Pop on the lid and simmer on a low heat for 5 minutes.
5. Pour in the dairy-free cream. Add the tarragon and salt and pepper. Stir well to combine and leave to gently bubble on a low heat whilst you sort out the mash.
6. Once the carrot and celeriac are soft, drain and shake out as much water as you can. Return the veg to the pan and mash, adding a little dairy-free milk if necessary, along with salt and pepper.
7. Turn the grill on high to heat up. Grab two individual dishes and spoon the creamy mushroom mix into the base of each. Top with the mash then pop under the grill for a couple of minutes to lightly brown.
8. Serve in the bowls with extra greens or broccoli on the side.

Magnificent mains

The recipes in this section take a little longer than those in the previous section, but none should take over an hour so they're not *that* complicated. I've included a few options for Sunday lunch or entertaining; socialising is still important, even when you're eating for health.

Leftovers are super-useful, creating a meal for a busy weekday night, so increase the ingredient amounts if you want to take advantage of this, especially if you are feeding hungry tummies. When my kids were at home, we never seemed to have leftovers, no matter how big the original dish was.

Vegetable curry with chickpea dumplings
Serves 4

These dumplings are divine! Inspired by a delicious recipe from Vegan Richa (www.veganricha.com), I've adapted them slightly to avoid the use of saturated fat, and they work like a treat every time. Light and fluffy, the flavour complements the spicy veggies underneath and avoids the need to cook extra rice, unless you're hungry of course, then feel free to serve with wholegrain basmati on the side.

I've not been prescriptive with the vegetables here so use whatever you like, enjoy or have in the fridge. Make sure it's a mix though to ensure you have a rainbow on your plate. If you must avoid tomatoes, omit them and replace with water. It won't be quite as rich but if it means you can still enjoy this delicious recipe then it's worth it.

Ingredients
For the curry:
1 onion
1 fat clove garlic
2-cm piece fresh ginger
750 g mixed vegetables

1 x 400-g tin tomatoes plus ½ can of water
   or 400 ml water (with extra if needed)
1 tsp ground cumin
¼ tsp turmeric powder
1 tsp garum masala
1 tbsp dried fenugreek leaves (optional but good)
1 good pinch chilli flakes
black pepper

For the dumplings:
100 g gram (chickpea) flour
1 tsp baking powder
¼ tsp turmeric powder
1 tsp garum masala
salt and pepper
10 g chopped fresh coriander
30 g red onion (optional but good)
180 g dairy-free yoghurt

Method
1. Start with the veggie curry. Peel the onion, garlic and ginger. Roughly chop then pop into a small blender pot with a little water. Blend to form a rough paste.
2. Prepare the veg you are using, dicing small. Put the veg that are quickest to cook in a separate pile.
3. Using a pan that can go into the oven, spoon in the paste and sauté over a medium heat for 5 minutes – add more water if necessary to prevent it burning and sticking.
4. Add the veggies that take longest to cook and stir into the onion mix.
5. Pour the tinned tomatoes and water, or just water, into the pan. Add the spices and stir well to combine.
6. Bring to the boil, then reduce the heat and simmer with the lid on until the veg start to soften. Add the remaining veggies to the pan and continue to simmer with the lid off until everything is cooked through and the fluid has evaporated a little. Turn off the heat.

7. Whilst the curry is simmering, make the dumpling mix. Place the gram flour, baking powder, spices, salt and pepper into a small bowl and add the dairy-free yoghurt. Stir well to combine, then mix in the fresh coriander and onion (if using). Stir again. The mix should be thick but easily droppable off the spoon. If it's too thick, add a little dairy-free milk. If it's too runny, add more gram flour.
8. Pre-heat the oven to 180°C. Add dollops of chickpea dumpling mix to the top of the veggie curry until it's used up. Place in the oven and bake for 15 minutes until the top is lightly browned.
9. Serve piping hot.

Walnut and white bean bake
Serves 4-6

I'm always creating different types of bakes to serve on a Sunday. There are so many combinations to choose from there's no need to be bored. This bake is a tasty combination of nuts and beans, with a few mushrooms added in for extra flavour and goodness. I love walnuts but you can use any nut you enjoy or have in the cupboard – hazelnuts are also an excellent choice.

If you are only cooking for two people, leftovers can be frozen or re-heated later in the week for a quick evening meal. If you must avoid even gluten-free oats, replace with some well-cooked rice.

Ingredients
1 medium onion
2 sticks celery
1 medium carrot
1 bay leaf
100 g mushrooms of choice
1 fat clove garlic
100 g walnuts
1 x 400-g tin white beans, drained and rinsed
1 heaped tbsp dried mixed or Italian herbs

50 g oats

salt and pepper

Method

1. Peel and roughly chop the onion or wash, trim and shred the leek. Wash, trim and finely dice the celery and carrot.
2. Heat 2 tbsp water in the base of a medium-sized pan. Add the onion or leek, celery, carrot and bay leaf. Sauté over a medium heat for 10 minutes until the veggies are soft, stirring from time to time. Add a little more water if the mix starts sticking to the pan.
3. Wipe the mushrooms clean and finely chop. Peel and grate the garlic. Add them to the pan and sauté for another 3 minutes or until the mushrooms start to soften.
4. In the meantime, pre-heat the oven to 180ºC. Line a 2-lb loaf tin with non-stick baking paper.
5. Place the walnuts in a food processor or small blender pot and pulse a few times – keep some texture. Roughly chop the white beans.
6. Once the veggies are soft, turn off the heat and remove the bay leaf. Add the dried herbs, walnuts, beans and oats to the pan. Season with salt and pepper and stir to combine, forming a stiff mixture. Taste and add more seasoning or herbs as needed.
7. Press the mix into the prepared loaf tin. Bake in the oven for 45 minutes, checking after 35 to make sure the top doesn't over cook – cover with tin foil or a baking tray if needed for the last 10 minutes.
8. Remove from the oven and leave to cool for 5 minutes. Remove from the tin by lifting it out with the baking paper.
9. Serve hot or leave to cool and store in the fridge in an air-tight container for up to 4 days. Can be served hot or cold.

Tempeh, hazelnut and apricot bake
Serves 4

Here's another bake suitable for Sunday lunch or seasonal celebrations. This combination of flavours popped into my head one day and I just had to try it, even though I thought it might be too random. Turned out the opposite was true – it's delicious! Every time I make this bake the feedback is 'ooooh, that's lovely'. I take that as a recommendation.

This has an autumnal feel to it, but the ingredients are available all year round. Whilst it partners perfectly with roast potatoes and accompanying veg, it's just as tasty cold with a salad on the side. Flexible, nutritious and tasty – what more could you want?

Ingredients
70 g dried apricots
2 tbsp ground flaxseed
4 tbsp water
1 small red onion
1 stick celery
1 medium leek
1 bay leaf
1 fat clove garlic
150 g hazelnuts
100 g tempeh
1 tbsp dried thyme
1 tbsp tamari or coconut amines
black pepper

Method
1. Pop the dried apricots in a small bowl and cover with hot water. Leave to soak whilst you prepare everything else.
2. Spoon the ground flaxseed into a bowl and add the water. Stir well and leave it to thicken.
3. Peel and finely chop the red onion. Wash, trim and shred the leek. Wash the

celery and finely chop. Peel and grate the garlic.
4. Heat 2-3 tbsp water in the base of a frying pan. Add the red onion, celery, leek and bay leaf. Sauté for 10 minutes until they're soft then turn off the heat.
5. Whilst the veggies are cooking, grate the tempeh and blitz the hazelnuts in a small blender pot so they're finely chopped (try not to turn them into a powder).
6. Line a 2-lb loaf tin with non-stick baking paper and pre-heat the oven to 180°C.
7. Drain the apricots and chop into small pieces.
8. Add the apricots, cooked veggies, tempeh, hazelnuts, thyme, tamari and black pepper to the gloopy flaxseed and stir well to combine. It should be a solid mix that sticks together when a little is pressed between your fingers.
9. Spoon the mix into the prepared loaf tin, pressing into the corners and flattening the top. Bake in the oven for 35-40 minutes until the top is lightly browned.
10. Remove from the oven and leave to set in the tin for 5 minutes or so.
11. Carefully remove from the tin using the baking paper and cut into slices.

Moussaka

Serves 4

If you avoid aubergine (eggplant), then this recipe is not for you as it is a key ingredient. The white potato can be subbed with sweet potato though, so do give this a try if that works for you.

I love moussaka but thought it was something I'd never eat again once I went plant-based. Fortunately, my lovely friend Mandy made it for me one day and opened my eyes to new possibilities. Never say never – it seems there's always a way to create an alternative.

There is a lot going on in this recipe. Each element can cook concurrently. Alternatively, make the lentil mix or cook the potato and aubergine earlier so you don't have to do too much at once. If you are entertaining, make this ahead and re-heat when you're ready to reduce the workload. It will taste even better too as the flavour develops over time.

Ingredients

2 large or 4 medium potatoes OR sweet potatoes
2 large aubergines

For the lentil sauce:
1 red onion
1 medium carrot
1 bay leaf
50 g mushrooms
1 clove garlic
1 tsp paprika
1 tsp dried oregano
1 pinch cloves
1 tbsp tomato purée
1 tbsp tamari or coconut amines
250 g cooked puy lentils
1 x 400-g tin tomatoes
100 ml veg stock or red wine
black pepper

For the bechamel sauce:
1 portion cashew cream (see page 301)
½ tsp garlic powder
4 tbsp nutritional yeast
1 pinch nutmeg
1 tbsp cornflour or tapioca flour

Method

1. Peel the potato and cut into slices. Pop into a pan of boiling water and cook until just soft – don't let them fall apart and go mushy. Drain and put to one side.
2. Wash the aubergine and cut into slices. Place on a baking sheet covered in non-stick baking paper. Pre-heat the oven to 180°C. Pop the tray in the oven and bake for 20 minutes or so until the aubergine has started to soften. Again, don't let it over-cook or it will collapse, and you won't be able to layer it. Remove the tray from the oven but leave the oven on, lowering the setting to 170°C.

3. *Make the lentil sauce.* Finely chop the onion, carrot and mushrooms. Grate the garlic. Heat 2 tbsp water in the base of a medium-sized pan and add the onion, carrot and bay leaf. Sauté for 5 minutes then add the mushrooms and garlic. Cook for another 2 minutes. Pour in the tinned tomatoes, tomato purée, herbs, stock or wine and tamari. Bring to a gentle boil then reduce the heat and simmer for 15 minutes. Add the cooked puy lentils and simmer for another 5 minutes. Turn off the heat and season.
4. *Make the bechamel sauce* by making the cashew cream and adding the other ingredients. Mix well to combine.
5. Once all the elements are ready, grab an oven-proof dish and spread a little olive oil over the bottom and sides. Start with a layer of potato followed by a layer of aubergine. Season and add a little extra dried oregano. Cover with the lentil mix then add a final layer of potato followed by aubergine. Pour the bechamel sauce over the top.
6. Pop the dish onto a baking tray and return it to the oven. Bake for 30 minutes then check to make sure the top isn't too brown. If it is, cover with foil once it's set and bake for another 10 minutes.
7. Leave to cool for 15 minutes or so before serving.

Comforting root vegetable stew and herby dumplings
Serves 3-4

Stew with dumplings is one of my favourite winter warmers. As a child, the stew would have been meat-based, but I explored (and stuck with) veg-based options during my earliest forays into vegetarianism in my early 20s.

This recipe uses a range of root vegetables readily available during the winter months. For texture, keep the mini onions whole and choose small Brussels sprouts wherever possible to again keep whole. Thyme, sage and rosemary complement the stew beautifully, best used in the dumplings though. Stick to dried mixed herbs in the body of the stew. To boost the protein profile, add kidney or borlotti beans before you add the dumplings if you so wish.

Ingredients
For the stew:
1 large leek
8 mini onions or shallots
1 large parsnip
2 medium carrots
½ medium celeriac
2 cloves garlic
300 ml vegetable stock
1 tbsp dried mixed herbs
black pepper
1 tbsp nutritional yeast (optional)
200 g Brussels sprouts
1 x 400-g tin kidney or borlotti beans, rinsed and drained
1 tsp cornflour

For the herby dumplings:
70 ml dairy-free milk (ideally soya)
1 tsp lemon juice
100 g gluten-free flour mix (ideally self-raising)
50 g gram or green pea flour
1 tsp baking powder
1 pinch salt and black pepper
2 tbsp chopped fresh herbs of choice or 1 tbsp dried herbs

Method
1. Trim, wash and shred the leek. Remove the outer onion leaves but leave whole. Peel and dice the parsnip, carrot and celeriac. Remove outer leaves on the Brussels sprouts and wash well. Peel and grate the garlic.
2. Use a medium-large shallowish pan with a tight lid. Heat 2-3 tbsp water in the bottom and add the leek, mini onions, parsnip, carrot and celeriac. Pop on the

lid and sweat over a medium-low heat for 5 minutes. Add the garlic and sweat for another 2-3 minutes.
3. Pour 250 ml veg stock into the pan. Add the dried herbs, black pepper and nutritional yeast (if using). Bring to the boil then reduce the heat and leave to simmer with the lid on for 20 minutes.
4. Whilst the veggies are cooking, make the dumplings. Pour the soya milk into a small bowl and add the lemon juice. Leave to curdle for 2-3 minutes. In a separate bowl, combine the flours, baking powder, seasoning and herbs. Pour in the curdled milk and stir to form a soft dough. Gently roll into 8 small balls.
5. Add the Brussels sprouts and drained tinned beans (if using) to the stew. Mix the final 50 ml veg stock and cornflour together in a small bowl and pour into the stew. Stir well – this will help it thicken slightly.
6. Carefully drop the dumplings onto the surface of the stew, pop the lid back on and let them steam for 15-20 minutes.
7. Once the dumplings are firm, remove the pan from the heat and serve.

Shiitake mushrooms and smoked tofu noodle bowl
Serves 2

This delightful noodle bowl has a lot of ingredients; when they come together the flavour is immense. Preparation takes more time than cooking but once you have everything chopped and grated, it's ready in under 20 minutes. Just make sure you're the one who doesn't have to clear up afterwards.

Ingredients
2 shallots or ½ onion
5 spring onions
1 red chilli (optional)
2 cloves garlic
2-cm piece fresh ginger
80 g seasonal greens
½ head broccoli
150 g shiitake mushrooms

600 ml vegetable stock
2 tbsp tamari or coconut amines
2 star anise
1 tsp fennel seeds
1 small square nori
2 small nests brown rice noodles
150 g smoked tofu

To garnish:
2 tsp sesame seeds
2 tsp sesame seed oil (optional)
lime wedges
black pepper
fresh coriander leaves

Method
1. Peel the shallots or onion and slice. Wash the spring onions, trim the ends and slice at an angle. Slice the chilli into rings, removing the seeds if you don't like it hot. Peel and grate the garlic and ginger. Wash the seasonal greens, remove any hard stems and finely shred the leaves. Separate the broccoli flowers from the stem. Chop both into small pieces. Wipe the mushrooms clean with some kitchen roll and roughly chop. Drain and cube the smoked tofu.
2. Add 2 tbsp water to the base of a large pan. Tip in the shallots/onion, spring onions and the chopped broccoli stems. Stir fry for 4-5 minutes until they start to soften. Add the garlic and ginger and cook for another 2-3 minutes.
3. Pour in the stock and add the fennel seeds, star anise, chilli and tamari. Crumble the nori and add it to the pan. Bring to a gentle bowl then reduce the heat and simmer for 10 minutes.
4. Add the broccoli flowers, sliced greens, mushrooms and noodles to the pan. Simmer for 5 minutes and then add the cubed tofu. Simmer for another 2 minutes.
5. Turn off the heat and serve in 2 deep bowls, making sure you use up all the broth. Garnish with sesame seeds, sesame oil, black pepper and fresh coriander and serve with lime wedges on the side.

Broccoli and kale tart
Serves 4

Gluten-free pastry can be a bit of a disappointment, so this tart does away with it completely by using soft, cooked quinoa to form the crust. It sounds a bit mad, but it works really well. Adding more water than normal to dried quinoa makes it super-sticky, exactly what we want for a simple pastry. Make sure you use a loose-bottomed non-stick tart tin though, ideally with smooth sides rather than fluted, otherwise the quinoa will get stuck where you don't want it to.

I love this combo of broccoli and kale, especially when magnificent purple sprouting is in season. Feel free to swap for whatever you like or have – I can highly recommend asparagus in this mix. It tastes fab hot or cold, especially the day after making once the flavours have had time to develop.

Ingredients

For the quinoa crust:
150 g quinoa, colour of choice
400 ml vegetable stock
3 tbsp ground flaxseed
black pepper
extra water as needed

For the filling:
1 medium red onion
1 medium head broccoli or bunch purple sprouting broccoli
2-3 handfuls kale or cavolo nero
300 g silken tofu
2 tbsp nutritional yeast
¼ tsp garlic powder
1 pinch ground turmeric
1 pinch salt and black pepper

Method

Make the quinoa crust:
1. Pour the quinoa into a sieve and rinse under a running tap. Pour the veg stock into a small saucepan with a lid and bring to the boil.
2. Add the quinoa to the boiling stock, pop on the lid and reduce the heat. Allow to simmer for 10-15 minutes until all the stock is absorbed and the quinoa is soft. Turn off the heat and leave to cool for a while.
3. Once the quinoa is cool enough to handle and is slightly sticky, add the ground flaxseed and stir well to combine. The mix should start sticking together when you press it between your fingers. Add 2-3 extra tbsp water if you need, to make this happen. Season with black pepper.
4. Pre-heat the oven to 200°C.
5. Tip the quinoa mix into a 20-cm loose-bottomed tart tin. Spread out and press it into the base and the edges with your hands. This may take a few minutes to get it spread out equally and pressed into the corners.
6. Place in the oven and bake for 20-25 minutes until the sides start to brown and the base feels firm to the touch.

Make the filling:
1. Whilst the pastry is baking, slice the onion and wash and chop the broccoli and kale into bite-sized chunks.
2. Heat 2-3 tbsp water in a large frying pan and sauté the onions with a pinch of salt. Once they start to soften, add the broccoli and chopped kale. Pop a lid over the top and steam cook for 3-4 minutes. Turn off the heat and remove the lid so they don't over-cook and lose their vibrant colour.
3. Pop the silken tofu, nutritional yeast, garlic powder, turmeric, salt and pepper into a small high-speed blender jug and blend for a few seconds to make a thick, creamy sauce.

Make the tart:
1. Pour the tofu mix into the pan of cooked vegetables and stir well to combine.
2. Spoon the mix into the quinoa base and flatten the top.
3. Pop back into the oven for another 15 minutes or so until the filling is set and the top starts to brown.

4. Remove from the oven and eat hot or leave to cool and store in the fridge for up to 3 days.

Cumin and turmeric traybake
Serves 2

I love a traybake and make one nearly every week. It's a super-easy way to create a tasty, colourful meal that doesn't need much attention. It's also a great way to use up left-over veg you're not sure what to do with. Alternatively, use a mix of frozen veg – great for portion control and time saving as someone has prepared it all for you.

This traybake features vibrant yellow turmeric and flavoursome cumin seeds topped with a tongue-tingling tamarind sauce. Feel free to use whatever vegetables you have or enjoy, I just like the combination below. If you need to avoid tofu, then add some cooked beans, peas or lentils near the end or scatter sprouted beans or lentils on the top before serving. The tamarind sauce can be made earlier – it stores in the fridge for up to 5 days and is very moreish, so you'll find lots of ways to use it.

Ingredients
½ red onion
½ medium cauliflower
½ head broccoli
1 medium red pepper
1 medium sweet potato
2 tsp cumin seeds
1 tsp ground turmeric
1 tbsp extra-virgin olive oil
200 g smoked tofu

For the tamarind sauce:
125 ml water
75 g pitted dates

1 tbsp tamarind paste
¼ tsp chilli powder
¼ tsp ground cumin
1 pinch asafoetida (optional)
salt to taste

Method
1. Pre-heat the oven to 180°C.
2. Slice the onion. Chop the cauliflower and broccoli into small pieces and wash under a running tap. Wash and chop the pepper into bite-sized pieces. Peel and chop the sweet potato into bite-sized pieces.
3. Scatter the cumin seeds over the base of a large oven-proof dish. Pop the prepared veggies into a large bowl and sprinkle the turmeric over the top along with a glug of extra-virgin olive oil. Stir well to coat then tip into the baking dish.
4. Place the dish in the oven and roast for 15 minutes. Dice the smoked tofu small. Turn the veg with a large spoon and cook for another 10 minutes before adding the tofu. Return to the oven for another 5 minutes.
5. Whilst the veggies are cooking, make the tamarind sauce. Pour the water into a small pan and add the dates. Pop on the lid and bring to the boil. Reduce the heat and simmer for 10 minutes until the dates are super-soft and hydrated. Turn off the heat and leave to cool.
6. Pop the dates into the small bowl of a food processor or hand blender. Blend to a paste, adding more water if it's too thick. Add the remaining ingredients and blend again to combine. Check the flavour and add more spices or salt as needed.
7. Once the traybake is golden brown, remove from the oven. Serve over a bed of wholegrain rice or quinoa, or on its own, with the sauce drizzled over the top.

Sesame-baked butternut squash rings with smoky chickpeas
Serves 4

Sometimes, it's worth going to that bit extra effort to create dishes that both look and taste amazing. These sesame-crusted squash rings look impressive and, when paired with deliciously smoky chickpea stew, make a wonderful celebration meal, or something special for the weekend.

You only need the 'bulb' end of the butternut squash for this recipe; you can use the leftovers in soup or curry another day. You need two squash to feed four so make sure you get a good-sized ring. Feel free to use alternative beans; black beans or rarer pink flamingo peas make great options. You can make the filling mix the day before if you wish to re-heat before serving, saving you time on the day and allowing the flavours to develop. Serve these with seasonal veg or a couple of seasonal salads from the section above; the beetroot and watercress (page 212) is a great one to match, or balance some lightly steamed tender-stem broccoli on top.

Ingredients
For the squash rings:
2 butternut squash
2 tbsp gram (chickpea) flour
4 tbsp water
4-6 tbsp sesame seeds

For the chickpea filling:
1 small onion
½ red bell pepper (optional)
4 medium mushrooms
1 clove garlic
150 ml passata
240 g cooked chickpeas or pink flamingo peas
1 tsp ground cumin
1 tsp smoked paprika

1 tsp dried thyme
2 big handfuls spinach or seasonal greens
salt and pepper to taste
fresh coriander leaves or parsley to garnish

Method
1. Pre-heat the oven to 180°C and line a large baking sheet with non-stick baking paper.
2. Remove the neck and bottom of the squashes and cut four 2.5- to 3-cm wide rings from each one (so you have 8 in total). Peel off the skin and remove the seeds and slimy bits on the inside.
3. Whisk the gram flour and water together in a bowl wide enough to dip the squash in and scatter the sesame seeds onto a plate.
4. Dip a squash ring into the flour mix then press it into the sesame seeds so they stick. Make sure the ring is coated then place on the baking tray. Repeat another 7 times then place the tray in the oven and bake for 45-50 minutes until the squash is soft but firm and the seeds lightly browned.
5. Now prepare the chickpea filling. Peel and finely slice the onion. Wash and finely chop the red pepper if using. Wipe the mushrooms clean and finely chop. Peel and grate the garlic.
6. Heat 2-3 tbsp water in the base of a pan and add the onion and red pepper. Sauté for 5 minutes until they start to soften. Add the mushrooms and garlic and cook for another 4 minutes.
7. Pour in the passata followed by the chickpeas and spices. Add a little water if the mix is a bit thick, but not too much as you don't want too much fluid. Bring to the boil then reduce the heat and simmer for 10 minutes.
8. Wash and shred the spinach then add to the pan. Simmer for 1 minute then turn off the heat. Season with salt and pepper as needed.
9. The sesame squash rings are ready when easily pierced with a knife and the seeds golden brown. Remove from the oven.
10. To serve, place two rings in the middle of a plate and fill with the chickpea mix. Garnish with coriander or parsley and serve immediately.

Roasted cabbage slices, aromatic millet and tahini dressing
Serves 2

I always get funny looks if I start praising the amazing flavour of roasted cabbage, but don't knock it until you've tried it. The natural sugars lightly caramelise in the heat, creating a deliciously savoury and satisfying flavour. The tasty tahini sauce complements it perfectly along with cooked millet embellished with fresh herbs and glistening drops of pomegranate seeds. Simple to make, but it creates quite the discussion over a special lunch or evening dinner party.

If you don't like or have millet, swap for quinoa, amaranth or my favourite, red rice. Amaranth takes longer to cook and can easily tip over into mushiness, so take great care if using it.

Ingredients
120 g millet
375 ml vegetable stock or water
1 bay leaf
½ medium savoy cabbage
1 tbsp extra-virgin olive oil
1 pinch salt and black pepper
2 tbsp mixed fresh herbs – coriander, parsley, chives etc
2 tbsp mixed seeds – pumpkin, sunflower, sesame
salt and pepper to taste
2 tbsp pomegranate seeds

For the tahini dressing:
3 tbsp tahini
60 ml water
2 tbsp lemon juice
½ tsp garlic powder
salt and pepper to taste
½ tsp cumin powder and 1 tbsp maple syrup (optional but good)

Method
1. Pour the vegetable stock into a pan and add the bay leaf. Bring the stock to the boil. At the same time, place the millet into a large frying pan and lightly toast over a medium heat for a few minutes until it starts releasing toasty aromas.
2. Carefully pour the toasted millet into the simmering stock – take care as it will bubble up. Reduce the heat, pop on the lid and leave to simmer for 15 minutes until all the stock has been absorbed.
3. Whilst the millet is cooking, pre-heat the oven to 180°C. Line a baking sheet with non-stick baking paper.
4. Cut the cabbage half into 4 equal slices. Remove any hard bits of the core but leave it intact as much as possible to prevent the slice collapsing. Rinse the slices under running water.
5. Brush the olive oil over each cabbage slice then place them on the baking tray and pop in the oven to roast for 20 minutes, turning halfway through.
6. Finely chop the herbs and put to one side.
7. Make the tahini sauce by putting all the ingredients into a small blender pot and blending until smooth. Check the flavour and add more seasoning, lemon or other flavourings as needed.
8. Once the millet is cooked, turn off the heat and transfer to a bowl so it doesn't over-cook. Remove the bay leaf and stir in the fresh herbs, keeping a few to garnish, and mixed seeds. Season with salt and pepper.
9. To serve, spoon the herby millet onto the middle of a plate or bowl. Sprinkle most of the pomegranate seeds on the millet then arrange cabbage slices on top. Drizzle tahini dressing over the cabbage and garnish with the remaining herbs and pomegranate seeds. Eat piping hot.

Baking

Cake has always been my favourite thing to eat. When I discovered an intolerance to dairy, my first question was 'how am I going to eat cake?' Fortunately, I soon discovered super-tasty, alternative ways to bake fully plant-based that worked every time. Plus, they're much less complicated than 'traditional' baking – a double win.

All the cakes and bakes in this section can be made with gluten-free flours, although feel free to use whole wheat or even barley flour if you can tolerate or prefer it. The recipes have a reduced sugar content too, with some completely avoiding added sugar. They're certainly not as sweet as many bakes, particularly shop-bought, but once your taste-buds have adjusted, you'll appreciate the flavour of the ingredients without the sickly sweetness.

Baking fully plant-based requires a slightly different methodology, so I have created my 'Sensitive Foodie Guide to Baking' easily accessible on my website https://thesensitivefoodiekitchen.com/the-sensitive-foodie-guide-to-baking/.

There's a mix of cakes, bakes and biscuits in the section, with plenty more options in my first book and on the website, in case you need more ideas and inspiration.

Apple, apricot and oat bars
Makes 8 large bars or 12 smaller ones

Apples, apricots and oats make the perfect combination and come together rather beautifully in these tasty bars. With a highly productive apple tree in my garden, I am always creating new recipes to use them up. I make huge saucepans of stewed apples, turning them into apple sauce that I freeze in small blocks. This means we can have gorgeous bars like these throughout the autumn and winter until the stash is used up.

Cinnamon contains antioxidant polyphenols alongside compounds that help move free sugars out of the bloodstream into cells, helping to support balanced blood sugar. It's also the perfect taste partner to apples.

Keep these bars in an air-tight container in a cool place or fridge for up to 4 days.

NB: the dates need a good soaking beforehand, so remember to do that earlier in the day.

Ingredients
120 g de-stoned dates (pre-soaked as below)
140 g soft dried apricots
300 g oats, split into a 200-g and a 100-g portion
1 tbsp cinnamon powder
1 pinch nutmeg
1 pinch salt
55 g flaked almonds split into a 40-g and a 15-g portion
300 g apple sauce
1 tsp vanilla essence

Method
1. Place the dates in a large bowl and cover with boiling water for at least 30 minutes, ideally 1-2 hours.
2. Chop the apricots into little pieces.
3. Pre-heat the oven to 180°C. Line a 20x20-square baking tin with non-stick baking paper.
4. Place the 200-g portion of oats, spices, salt, chopped apricots and the 40-g portion of flaked almonds into a large bowl.
5. Drain the soaking dates but retain the water. Pop the dates into a high-speed blender jug with 50 ml soaking water and blend for 30 seconds until they're partially broken down into a thick paste.
6. Add the 100-g portion of oats, apple sauce, vanilla essence and another 50 ml of the soaking water to the blender pot and blend to a smoothish paste.
7. Pour this thick paste into the dry ingredients and stir well to combine. The mix will be thick but shouldn't be dry. If it is, add a little more water.

8. Transfer the mix to the baking tin, spreading it out into the corners and flattening the top. Sprinkle the remaining 15-g portion of flaked almonds on the top and gently press them into the mix.
9. Bake in the middle of the oven for 20 minutes then turn the tin and bake for another 10 minutes until the mix is firm and lightly browned on top.
10. Remove from the oven and leave to rest in the tin for 5 minutes before lifting it out on the baking paper, carefully removing it and leaving it on a cooling rack. Once fully cool, cut into 8 or 12 slices.

Black bean chocolate brownies

Makes 9 squares or 12 smaller rectangles

The first time I heard black bean brownies mentioned, I was very sceptical. I couldn't get my head around what the texture would be like. As seeing is believing, I of course had to make them and was happily surprised by the flavour and super-gooey centre. This is now one of the recipes I teach to medical students and love to see their surprised faces when they taste them for the first time.

The key to getting the right gooeyness is baking time. Too long and the mixture dries out. Too short and it just oozes everywhere. The ideal time is when the top has set but there is still some give when you press it with your finger. It feels a little undercooked but carries on setting when you remove it from the oven. Be brave and you'll get it right!

I add chocolate chips when I'm making these for other people but leave them out when I'm going to indulge as chocolate contains high levels of saturated fat. Adding a few raisins or finely chopped walnuts adds extra texture or crunch.

Ingredients
1 x 400-g tin black beans
2 tbsp ground flaxseed
60 g nut butter of choice
2 tsp vanilla essence

The plant-based whole-food recipes

100 ml soya milk (or dairy-free milk of choice)
1 tbsp lemon juice
45 g self-raising gluten-free flour
60 g cocoa powder
1 tsp baking powder
100 g coconut sugar
90 g dairy-free chocolate chips (optional)
50 g chopped walnuts or raisins (optional)

Method

1. Pre-heat the oven to 180ºC. Line a 20x20 baking tin with non-stick baking paper. Drain and rinse the black beans.
2. Tip the ground flaxseed into a large bowl. Add 4 tbsp water, the nut butter, vanilla essence, 60 ml soya milk and 1 tbsp lemon juice. Mix well to combine.
3. Add the black beans to the mix. Grab a stick blender or potato masher and mash the beans into the mix (or use a food processor to make it easier). The mix can have a few lumps – no need to make it smooth. It will be thick and gloopy.
4. In a separate bowl mix the flour, cocoa powder, baking powder and sugar together.
5. Tip the flour mix into the mushy bean mix along with the chocolate chips (if using), raisins or walnuts and the remaining soya milk. Using a large spoon, stir everything together making sure you scoop up all the mix from the bottom of the bowl. If the mix is too dry, add a little more soya milk so it drops easily off the spoon.
6. Quickly spoon the mix into the prepared baking tin. Spread out to the corners and give it a good tap on the worktop. Place in the middle of the oven for 15 minutes.
7. Check the tin – if the top is still very bouncy and a skewer or knife comes out with lots of mix on it, pop it back in the oven for up to 5 more minutes. Don't over-bake or you won't get the soft, sticky centre.
8. Remove from the oven and leave the brownies to settle in the tin for 5 minutes before turning them out onto a cooling rack.
9. Cut into 9 or 12 pieces. Sieve extra cocoa powder over the top to decorate if you wish. Store in an airtight container for up to 4 days, or freeze.

Pear and ginger muffins
Makes 12

Pear and ginger are a delicious combination and really make these muffins sing. This recipe contains less sugar and fat than your average muffin. The lower fat levels do create a little problem – they can stick to the wrapper, but only for a few hours after baking. Once they've fully cooled down and rested, the paper peels off with no problem. An odd but solvable problem; you just need patience. If you're lacking in that, feel free to eat whilst they're still warm but be prepared to nibble the wrapper too.

These muffins keep in an air-tight container for 3 days and freeze well.

Ingredients
3 small ripe pears
285 g self-raising gluten-free flour
1 tsp baking powder
80 g coconut sugar
3 tsp ground ginger
1 pinch salt
220 ml dairy-free milk (soya works best)
1 tbsp lemon juice
90 ml extra-virgin olive oil
1 tsp vanilla essence

Method
1. Pre-heat the oven to 180°C and line a 12-hole muffin tin with wrappers.
2. Carefully peel, core and chop the pears into small pieces.
3. Place the flour, baking powder, coconut sugar, ground ginger and salt into a large bowl.
4. In a separate bowl, pour the dairy-free milk, lemon juice, olive oil and vanilla essence and mix well to combine.
5. Pour the wet mixture into the dry and quickly combine together with a large spoon, scraping the flour off the bottom of the bowl. Add the pears and swiftly mix in.

6. Quickly spoon the mix into the muffin wrappers so they are three-quarters full and pop in the middle of the oven to bake for 18-21 minutes until the muffins have risen and spring back when the top is pressed.
7. Transfer to a cooling rack and leave to cool.

Sticky date and ginger cake

Makes 9 squares or 12 smaller rectangles

If you're a ginger fan, here's another delicious bake packed with its wonderfully warming flavour. As mentioned earlier in this book, ginger is about so much more than just flavour. Renowned as a calmative for nausea or indigestion, ground ginger can also act as a natural form of pain relief, particularly for period pains – the perfect excuse for eating cake in case you needed one. Crystallised ginger packs a lot of sugar; there's only a little in this bake but feel free to leave it out if you prefer. This cake is delicious warm or cooled with a dollop of dairy-free yoghurt on the side if you so wish.

Ingredients
150 g dates
250 ml dairy-free milk
125 ml water
½ tsp bicarbonate of soda
250 g self-raising gluten-free flour
1 tsp baking powder
2-3 tsp ground ginger
1 tsp ground cinnamon
1 pinch salt
50 g crystallised ginger (optional but very good)
75 ml maple syrup
100 ml mild olive oil
1 tsp vanilla essence

Method
1. Chop the dates and pop them in a small pan with the dairy-free milk and water. Bring to the boil then reduce the heat and gently simmer for 10 minutes.
2. Turn off the heat and leave to cool for a few minutes before adding the bicarbonate of soda. Whisk it in carefully as the mix ferociously bubbles up. Leave it to cool whilst you get everything else ready.
3. Pre-heat the oven to 180°C and line a square 20x20-cm baking tin with non-stick baking paper. Chop the crystallised ginger into tiny pieces (if using).
4. Place the flour, baking powder, spices and salt into a large bowl with the crystallised ginger.
5. Add the maple syrup, oil and vanilla essence to the cooled date mix and stir well to combine.
6. Pour the wet date mix into the dry and stir quickly to bring it all together. Pour the combined mix into the prepared tin, tap it on the worktop to level it and place in the middle of the oven. Bake for 25 minutes.
7. Once baked, remove from the oven and leave to rest in the tin for 5 minutes before transferring it to a cooling rack. Leave to cool then cut into squares or rectangles and store in an air-tight container for up to 4 days. Freezes well.

Cherry Bakewell flapjacks

Makes 9 squares or 12 rectangles

I've already mentioned that I'm partial to a flapjack and love creating new flavour combinations whilst keeping the same core gut-loving ingredients of nuts and seeds. I've used frozen cherries in this recipe as they are available all year round and are softer than fresh. They also come without stones, which makes chopping them a little easier. If you happen to have fresh cherries to hand, then feel free to use them.

Ingredients
150 g frozen cherries, defrosted
200 g whole oats
50 g ground almonds
50 g flaked almonds

25 g pumpkin seeds
1 tsp almond essence
3 tbsp maple syrup
2 tbsp ground flaxseed
4 tbsp dairy-free milk

Method
1. Chop the defrosted cherries into small pieces. Keep any juice left in the bowl.
2. Pre-heat the oven to 160°C. Line a 20x20-cm square baking tin with non-stick baking paper.
3. Place the oats, almonds and pumpkin seeds together in a large bowl. Mix well then add the chopped cherries and mix again.
4. In the bowl with the cherry juice, add the almond essence, maple syrup, ground flaxseed and dairy-free milk. Mix well to combine and leave to thicken for 3-4 minutes.
5. Pour the wet ingredients into the dry, then mix well to make sure everything is combined.
6. Tip the mix into the prepared baking tin and spread out evenly, pressing into the edges and ensuring the top is flat and pressed down.
7. Pop the tin in the oven and bake for 15 minutes or until the top is lightly browned.
8. Remove from the oven and leave to cool in the tin. After 10 minutes, mark out 9 large squares or 12 smaller rectangles, then leave to cool completely.
9. Remove the flapjacks from the tin using the baking paper. Finish cutting the flapjacks into squares or rectangles and peel off the baking paper. Store in an air-tight container in a cool place.

Spiced cookies
Makes 8

I make these lovely, spiced cookies in the lead up to Christmas, but to be honest you can make them any time of the year; adjusting the spice levels makes them seasonally appropriate. Delicious on their own, they also make a tasty accompaniment to stewed fruit, mousse or even rice pudding.

The baking time is crucial. Too short and they're horribly under done but over bake and they're so tough you might fear for your tooth enamel. I found 8 minutes is just about perfect with a turn halfway through. Do be mindful that everyone's ovens are different, so watch carefully the first time you make these and note down your bespoke timing.

I've added cornflour into the recipe to support a gluten-free flour mix. Gluten is the glue that holds baked goods together. Some flour mixes contain gum designed to act as the binding agent; try to find one with this added or add xanthum gum yourself, if you can tolerate it, of course.

Ingredients
225 g gluten-free flour
1 tbsp cornflour
1 tsp baking powder
1 pinch salt
1 tsp cinnamon
1 tsp ground ginger
1 pinch nutmeg
1 pinch ground cloves
60 g coconut sugar or molasses
3 tbsp tahini or almond butter
6 tbsp dairy-free milk
extra flour for rolling out

Method
1. Place the flour, cornflour, baking powder, salt and spices into a large bowl and mix well to combine.
2. In a separate bowl, add the sugar, tahini or nut butter and dairy-free milk. Beat together with an electric whisk to create a smooth mix.
3. Pre-heat the oven to 180°C and line a large baking tray with non-stick baking paper.

4. Sieve the flour mix into the sugar mix and bring together into a dough, first with a spoon and then your hands. Gently press it together but don't try to knead it.
5. Sprinkle extra flour onto the worktop and place the dough on top. Carefully press it down to flatten it a bit then place a sheet of non-stick baking paper on top. Roll out the dough with a rolling pin to 2.5-cm thickness.
6. Using a round or shaped cookie cutter, cut out cookies and transfer to the baking sheet. Bring any excess dough together, roll and cut out again until it's all used up.
7. Place the tray in the middle of the oven and bake for 8 minutes, turning once half way through to get an even bake.
8. Remove the tray from the oven and transfer the cookies to a cooling rack. Leave to cool fully and store in an air-tight container for a maximum of 3 days.

Sweet carrot scones

Makes 6

As butter is a key ingredient of scones, I was disappointed to think I might never be able to eat them again. Trying to find an alternative was a challenge, but once I realised that certain vegetables could be used in baking, carrots came to the rescue. You'll need to make the carrot purée ahead of time, so bear that in mind when planning your bake.

Of course, puréed carrot is very different to butter in texture, flavour and, well, everything. But it works well as a binding agent, provides some sweetness and creates a relatively light baked scone. I have added a little sugar to this recipe as scones are a treat, but feel free to leave it out if you prefer. I've tried other options and decided substitutes don't work. Sometimes it's sugar or no sugar; nothing else will do.

Ingredients

1 medium carrot to make 80 g carrot purée
225g gluten-free self-rising flour
1 tsp baking powder

½ tsp golden ground flaxseed
1 pinch salt
30 g sugar (optional)
1 tbsp mild olive oil
5 tbsp dairy-free milk of choice plus extra for brushing the top
30 g raisins (optional but adds to sweetness)

Method

1. *First, make the carrot purée.* Peel a medium-sized carrot, chop it into small pieces and pop it in a steamer basket. Steam for 10 minutes until soft then turn off the heat. Leave to cool in the steamer basket. Once completely cool, transfer to a small blender pot and add a little water. Blend to smooth – you may have to add a little more water but do so carefully as you want a thick purée, not a watery orange sauce.
2. Pre-heat the oven to 200ºC. Line a baking tray with non-stick baking paper.
3. Add the flour, baking powder, salt, ground flaxseed and sugar together in a large bowl and mix well.
4. Mix the carrot purée, olive oil and dairy-free milk together in a bowl. Make sure they are well combined.
5. Pour the wet ingredients into the dry and cut in with a knife until the two mixtures start to combine. Add the raisins if using, then bring it all together with your hands to make a soft dough.
6. Remove the dough from the bowl and knead gently on the worktop until the raisins are well distributed. Carefully flatten the dough with your palm until it's spread a bit and 3-cm thick. You can use a rolling pin if you like, but I find hands work best.
7. Using a 7-cm wide cookie cutter, cut out your scones and place onto the baking tray. Re-knead the dough and flatten 2-3 times until you have used it all up.
8. Brush the tops with the extra dairy-free milk. Bake in the oven for 14-18 minutes until lightly golden on top and firm on the bottom. Remove from the oven and leave to cool on a tray.
9. Eat whilst still warm with a dollop of raspberry chia jam (page 285) or store in an air-tight container for 2 days. These freeze well so make a batch and take out one or two as you need them.

Plum and cardamom cake
Makes 10 slices

Plum season runs from mid-summer to late autumn and, in a good year, they are abundantly available, especially if you have a productive tree in your garden. Deliciously sharp but sweet, there are plenty of varieties to try, although Victoria plum is still, and always will be, my favourite.

Delicious raw as a snack or dessert, these tasty fruits provide sweetness and moisture to bakes. Often paired with cinnamon, I find I prefer them with cardamom for a deeper, more exotic flavour. An underrated spice, cardamom contains its own array of polyphenols and other antioxidants and has mood-enhancing properties, so it's not just cake that brings a little happiness, but the spices within help too.

Ingredients
4 ripe medium-large plums
200 g self-raising gluten-free flour
1 tsp baking powder
½-1 tsp ground cardamom
80 g coconut sugar
250 ml soya milk or dairy-free milk of choice
1 tbsp lemon juice
1 tsp vanilla essence
3 tbsp olive oil

To top:
1 tsp coconut sugar
½ tsp ground cinnamon

Method
1. Wash the plums, remove the stones then chop three into small pieces and slice the other.
2. Pre-heat the oven to 170°C. Grease the base and sides of an 18-cm spring-form cake tin and cover the base with non-stick baking paper.

3. Place the flour, baking powder, salt, ground cardamom and coconut sugar into a large bowl and mix well to combine.
4. In another bowl, add the soya milk and lemon juice and let it curdle for 2-3 minutes before adding the vanilla essence and olive oil. Mix well.
5. Mix the coconut sugar and cinnamon for the topping together in a small bowl and put to one side.
6. Pour the wet mix into the dry and swiftly fold together using a large spoon, making sure you bring in the flour at the bottom of the bowl. Add the **chopped** plums and stir them into the mix.
7. Tip the cake mix into the prepared cake tin. Arrange the plum slices over the top in a pattern and gently press them into the mixture. Sprinkle the coconut cinnamon sugar over the top and place in the middle of the oven. Bake for 40-45 minutes until the top is lightly browned and a skewer comes out clean.
8. Remove from the oven and leave to rest in the tin for 10 minutes. Release the sides of the tin, remove the cake, peel off the baking paper from the bottom and leave on a cooling rack.
9. Eat slightly warm if desired or leave to cool completely and store in an air-tight container for up to 3 days.

Carrot and maple muffins
Makes 10

Discovering carrot cake as a teenager working in a health food café triggered my interest in plant-based eating, so it would be remiss of me not to include a carrot cake-style bake in this section. I am still a huge fan of carrot cake, but some recipes are loaded with sugar and fat. This version contains minimal amounts of both but retains the lovely moisture and spices I always associate with carrot cake.

Pecan nuts are rich and buttery and help provide some fat to the mix. Feel free to substitute them with walnuts or omit them if you prefer. I've used both mixed spice and cinnamon in this recipe, but if that's a bit much for you, cut back on the amounts or use just one. Soya milk is best for this recipe as it curdles well and makes the baking powder more reactive, ensuring you get a good rise. If you must avoid soya, use whichever dairy-free milk you prefer and expect less height in your muffins. You can also make this recipe oil free by replacing the olive oil with apple sauce. Again, the rise won't be as high, but the muffins will still taste gorgeous.

This mix works well as a whole cake instead of muffins if you prefer. Use a small 18-cm loose-bottomed cake tin and increase the baking time to ensure the middle section is fully baked.

Ingredients
220 ml soya milk
1 tbsp lemon juice
1 medium carrot
280 g gluten-free self-raising flour
1 tsp baking powder
2 tsp mixed spice
1 tsp ground cinnamon
1 pinch salt
30 g pecan nuts
50 g raisins or sultanas
80 ml maple syrup
100 ml olive oil, or apple sauce if oil free
1 tsp vanilla essence

To top:
2 tbsp maple syrup

Method
1. Pre-heat the oven to 180°C. Grab a 12-hole muffin tin and add muffin cases to 10 of the holes.
2. Pour the soya milk into a large jug and add the lemon juice. Leave to curdle for a few minutes. Peel and finely grate the carrot and add to the soya milk.
3. In a large bowl, combine the flour, baking powder, mixed spice, cinnamon and salt.
4. Finely chop the pecan nuts and split into 20-g and 10-g portions. Add the 20-g portion to the flour mix along with the raisins or sultanas.

5. Add the maple syrup, vanilla essence and olive oil or apple sauce into the soya-carrot mix and stir well to combine.
6. Put the 10-g portion of pecans in a small bowl and add the 2 tbsp maple syrup for the topping.
7. Pour the wet ingredients into the dry and quickly mix – don't worry if it's a bit lumpy, you want to retain the air, and the lumps will sort themselves out in the oven.
8. Spoon equal amounts of the mix into the muffin wrappers and add a little of the maple-pecan syrup onto the top of each muffin.
9. Tap the muffin tin on the worktop and place in the middle of the oven. Bake for 20-25 minutes, turning the tray halfway through.
10. Remove from the oven and leave to cool in the tray for 10 minutes before transferring to a cooling rack. Store in an air-tight container for up to 3 days or freeze for another day.

Almond and cardamom balls
Makes 12

Admittedly there's no baking here, but I love raw 'energy' balls and had to include at least one version in this book. I created this tasty combination for an online retreat I helped to run during the Covid lockdown. A common phenomenon now, but at the time it was a novel concept, and we had free range to recreate the retreat experience for people in their own homes. I ran live cooking classes, recorded several cooking videos and provided a selection of other whole-food plant-based recipes for attendees to try, including this one.

The cardamom flavour really comes through in these raw balls, pairing beautifully with the almonds. You could use cashews or macadamia nuts instead if preferred, or if you're nut free, replace with sunflower seeds.

These balls keep in the fridge for up to 5 days but also freeze well, so make a large batch and keep extras for when you need a little pick-me-up.

Ingredients

110 g dates
80 g whole almonds (skin on)
100 g gluten-free oats
80 g raisins
½ tsp ground cardamom
½ tsp ground cinnamon
1 pinch salt
3-4 tbsp ground almonds

Method

1. Place the dates in a bowl of boiling water for 10 minutes or so to soften then drain but retain a little of the soaking water.
2. Place the almonds into the bowl of a food processor and pulse a few times to break them down.
3. Add the drained dates, oats, raisins, spices and salt and blend until everything is broken down and sticks together. If the mix is too dry, carefully add a little of the retained soaking water but take care not to make it too sticky. Blend again.
4. Sprinkle the ground almonds onto a plate.
5. Remove a spoonful of the mix and roll it into a ball with your fingers. Roll each in the ground almonds to coat them, then place on another plate. Repeat until all the mix is used up.

Desserts

My sweet tooth loves dessert almost as much as cake, so I've added a selection of tasty, satisfying desserts that still fit the whole-food plant-based criteria. Life would be just a bit too sad without something sweet to enjoy.

Nearly all of my desserts use some kind of fruit, both raw and cooked. Fruit provides natural sweetness, more fibre and, even when cooked, some extra nutrients and magical polyphenols that support the body. When matched with other whole ingredients, you could almost say that dessert is health food – almost.

During the week, we tend to eat just fruit or fruit with dairy-free yoghurt, with desserts a treat at the weekend. If you're low in energy, creating a second course for a meal might just be too much – you can always persuade someone else to make it for you though.

Whenever we're invited to friends for dinner, I always offer to bring dessert just to help my hosts out. Usually, starters and mains are no problem for them, but desserts are often a challenge, even though all of mine are simple to make. It brings me great pleasure to see their surprised faces as they tuck in to a super-tasty 'free-from' dessert – free from anything dodgy maybe, but never free from flavour.

Rhubarb and strawberry crumble
Serves 4

We are big crumble fans in our house, and what's not to love? Super-tasty and flexible, you get softness, crunch and natural sweetness in every mouthful. Often seen as a warming winter treat, crumble using spring and summer fruits are just as delightful, especially on those cool, damp days. Of course, you can just sub whatever fruit is in season to make this an all-year-round dessert.

Traditional crumble recipes tend to have lots of refined sugar, flour and fats in the topping. This version relies on the natural sweetness of the strawberries to soften the rhubarb's sharpness - you can add a little maple syrup though if the rhubarb is really tart. If you have a glut of fruit, make extra crumble to pop in the freezer for later in the year.

Ingredients
4-5 stalks rhubarb
150 g strawberries
1 tbsp maple syrup
2 tbsp water
85 g oats (gluten-free if needed)
70 g buckwheat flour (or other gluten-free flour)
2 tbsp nut or seed butter of choice
1 tbsp maple or date syrup
1 tsp ground cinnamon

Method
1. Pre-heat the oven to 180°C.
2. Chop the rhubarb into chunks, slice the strawberries in half (if big) and place in a medium-sized oven-proof dish with the maple syrup (if using) and water. Ensure everything is mixed well together.
3. Mix the oats, buckwheat flour and cinnamon together in a large bowl. Add the nut butter and rub in using your fingertips until it's blended in and small chunks stick together. Add the maple or date syrup and a little water to help the mix stick. (You can do this in a food processor if you don't want crumble mix up your nails.)
4. Sprinkle over the top of the prepared fruit and pop in the oven for 20 minutes or so, until the fruit bubbles up a bit and the top is lightly browned and firm.
5. Leave to rest for a few minutes then serve with cashew cream, dairy-free ice cream or whichever accompaniment you choose.

Raspberry mousse
Serves 2

I do love a mousse but finding a quick, easy mousse recipe evaded me for some time. I did create a highly complicated one using aquafaba, the brine from tinned chickpeas, which tasted good but took up a lot of time. One day I started thinking about whether silken tofu would be a good base – it turned out to be just what I was looking for, first as a chocolate mousse then evolving into this gorgeously tasty raspberry one. If your ears pricked up at the word chocolate, just add cocoa powder to the mix.

This mousse doesn't have the firm set you'd get with double cream but it's light, satisfying and gives you an extra protein hit too. Make sure you only use silken tofu; other types just won't give you the same creamy, smooth texture. Enjoy this without garnish for a quick dessert or dress it up with whole fruits, cocoa powder or even a sprinkle of granola.

Ingredients
150 g silken tofu
80 g raspberries – fresh or defrosted
½ tsp lemon juice
1 or 2 tbsp maple syrup

Garnish with:
retained raspberries, other berries or seasonal fruit, mint, chocolate etc

Method
1. Keeping a few raspberries for decoration, place all the other ingredients except the decoration into a small blender pot and blend until smooth.
2. Spoon into ramekins or small dishes and place in the fridge for 2 hours. Decorate and serve chilled.

Chia chocolate pudding
Serves 2

Another super-simple mousse-like dessert, this time using the magic of chia seeds to provide some solidity. These need much longer to set than the raspberry mousse above, but preparing in advance means you need to do very little before serving.

Chia seeds are an excellent source of omega 3 fatty acids. When mixed with fluid, they swell, forming a thick, gloopy texture. As well as providing structure, this reaction also makes the healthy fats available for absorption. Match this with the polyphenols in cacao and berries, and this dessert does much more than just taste delicious.

Ingredients
15 g raw cacao powder (cocoa powder will also be fine)
30 ml maple syrup
1 tsp vanilla paste
180 ml dairy-free milk of choice
50 g chia seeds
100 g berries or fruit of choice, or a mix (passion fruit is good)

Method
1. Mix the cacao, maple syrup, vanilla paste, dairy-free milk and chia seeds together in a large jug and whisk to combine.
2. Place 90 g of the berries or whatever fruit you are using in the bottom of 2 serving dishes – large round glasses look good.
3. Carefully pour the chia mix over the fruit then chill in the fridge for a minimum of 4 hours.
4. Serve with the remaining fruit piled on top, and a dusting of cacao powder if you wish.

Raw blueberry lemon tarts
Makes 6 individual tarts or 1 large one

Raw desserts are delicious but usually contain coconut cream or milk for structure. These tasty tarts use a raw pastry base that is then filled with a super-thick cashew cream. It may look a little fiddly but trust me when I say this is easier than it might look and rewards you with wonderful flavours and admiration from your family or guest(s).

I find it easier to make this with individual tartlet tins. They must have a loose base though or you won't be able to get the tarts out of the tin; this is even more important for a large tin. A high-speed blender is too powerful for this recipe. A food processor provides much more control over speed and consistency.

Once you've made these tarts once, I guarantee you'll be doing it again as they are just gorgeous.

Ingredients
For the base:
150 g de-stoned dates
100 g gluten-free oats
90 g sunflower seeds or almonds
grated rind from ½ unwaxed lemon
1 pinch salt

For the filling:
150 g cashew nuts
2 tbsp maple syrup
1 tsp vanilla paste
juice 1 lemon and ½ lemon rind, grated
200 g blueberries
mint leaves to garnish (optional)

Method
1. Place the dates in a bowl of hot water and soak for at least 1 hour. Do the same to the cashew nuts for the filling in a separate bowl.
2. To make the base, place the oats and sunflower seeds or almonds into a food processor bowl and pulse a few times to break them down. Drain the dates (retain the soaking water) and pop them into the food processor along with the lemon rind and salt. Blend until the mix starts to stick together – add a little of the soaking water if it's too dry but take care not to make it wet.
3. Remove the base dough from the food processor and cut into 6 equal portions, rolling them into small balls, if making individual tarts, or roll to form one large ball.
4. Tear off 2 sheets of non-stick baking paper, laying one on the worktop. Pop a ball on top then lay the other sheet of baking paper over the top. Press down to flatten a bit with the palm of your hand then roll flat with a rolling pin to form a circle just wider than the tart tin. Remove the top sheet of baking paper, turn upside down over the tin and carefully peel away the bottom sheet, letting the mix drop into the tin. Press into the corners and trim the edges. Repeat if using small tins until they all have a base. Pop in the fridge to chill.
5. *Make a thick cashew cream* by draining the cashew nuts and popping them into the food processor bowl. Blitz to form a thick paste. Add the maple syrup, lemon juice, lemon rind and vanilla and blend again. The mix will still be too thick and lumpy so add date-soaking water a little at a time to form a really thick cream. Be careful not to add too much or it will run out of the 'pastry' cases.
6. Remove the base cases from the fridge and fill with the cashew cream. Cover the tops with blueberries, then chill in the fridge until you are ready to serve.
7. Just before serving, carefully remove the tarts from the tartlet tins (or tin) by pushing up the base from underneath. Lever the base away from the bottom of the tart and serve on a small plate with a garnish of mint leaves.

Raspberry Bakewell tart
Serves 6

Bakewell tart is an English dessert traditionally made with buttery shortcrust pastry filled with thick layers of jam and frangipane, often topped with a super-sweet layer of icing. Having such a sweet tooth, I used to love tucking into this tasty tart. Unfortunately, all the dairy and sugar inside did not love me back and once I started to use food as medicine, Bakewell tarts were off the menu.

That is, until I worked out how to make an alternative version. This Bakewell tart retains the lovely almond flavour and is still sweet even though it uses minimal sugar. The binding agent is aquafaba, chickpea brine (from a tin) or cooking water that has similar properties to egg white. It has a strong beany aroma but fortunately this isn't detectable in the final bake. Served slightly warm with a dusting of icing sugar (or not) and a drizzle of dairy-free cream, everyone enjoys this tasty tart whether they're plant-based or not.

Apologies if you must avoid almonds though, as I've not come up with a good alternative for you just yet. You could use an alternative nut or seed butter for the pastry, miss out the frangipane and make yourself a lovely jam tart instead.

Ingredients
For the pastry:
200 g gluten-free flour mix for pastry
1 tbsp cornflour
1 tbsp ground golden flaxseed
5 tbsp almond butter
up to 120 ml chilled water

For the frangipane:
200 g ground almonds
60 g coconut sugar
1 pinch salt
2 tbsp cornflour

½ tsp almond extract
½ tsp vanilla essence
6 tbsp aquafaba
1 tbsp dairy-free milk

For the jam:
1½ tbsp chia seeds
200 g raspberries, fresh or frozen
1 tbsp maple syrup (optional if your raspberries are ripe and sweet)

Method
1. *Make the pastry:* Sieve the flour and cornflour into a large bowl. Add the ground flaxseed and stir well to combine. Rub the almond butter into the flour with your fingertips to form small breadcrumbs. Add 90 ml of the chilled water and bring together with a spoon, then your fingers, to form a soft dough. Add extra water a little at a time if it's too dry but be careful not to make it soggy. Form a ball then place in the fridge to rest.
2. *Make the frangipane:* Mix the ground almonds, coconut sugar, salt and cornflour together in a large bowl. Add the almond extract, vanilla essence, aquafaba and dairy-free milk and mix well to form a thick paste.
3. *Make the chia jam:* Pop the chia seeds into a small blender and blitz for a few seconds to break them down. Tip the raspberries into a small pan and add the maple syrup. Simmer the fruit for 5 minutes or so until it starts to break down and lots of juice is released. Turn off the heat and stir in the chia seeds. Leave to cool – it will soon start to thicken.
4. *Make the tart:* Pre-heat the oven to 180°C. Grab 6 loose-bottomed tart tins and lightly grease with olive oil. Remove the pastry from the fridge and cut into 6 equal portions. Place one ball onto a sheet of non-stick baking paper and cover with another sheet. Gently roll the pastry out into a round big enough to fill the tin. Carefully peel off the baking paper and drop into a tart tin. Press the pastry into the edges and patch where needed. Trim the top. Repeat until all the cases are filled.
5. Spoon the raspberry chia jam into the base of the tarts then cover with frangipane. Place the tarts on a large baking tray and pop in the oven. Bake

for 15-20 minutes until the top is lightly browned, turning the tray halfway through.
6. Serve warm or chilled with a sprinkle of icing sugar on top if desired.

Blackberry and apple tray bake
Makes 12 squares

Autumn brings us apples and blackberry-laden bushes just begging to be picked. Both these seasonal fruits contain a wonderful selection of fibre and polyphenols that the microbiome just adores. They taste mighty fine too.

This dessert is a simple traybake that makes the most of this wonderful pairing. Both apples and blackberries freeze well, so it's a dessert that can be enjoyed well into the winter and a way to make sure the most is made of this seasonal glut.

Ingredients
250 g eating apples
500 g self-raising gluten-free flour
1 tsp baking powder
1 pinch salt
2 tsp ground cinnamon
100 g coconut sugar
200 g blackberries
400 ml soya milk (or dairy-free milk of choice)
2 tbsp lemon juice
100 ml maple syrup
100 g apple sauce
90 ml mild olive oil
2 tsp vanilla essence
80 g blackberries to top

Method

1. Line a 35x26-cm rectangular cake tin with non-stick baking paper. Pre-heat the oven to 180°C.
2. Wash, de-core and finely chop the apple into small pieces.
3. Sieve the flour, baking powder and salt into a large bowl. Add the sugar and chopped apple and stir well to combine. Wash both sets of blackberries but don't add them just yet.
4. In a large jug, add the dairy-free milk, lemon, maple syrup, apple purée, olive oil and vanilla essence. Stir well to combine.
5. Pour the wet mix into the dry and quickly stir to combine. Add the 200-g portion of blackberries and carefully fold these in before transferring the mix to the prepared baking tin, making sure it's spread into the edges.
6. Scatter the remaining blackberries over the top and gently press them into the mix so they can still be seen.
7. Place the tin in the middle of the oven and bake for 30-35 minutes, until the bake has risen and is lightly browned on top.
8. Remove from the oven and leave to cool slightly in the tin before cutting into squares. Serve warm or chilled with dairy-free cream, yoghurt or custard, as desired.

Baked crunchy nectarines

Serves 2

Simple desserts can be as tasty as the more complex ones, which is just as well when you're struggling with fatigue or when concentrating on a recipe with more than three ingredients is just too much for your brain to deal with. This sweet and tasty dessert can be baked in an air fryer if turning on the oven is a step too far.

Healthy granolas can be found in health food shops and some larger supermarkets – try to avoid ones that are packed with extra sugars and saturated fats. If you want to control the ingredients, it's easy to make your own version – there's a simple recipe on The Sensitive Foodie Kitchen website if you need a little inspiration https://thesensitivefoodiekitchen.com/tasty-oil-free-granola/.

I love this recipe with nectarines or peaches when they're in season. Apples, pears and plums work just as well, so feel free to use whatever is in season or you enjoy.

Ingredients
2 ripe nectarines (or fruit of choice)
4 tbsp granola
1 tbsp maple syrup

To serve:
Dairy-free yoghurt or ice cream of choice

Method
1. If using the oven, pre-heat to 170°C or prepare your air fryer as per instructions.
2. Cut the nectarines in half and remove the stones.
3. Pop the granola into a small bowl and add the maple syrup. Stir well to combine.
4. Place the nectarine halves onto an air fryer-compliant baking tin, or normal baking tin if using the oven. It's helpful to use a smallish one so the nectarine halves hold each other up.
5. Fill the nectarines with granola. Bake them for 15 minutes or until they are soft and the juices start to flow.
6. Serve hot with your topping of choice.

Baked 'cheesecake'
Serves 8-10

When I first started creating recipes as the Sensitive Foodie, I was very keen on raw cheesecakes. Indeed, there are three in my first book – all delicious of course but not suitable for anyone with autoimmune disease as they use coconut cream which is packed full of saturated fat. Coconut cream is perfect to create structure for a raw cheesecake, not so great for an anti-inflammatory diet – a shame as I love cheesecake.

Trying to work out how I could still enjoy cheesecake using whole ingredients, but no coconut oil or cream, took some time. Spurred on by my desire for desserts, I got there in the end. The result is not 'low fat' but it's lower in saturated fat and higher in healthier polyunsaturated fats in whole foods which makes the difference. It's also high in fibre so the sugars are released gradually. Most of all, it tastes like a baked cheesecake which means you don't miss out on a delicious dessert, even though it does take a while to make. You can spread this out over 2 days though and it's worth doing that to ensure you get a good set. It's a lot of effort, but I assure you it's worth it.

This recipe is soya heavy so if you avoid it, please move on to the next dish as this is not for you. You'll need to soak the cashew nuts before you start so factor this into your planning time. If you are nut free, replace the cashews with sunflower seeds. They will need 4 hours' soaking time and won't create the same creaminess but it's still a good option to ensure you can have a version that suits you.

As this is a vanilla baked cheesecake, I find vanilla paste provides a stronger flavour than essence so use that if possible. If not, just increase the amount of vanilla essence and don't skip the lemon as it's integral to the overall flavour. For the fruit, strawberry or raspberry is always my favourite. Passion fruit and mango make a lovely combination if you like to go tropical, but essentially use whatever you like or prefer.

Ingredients

For the base:
100 g gluten-free flour blend for pastry
20 g coconut sugar (optional but good)
1 pinch salt
35 g tahini or cashew nut butter
1 tbsp maple syrup
4 tbsp chilled water

For the cheesecake centre:
175 g cashew nuts
250 g silken tofu or very soft tofu

60 g soya yoghurt
85 ml soya milk
85 ml maple syrup
1 tsp vanilla paste or 2 tsp vanilla extract
1 lemon, juice and rind

For the fruit topping:
225 g fresh or defrosted fruit of choice
1 tbsp maple syrup
1½ tsp cornflour
2 tsp water

Method
1. Place the cashew nuts for the cheesecake centre into a bowl and cover with boiling water. Leave to soak for at least 30 minutes, ideally 2 hours.
2. Grab a 20-cm loose-bottomed baking tin and line the base and sides with non-stick baking paper. (Brush the sides with a little olive oil to help the paper stay in place.)
3. Make the base by placing the flour, coconut sugar and salt into the bowl of a food processor. Add the tahini or nut butter and maple syrup. Pulse the mix until everything is combined and forms a fine crumb.
4. Add 2 tbsp water and blend to bring the mix together, adding more water a little at a time so you get a soft but not sticky mix.
5. Grab a sheet of non-stick baking paper and tip out the mix. Bring it together with your fingers to form a soft ball then roll out to form a circle just bigger than the tin. Carefully tip the pastry into the bottom of the tin. Press into the corners and slightly up the side. If it breaks or cracks, just patch it with excess pastry or pinch together. Pop in the fridge to rest whilst you make the filling.
6. Pre-heat the oven to 180°C.
7. Make the filling: Rinse out the food processor bowl. Drain the cashew nuts then add all the 'cheesecake' ingredients to the food processor and blend together until smooth.
8. Remove the pastry from the fridge and pour in the cheesecake mix. Tap the tin on the worktop to expel any bubbles then transfer to the oven. Bake for 35

minutes in the middle of the oven or until the mix has set. It shouldn't wobble in the middle when moved and be very lightly browned on top. If it needs a little longer, cover with some foil to prevent over-browning.
9. Remove from the oven. Leave to cool in the tin then chill for 4 hours or overnight.
10. *Make the fruit topping:* If using berries, place the fruit in a small pan over a low heat. Cook gently until the fruit is soft and juices leak into the pan. Mix the cornflour and water together in a small bowl. Pour into the pan and stir continuously until the fruit mix thickens. Turn off the heat and leave to cool. Spoon the mix over the top of the set cheesecake. Chill for 30 minutes until the topping has set, then cut into slices and serve.
11. If you are using mango and passion fruit, mash some of the mango and chop the rest. Mix with the passion fruit pulp and spoon over the top just before serving.

Ginger and pear rice pudding
Serves 2

We're back to my favoured combination of pear and ginger for a tasty twist to this traditional dessert. Rice pudding is the ultimate comfort food. Pear adds sweetness and the ginger supports digestion and soothes pain. This pudding can be made on the hob, but I find it's so easy to burn the pan it's better to bake low and slow in the oven. Not only is it more successful but it means you can go off and do other things whilst it cooks instead of holding a hob-side vigil. Feel free to use other fruit; frozen berries are particularly good.

Ingredients
60 g pudding or basmati rice or flaked red rice
1½ tbsp maple syrup
1-2 tsp ground ginger
600 ml dairy-free milk of choice
2 ripe pears

To serve:
2 tsp sliced almonds (optional)

Method
1. Pre-heat the oven to 160°C.
2. Rinse the rice under a running tap then tip into an oven-proof dish that has a lid.
3. Add the maple syrup, ground ginger and dairy-free milk. Mix well then pop on the lid and place in the middle of the oven to bake for 45 minutes.
4. Peel the pears, de-core and chop them into small pieces. Add to the rice pudding then bake for another 20 minutes or until the rice is soft and swollen.
5. Serve hot with a scattering of sliced almonds if desired.

Apple and salted caramel slice
Serves 9-12 (depending on size)

I discovered that dates make the perfect plant-based caramel early on in my plant-based adventures. Gorgeous in itself, but then I realised a little salt turned it into salted caramel – even better. Match that with sweet apples and a crunchy crumble topping and you get a deliciously sticky, sweet but still healthful dessert that you'll want to make time and again. It will also surprise your guests as they won't believe it's made with healthful, whole ingredients.

Unless you are using gloriously sweet but very expensive Medjool dates, you'll need to factor in soaking time for your dates. A couple of hours is ideal but if you're short of time, 10 minutes' minimum will do. Serve warm or cooled with dairy-free cinnamon ice cream or dollops of thick dairy-free yoghurt. These tasty slices keep in the fridge for up to 4 days and also freeze well, ideal for batch cooking.

Ingredients
For the caramel:
280 g de-stoned dates
2 tsp vanilla essence
250 ml dairy-free milk
¼ Himalayan salt

For the base:
270 g gluten-free flour
1½ baking powder
100 g coconut sugar
150 g oats
1 pinch salt
170 g nut butter of choice

For the filling:
3 medium eating apples
50 g walnuts or pecan nuts (optional but good)

Method

1. *Make the caramel:* Soak the dates in hot water for a minimum of 10 minutes to let them soften. Drain but reserve the soaking water. Place the drained dates in a food processor bowl. Add the vanilla essence, dairy-free milk and salt and blend until smooth. Taste and add a little more salt if needed.
2. *Make the base:* Line a 33x22-cm baking tin or dish with grease-proof paper. Pre-heat the oven to 170°C. Place the flour, baking powder, coconut sugar, oats and salt in a large bowl and mix together well with a spoon. Add the almond or butter alternative of choice and rub in with your fingertips to make a sticky breadcrumb-like mixture. Add 5 tbsp of the reserved date water and bring together into a soft dough. If the mix is too dry, add a little more date water with care – you don't want it too wet.
3. Cut off one-third of the dough and put it to one side. Press the remaining dough into the base of the prepared dish or tin, spreading it out as evenly as possible. Pop in the oven to bake for 10 minutes then remove and leave to cool slightly.
4. Make the filling and finish off: Wash the apples, de-core them and cut into thin slices. Chop the walnuts or pecans if using. Scatter half the apple slices over the slightly cooled base. Drop two-thirds of the salted date caramel over the apples then cover with the remaining slices. Add the remaining caramel and scatter the nuts over the top. Finally, drop pieces of the remaining dough on top, roughly covering the filling.

5. Place back in the oven and bake for 30 minutes until the top is lightly browned and the apples soft when pricked with a knife. Remove from the oven, leave to settle for 5 minutes, then serve.

Sauces and dressings

A little bit of sauce or dressing can liven up the simplest of dishes with minimal effort. Every recipe in this book provides a range of body- and gut-loving nutrients, including these sauces and dressings. Everything counts in a whole-food plant-based diet, including the little bits that brighten up a dish.

I try to avoid expensive kitchen equipment to ensure this way of eating is accessible to all budgets. Most of these sauces do need either a high-speed blender or a small blender pot that attaches to a stick blender. Fortunately, there are some reliable low-cost versions available to buy new or keep an eye out on online marketplaces as there are often good bargains to be found. Make sure you check it all works first though.

White bean sauce
Serves 2-4

Sometimes you just need a quick and easy sauce for pasta or roasted veggies – this white bean sauce hits the spot, with not a tomato in sight. Adjust the amount of dairy-free milk to make it thick and creamy or more pourable. I love this with a selection of lightly cooked veg and pasta for a quick evening meal.

If you like and can tolerate miso, add that instead of nutritional yeast for a deeper savoury flavour and don't forget the lemon juice – it lifts the flavour marvellously.

Ingredients
1 x 400-g tin of cannellini beans
80-120 ml dairy-free milk of choice
1 clove roasted garlic or ½ tsp garlic powder
4 tbsp nutritional yeast or 1 tsp miso
1 tbsp lemon juice
salt and pepper to taste

Method
1. Add all the ingredients to a blender pot and blend until smooth.
2. Check the flavour and add more garlic, nutritional yeast, lemon juice or seasoning as needed.
3. Warm through gently or stir into pasta etc.

Sweet and sour sauce

I love Chinese sauces but when you look at the ingredients list on the ones available in the supermarkets, there are a lot of additives that are not conducive to gut health. So, to avoid all those chemicals, I create my own versions – equally delicious but with minimally processed ingredients. If you're using tinned pineapple, omit the maple syrup as it should be sweet enough.

Just pour over stir-fried veggies and tofu, cook for a couple of minutes and it's ready to serve.

Ingredients
200 g fresh or tinned pineapple
5 tbsp apple cider vinegar
2 tbsp tamari or coconut amines
1 tbsp tomato purée
1 heaped tbsp cornflour

Method
1. Place all the ingredients into a high-speed blender jug and blend until smooth.
2. Use immediately.
3. Store any leftover sauce in a jar in the fridge. Use within 3-4 days.

Tamarind stir-fry sauce
Serves 2

Tamarind provides a delightful sour taste that gives depth to lots of different types of sauces. Buying the pulp to extract the tamarind 'juice' is hard work though, so I keep a small jar of concentrated tamarind, bought from the health food shop or ethnic stores, in the fridge for when I need it. This is 100% tamarind, different to most tamarind pastes found in supermarkets that contain added sugar, salt and oils. Always check the label.

This sauce for stir fries provides an intense flavour that complements rainbow veggies perfectly. Double the amounts to serve a hungry family or to keep extra in the fridge for later in the week.

Ingredients
1 dsp tamarind concentrate
½ tsp garlic powder or 1 clove grated fresh garlic
2 tbsp water
1 tbsp maple syrup
1 pinch chilli flakes
salt and black pepper to taste
1 tsp cornflour

Method
1. Put the tamarind paste into a small bowl and add the water. Stir well to create a looser paste.
2. Add all the remaining ingredients except the cornflour and stir well to combine. Add more water if it's too thick – you want it a pouring consistency.
3. Just before you're ready to use it, add the cornflour and whisk well to combine.

Lemon and herb dressing
Serves 4

This tasty dressing contains anti-inflammatory omega 3 fatty acids in the flaxseed oil. The lemon adds freshness but also helps you to absorb nutrients from any green veggies added to it. Fresh herbs all contain anti-inflammatory nutrients as well as gut-loving compounds. If you can, grow your own at home for lower costs and freshness – even a couple of pots on the windowsill can produce fresh herbs all year round.

Ingredients
1 unwaxed lemon, juice and grated rind
3 tbsp cold pressed flaxseed oil
½ tsp Dijon mustard (optional)
2 tbsp chopped fresh herbs – I use basil, oregano and chives
salt and pepper to taste

Method
1. Place all the ingredients in a clean jar with a lid and shake well to combine.
2. Check the flavour and add more seasoning if required.
3. Serve on salad or cooked vegetables with a spoon so you distribute equal amounts of chopped herbs.
4. Keep leftovers in the fridge.

Turmeric ginger tahini dressing
Serves 2

I love this zingy, nutrient-packed dressing, perfect for drizzling over salads, cooked vegetables or bakes. It can even be used as a mayo for coleslaws or other salad mixes. Use more or less ginger depending on your taste-buds. Fresh is preferable to dried ginger, although if that's all you've got then try it. Alternatively, leave out the ginger completely and have a turmeric dressing instead.

Ingredients

2-cm knob fresh ginger

50 g tahini

2 tbsp water

2 tbsp lemon juice

1 tbsp maple syrup

¼ tsp garlic granules (optional)

¼ tsp ground turmeric

black pepper

1 pinch salt

Method

1. Peel and finely grate the ginger.
2. Pop it into a small blender pot with the remaining ingredients and blend to form a thick but pourable dressing.
3. Check the flavour and add more lemon, ginger, salt or pepper as desired and blend again.
4. Store in the fridge for up to 4 days.

Leafy green sauce

Serves 2

Another super-tasty sauce, this time vibrant green instead of yellow. Pour over cooked or roasted vegetables, savoury bakes or pasta. You can use a home-made cashew cream as the base or a store-bought dairy-free cream if you're short on time. Mix up the greens depending on the season or personal tastes. Kale is a little too fibrous for this sauce, even with a high-speed blender giving it a good blast but feel free to use that if it's all you have. Whatever leaf you use, remember to add the lemon juice; it lifts the flavour as well as helping you to absorb all the nutrients.

Ingredients

100 ml dairy-free cream (cashew cream, Oatley, Alpro etc)

100 g green leaves – spinach, watercress, coriander, Swiss chard etc

1 pinch garlic powder (optional)
1 small lemon, juiced
salt and pepper to taste

Method
1. Pop all the ingredients into a small blender pot and blend until smooth.
2. Check the flavour and add more lemon or seasoning as needed.
3. Use immediately or store in a jar in the fridge for 2 days.

Elderflower dressing
Serves 4

Elderflowers are synonymous with spring and summer; this lovely, refreshing dressing is perfect for seasonal salads, making the sun shine on your plate even if it's raining outside. There is a little apple cider vinegar in this recipe – if you can't tolerate it just use extra lemon juice.

Ingredients
2 tbsp elderflower cordial
1 tbsp apple cider vinegar
1 tbsp lemon juice
2 tbsp cold-pressed flaxseed oil/extra-virgin olive oil
salt and pepper to taste

Method
1. Put all the dressing ingredients into a small jar and mix to combine.
2. Check the flavour and add more lemon, vinegar or seasoning as needed.
3. Keep in the fridge until you're ready to use for up to 1 week. Shake well before using.

Simple cashew cream
Serves 4

This simple cashew cream recipe is the only duplicate from my first book. I've repeated it as it's an essential basic of any whole-food plant-based kitchen. Easy, versatile and simply delicious, once made, you can add both sweet and savoury elements and it can be used raw and heated.

If you can't tolerate cashews, almonds work too (use blanched) or if you are nut free, try it with sunflower seeds. Both will need a longer soaking time, and sunflower seeds leave the cream with a slight grey tinge but still tasting good. This recipe creates a single cream consistency; if you want something a bit thicker, reduce the amount of water used.

Ingredients
150 g cashew nuts
300 ml water (plus water for soaking nuts)
To make sweet cream, add a dash of maple syrup and vanilla essence. For savoury, add nutritional yeast/mustard/garlic powder/salt and pepper/fresh herbs etc

Method
1. Place the cashew nuts in a large bowl, cover with warm water and soak for at least 30 minutes, ideally 2 hours.
2. Drain the nuts and place them in a high-speed blender with the clean water.
3. Blend on high until smooth and creamy.
4. Use immediately or store in a jar in the fridge for up to 3 days.

Raw chocolate sauce
Serves 2

Cacao contains some wonderful polyphenols and is a great source of magnesium. It also tastes awesome. Chocolate products, though, contain high amounts of saturated fat in the cocoa butter, making it one to avoid when eating for autoimmune disease. Fortunately, all is not lost, as can be seen in the baking and dessert sections. This raw chocolate sauce is another recipe to add to the 'Hooray I can eat chocolate' list. Super-simple to make, it's silky smooth and full of deep chocolatey flavour – perfect for pouring on desserts or cakes or for dipping strawberries in. Lovely!

Ingredients
30 g raw cacao powder
4 tbsp maple syrup
1 tsp vanilla essence

Method
1. Place all the ingredients into a small bowl. Stir well to combine using a small balloon whisk – it will take 2-3 minutes to mix.
2. Use immediately or store in a small jar in the fridge for up to 3 days (although it won't last that long!).

Raspberry sauce
Serves 4

Desserts don't have to be complicated. This yummy raspberry sauce is lovely poured over dairy-free yoghurt, pancakes or home-made ice cream. I use frozen raspberries out of season as they release lots of juice. If you have a glut of fresh raspberries, heat is not needed. Just blend and sieve them (if you don't want the seeds) and use straight away. You can use mixed frozen fruit instead if you can't find raspberries.

Ingredients
300 g frozen raspberries or mixed berries
1 tbsp maple syrup
1 tsp lemon juice
1 tsp cornflour

Method
1. Pop the raspberries into a small pan with the maple syrup and bring to a simmer over a medium heat. Mash the berries once soft to release more juice. Simmer for 2-3 more minutes.
2. In a small bowl mix the cornflour with a little of the berry juice to make a paste. Pour it into the raspberry mix with the lemon juice and stir constantly with a wooden spoon until it thickens a little.
3. Turn off the heat and leave to cool. Use straight away or keep in the fridge for up to 4 days.

Spreads and breads

This last section contains a selection of super-tasty dips and spreads to brighten up your lunch or impress guests when they come to visit, worried about what might be served. All the breads are gluten free and can be frozen, so if you are the only one enjoying them, you can be confident that you won't have to worry about eating everything in one go. Unless you want to, of course.

Turmeric hummus
Serves 4

Hummus is a mainstay of my whole-food plant-based diet, so I had to include at least one recipe for it before I tempt you with some alternatives. Super-easy to make, this vibrant yellow hummus is packed with the anti-inflammatory benefits of turmeric, so it needs a bigger than average grinding of black pepper. If you have some to hand, fresh turmeric adds a different dimension flavour-wise, but it can leave you with very stained fingers, so ground turmeric powder is just as good.

Sprinkle the top with freshly chopped red chillis if you can tolerate them and a scattering of fresh coriander; both make the colours sing. A teaspoon of harissa roughly stirred in is another tasty option.

Ingredients
1 x 400-g tin chickpeas or 260 g home-cooked chickpeas
2 tbsp tahini
2 tbsp extra-virgin olive oil, cold-pressed flaxseed oil, or water if oil free
2 cloves roasted garlic or 1 raw garlic, grated
1 lemon, juice only
1 tsp fresh grated turmeric or ½ tsp dried turmeric powder
½ tsp ground paprika
salt and black pepper

To garnish:
chopped red chillis, fresh coriander, 1 tsp harissa, 1 tsp sesame seeds (all optional)

Method
1. Drain the chickpeas and rinse well.
2. Place all the ingredients except for the garnish into a food processor and pulse until everything is well broken down. If the mix is a bit lumpy, add a little water and blend to get the level of smoothness you desire.
3. Check the flavour and add more seasoning or lemon juice if needed.
4. Transfer to a serving dish, garnish and dip in.
5. Store in the fridge for up to 4 days.

White bean, thyme and roasted garlic dip
Serves 4-6

A great alternative to hummus, this delicious dip is perfect as an impressive starter if you're entertaining or just fancy something a bit different for lunch. Use up leftovers as a topping for roasted veg or a baked sweet potato.

I try to keep some roasted garlic in the fridge to make dishes like this. It's easy to do – when the oven is on, wrap a bulb of garlic in some foil and pop in the oven for 30 minutes or so until the cloves are squashy when squeezed. Leave to cool before popping in the fridge in an air-tight container, removing cloves as you need them.

Ingredients
1 x 400-g tin cannellini beans
½ lemon – juice and grated rind
5-6 sprigs fresh thyme or lemon thyme
4 cloves roasted garlic
1-2 tbsp extra-virgin olive oil
salt and pepper

To garnish:
extra thyme and extra-virgin olive oil (optional)

Method
1. Drain the beans and rinse well under running water. Leave to drain.
2. Pick the thyme leaves off the woody stems and roughly chop. Peel the roasted garlic cloves, discarding the skin.
3. Place all the ingredients except those for the garnish into a food processor and blend til smooth.
4. Taste and add more salt, pepper or lemon as needed.
5. Transfer to a small bowl and keep in the fridge for up to 3 days. Garnish with extra olive oil and thyme leaves before serving.

Smoky red lentil dip
Serves 4-6

This is another amazingly simple but super-tasty hummus alternative that will impress dinner guests, family or just yourself. This takes a little longer than the white bean dip above but is still super-simple. Adjust the flavour to suit your taste-buds; feel free to add a little chilli if you enjoy a bit more of a spicy kick.

Ingredients
100 g split red lentils
230 ml vegetable stock
1 bay leaf
3 cloves roasted garlic
½ lemon – juice only
1 tbsp tomato purée (leave out if you avoid tomatoes)
½-1 tsp smoked paprika or hot Spanish smoked paprika
1-2 tbsp extra-virgin olive oil
salt and pepper

Method
1. Rinse the lentils in a sieve under running water whilst the vegetable stock comes to the boil in a small saucepan. Add the bay leaf to the stock and carefully tip in the lentils.
2. Pop on the pan lid and reduce the heat so the lentils simmer for 15-20 minutes until they are soft and the stock is absorbed. Remove from the heat and leave to cool.
3. Once the lentils are cool, remove the bay leaf and place the lentils into a food processor along with the other ingredients.
4. Blend until smooth. Check the flavour and add more salt, pepper, lemon or paprika as needed.
5. Transfer to a bowl and store in the fridge until you're ready to serve for up to 3 days. Garnish with a sprinkle of smoked paprika before serving.

Green pea dip
Serves 4

This pea dip is super-cheap to make and carries a beautifully fresh flavour. Leave out the raw onion if you wish and/or add mint or coriander leaves if you have some to hand. If you don't have soya yoghurt, add a little soya cream or, if not, soya milk to moisten the mix and extra lemon to keep it tart.

Ingredients
150 g frozen peas
2 tbsp red onion or 2-3 spring onions
1 tbsp fresh coriander or mint leaves (optional)
2 tbsp unsweetened soya yoghurt
2-3 tbsp lemon juice
salt and pepper to taste
sprinkle chilli flakes to garnish (optional)

Method
1. If you use a microwave, pop the peas in a microwave proof bowl, cover with water and cook on high for 6 minutes until well cooked. Drain and leave to cool. Alternatively, place the peas in a pan with boiling water. Simmer for 5 minutes until they are well cooked but still a fresh green colour. Drain and cool. Whilst the peas are cooking, finely chop the onion, if using
2. Once the peas are cold, place them in a small blender pot. Add the red onion, coriander or mint (if using), soya yoghurt, lemon juice, salt and pepper. Blend until everything is combined and a rough spread is formed. Check the flavour and add more lemon juice or seasoning as needed.
3. Transfer to a small dish and sprinkle chilli flakes on top if using.
4. This dip will keep in an air-tight container in the fridge for up to 3 days.

Melty vegan 'cheese'
Serves 3-4

This is a super-tasty mix that can be used for pouring on top of roasted vegetables, topping a baked potato, a hot fondue-esque dipping sauce or even spread over toast to create a type of Welsh rarebit. Add more nutritional yeast if you desire. Chilli flakes make a tasty addition too. Once cooled, the mix sets but remains squashy. You can slice it to put in sandwiches or wraps if you desire.

Ingredients
70 g cashew nuts
250 ml water
4 tbsp cornflour/tapioca flour
4 tbsp nutritional yeast
¼ tsp garlic powder
¼ tsp salt

Method
1. Place all the ingredients into a high-speed blender and blend until smooth.
2. Pour into a small saucepan and place over a medium heat. Stir constantly as the

mix thickens very quickly.
3. Continue stirring to prevent lumps forming. Once thick and gooey, turn off the heat.
4. For hot melty cheese or dipping sauce, use immediately. Otherwise, continue to stir until the mix has cooled. Whilst warm and pliable, pour into a container and store in the fridge.

'Ricotta' two ways
Serves 4

One of my favourite flavour combinations is spinach and ricotta. I really missed it when I went dairy free, so I made it my mission to find a good alternative. In the end, I came up with not one but two versions, both super-creamy and delightful. The tofu ricotta adds an extra serving of plant protein and can be made nut free by replacing the cashews with sunflower seeds.

Use the mix to stuff pasta tubes, wraps or on top of veggies. It can also be used as a sauce for lasagne and even in the moussaka recipe in the mains section. Both options store in the fridge for a maximum of 3 days.

Ingredients

For the almond ricotta:
100 g blanched almonds
125 ml water
2 tsp nutritional yeast
½ tsp Himalayan salt
2 tsp lemon juice

For the tofu ricotta:
80 g cashew nuts or sunflower seeds
300 g silken or soft tofu
3 tbsp nutritional yeast
1 tsp salt
3 tbsp lemon juice
¼ tsp garlic powder (optional)

Method
1. For the almond ricotta, soak the nuts for 8 hours or overnight. For the tofu ricotta, soak the cashews for 2 hours or sunflower seeds for 4 hours.
2. Drain the nuts or seeds and rinse well.
3. For each recipe, place all the ingredients into a food processor (preferred) or high-speed blender and blend til smooth. You may need to scrape the sides down a few times to bring things together and blend again.
4. Check the flavour and add more seasonings if desired.
5. Stores in the fridge for up to 3 days.

Mushroom paté
Serves 4-6

Mushrooms mixed with umami tamari and roasted garlic form a deliciously rich whole-food version of paté. What's great about this recipe (apart from the flavour) is that the texture is supported by either walnuts or cooked brown lentils, adding more protein and fibre, plus omega 3 if the walnut option is chosen. Woodland mushrooms are lovely in this paté, but chestnut or even white mushrooms are fine. Lay them gill side up on a sunny windowsill for 15 minutes or so and they'll even make some vitamin D for you.

Unlike some dishes, the flavour fades rather than develops so this paté is best eaten on the same day it's made, or the next at a push. Feel free to use garlic powder rather than roasted garlic. I prefer roasted as it's sweeter but full flavoured. If you're a garlic fiend, feel free to add as much as you like but be careful if you're sharing it with others who might not share your passion for it.

Ingredients
200 g walnuts or cooked brown lentils
1 small onion or medium-sized shallot
1 bay leaf
150 g mushrooms of choice
2 cloves roasted garlic or ½ tsp garlic powder
2 tbsp tamari or coconut amines

2 tbsp lemon juice

salt and pepper

Method
1. If you are using walnuts, pre-heat the oven to 160°C. Pop the walnuts onto a baking tray and lightly toast for a few minutes – you want them releasing their lovely aromas rather than dark brown. Remove from the oven and leave to cool.
2. Finely chop the onion or shallot. Wipe the mushrooms clean and finely chop.
3. Add 2-3 tbsp water to the base of a small pan and add the onion or shallot and the bay leaf. Sauté for 5 minutes over a medium heat then add the chopped mushrooms. Cook for another 5 minutes until the onion is soft and the mushrooms have released their juices. Leave to cool for a few minutes, then remove the bay leaf.
4. Smash the roasted garlic.
5. Add the onion, mushrooms, walnuts or lentils, smashed garlic, tamari, lemon juice, salt and pepper to a small food processor bowl and blitz to combine. Leave a little texture if you like but you want it pretty smooth. Check the flavour and add more tamari, lemon juice or seasoning as desired.
6. Transfer to a small bowl before serving. Tastes lovely with warm sweet potato flatbread.

Sweet potato flatbread
Makes 3

I've not been able to eat 'normal' bread for 16 years now and whilst I can't say I miss it, I do enjoy creating tasty alternatives that I *can* eat. Sweet potato plays the role of binding agent in these simple flatbreads; the extra anti-inflammatory compounds are a bonus.

These flatbreads work best with ancient grains like emmer or spelt but you can be successful with a gluten-free flour mix as well. Make sure there's some xanthum gum in there to stop the bread collapsing. If you prefer to avoid that, add a little cornflour or gram flour to support the structure. The sweet potato can be steamed or baked the day before so it's ready to use when you want to make these breads.

These flatbreads are best eaten on the day they're made (hence the smaller amount of ingredients). If you want to make them in bulk, then just double the recipe and pop the extras in the freezer. Defrost and warm through again before eating.

Ingredients

100 g cooked sweet potato
150 g wholewheat or gluten-free flour
1 tsp baking powder
1 pinch salt
2 tbsp dairy-free yoghurt of choice
water if needed

Method

1. Place the cooked sweet potato into a small blender pot, add a little water and blend until smooth.
2. Place the flour, baking powder and salt into a large bowl and mix well.
3. Add the sweet potato and dairy-free yoghurt to the flour and mix in, first using a spoon and then your hands as it comes together into a soft dough. If the dough is dry, add a tiny bit of water but take great care not to add too much – it doesn't want to be sticky.
4. Gently knead for a couple of minutes until everything is combined and the dough is smooth.
5. Tear off a piece of non-stick baking paper and lightly dust it with a little extra flour. Cut the dough into three equal-sized pieces.
6. Place one of the pieces onto the floured baking paper, squash it a little with your hand then gently roll flat with a rolling pin until it's half 1-cm thick. Don't make it too thin or it won't peel off the paper.
7. Place a large non-stick frying pan onto the hob over a medium heat. Pick up the flatbread on the baking paper and turn it upside down and carefully peel it off into the pan.
8. Cook on one side for 2-3 minutes until it starts to bubble and brown slightly. Carefully turn it over onto the other side and cook for another 2-3 minutes. Transfer to a warm plate and cover with a tea towel whilst you repeat the steps above twice more with the remaining dough.

Buckwheat bread
Makes 12 slices

The original recipe for this tasty bread is oat and buckwheat, one that gets regular feedback on my website, and one I still tend to go for. However, oats are not for everyone, so I wanted to see if this loaf would be as good with just buckwheat – it is. Using a mix of buckwheat flakes and flour, it's lightly textured and full of flavour, much less dense than using soaked buckwheat groats which was the recipe I started with years ago.

Store this loaf in the fridge or a cool place; buckwheat ferments quite readily, forming a funky taste and aroma that haunts your mouth and nose.

Ingredients
40 g buckwheat flakes
1½ tbsp chia seeds
100 ml water
340 g buckwheat flour
115 g buckwheat flakes
1½ tsp baking powder
1 tsp salt
3 tbsp ground flaxseed
3 tbsp pumpkin seeds
3 tbsp sunflower seeds
375 ml water
1 tbsp sunflower seeds extra for top of the loaf

Method
1. Mix the 40 g portion of buckwheat flakes and chia seeds with the 100 ml water and leave to thicken for a few minutes.
2. Line a 2-lb baking tin with non-stick baking paper and pre-heat the oven to 200°C.
3. Place the buckwheat flour, 115 g portion buckwheat flakes, baking powder, salt, ground flaxseed and other seeds in a bowl and mix to combine.

4. Add the thick buckwheat/chia seed paste and 290 ml water. Stir well to bring together into a sticky but not wet mix. Add more water if needed.
5. Transfer the mix to the prepared baking tin, pressing into the sides and flattening the top. Sprinkle the extra seeds over the top and gently press into the mix.
6. Place the tin in the middle of the oven and bake for 30-35 minutes until the top is lightly browned and the bottom sounds hollow when you tap it.
7. Remove from the oven. Lift the loaf out of the tin with the baking paper and transfer to a cooling rack.

Red lentil bread

Makes 12 slices

This tasty loaf is an excellent high-protein option that fills up the hungriest of tummies. Red lentils can be seen as the 'gateway' lentil when it comes to dealing with the side effects of pulses as they have been split and their tough outer coating removed; the skin is often the culprit for excess gas as the microbiome go wild for it. They are also much easier to cook and blend well into a gloopy bread mixture when soaked for a while.

Unlike the buckwheat bread above, soaking time does need to be factored in. Two hours is enough, but I tend to pop the lentils in water just as I go to bed, then they're more than ready the next morning. Once the soaking is done, it's a pretty quick bake.

This bread keeps for 3 days but it freezes well. Cut into slices, then separate each slice with a small piece of non-stick baking paper before you pop it in the freezer. Sounds like a faff but it will ensure you can take out just one or two slices as needed rather than defrost the whole loaf.

Ingredients
340 g red split lentils
300 ml water
100 g gram (chickpea) or green pea flour

2 tbsp ground flaxseed
1 tsp salt
1 tbsp baking powder
2 tbsp psyllium husk
60 g mixed seeds
1 tbsp lemon juice
1 tbsp mixed seeds to top (optional)

Method
1. Rinse the red lentils under running water than place into a large bowl, cover with water and leave to soak for at least 2 hours.
2. Pre-heat the oven to 200°C. Line a 2-lb baking tin with non-stick baking paper.
3. Drain the soaked lentils and place in a food processor with the water. Blend until smooth then pour into a large bowl.
4. Add the gram flour, ground flaxseed, salt, baking powder and psyllium husk. Stir together to combine then add the mixed seeds and lemon juice. Stir again, making sure everything is well combined.
5. Pour the mix into the prepared loaf tin and tap it on the work top. Sprinkle the extra seeds on top, gently pressing them into the mix.
6. Place in the middle of the oven and bake for 40-45 minutes until the top is lightly browned and a skewer comes out clean.
7. Transfer to a cooling rack and leave to cool fully before slicing.

APPENDICES

Appendix 1: Types of fibre — 318
Appendix 2: Different groups of phytonutrients — 320
Resources — 321
References — 325

Appendix 1

Types of fibre

Table A1: Types of fibre

Type of fibre	Soluble or insoluble	Where it's found	What it does
Cellulose, hemi-cellulose	Insoluble	Nuts, whole grains, seeds, skins of fresh produce	Nature's 'brillo pad', keeps bowels active, preventing constipation; reduces risk of diverticulitis and can help with satiety and weight loss
Inulin, oligofructose	Soluble	Onions, beets, chicory root	Prebiotic, supporting beneficial bacteria and immune function
Lignin	Insoluble	Flaxseed, rye and some green leafy veg	Supports heart health, immune function
Mucilage, beta-glucans	Soluble	Oats, beans, peas, barley, flaxseed, berries, soyabeans, bananas, apples, carrots, okra	Helps lower LDL cholesterol, supports heart health, reduces risk of diabetes
Pectin and gums	Soluble (some insoluble)	Fruit, berries, seeds. Often extracted and used in processed foods	Prebiotic. Can slow transit time; lowers blood cholesterol levels
Psyllium	Soluble	Found in seeds from rush plants, husks of Psyllium plants	Prevents constipation; lowers cholesterol
Resistant starch	Soluble	Found in cell walls of plants, particularly in green bananas, oatmeal and legumes	Prebiotic. Increases satiety, controls blood sugar levels, increases insulin sensitivity

Appendix 1

Some fibres are extracted from whole foods and added to processed foods, either to aid binding and texture, or to boost fibre content. Remember, refining foods removes natural fibre. When fibre is added back in it may be in an extract form or in different amounts to what is found in nature. This can have a negative effect, leading to bloating, stomach cramps and increased transit times or act as hidden gluten, which can trigger an inflammatory reaction.

Fibres to watch out for are gums, polydextrose polyols used as bulking agents and sugar substitutes (dextrose, sorbitol and citric acid), modified starch (of which there are many highly chemical options) and wheat dextrin, a soluble fibre extracted from wheat starch and used in many processed foods.

Appendix 2

Different groups of phytonutrients

Table A2: The main types of phytonutrients

Group name	Description
Polyphenols	The largest group of phytonutrients. Contains four different types – phenolic acids, flavonoids, tannins and lignans. Polyphenols you may be familiar with include curcumin, quercetin, resveratrol and the powerful group of flavonoids called anthocyanins
Carotenoids	Another large group, many acting as precursors to vitamin A. Lycopene is in this group although it's not connected to vitamin A, unlike beta-carotene
Glucosinolates and thiocynates	A large group of sulphur-containing biologically active compounds
Limoninoids	A small group found mainly in citrus fruit
Sterols	A small group with a similar structure to cholesterol in animals that helps to reduce blood cholesterol levels. Campesterol is one type

Resources

For a full list of autoimmune conditions with a summary explanation for each, go to the directory on the Autoimmune Association website: https://autoimmune.org/disease-information/

If you haven't already found my website packed with more recipes and information, then head over to: www.thesensitivefoodiekitchen.com for a browse.

Recommended reading

Dr Monica Aggarwal and Dr Jyothi Rao. *Body on Fire: How Inflammation Triggers Chronic Illness and the Tools We Have to Fight It*. Healthy Living Publications, Tennessee, USA; 2020.

Dan Buettner. *The Blue Zones: 9 Lessons for Living Longer from the people who've lived the longest, Second Edition*. National Geographic; 2008.

Dr Nitu Bajekal and Rohini Bajekal. *Living PCOS Free: How to regain your hormonal health with Polycystic Ovary Syndrome*. Hammersmith Health Books; 2022.

Dr Will Bulsiewicz. *Fibre Fuelled: The Plant-Based Gut Health Plan to Lose Weight, Restore Health and Optimise Your Microbiome*. Vermillion, Penguin Random House; 2022.

Brenda Davis, Vesanto Melina and Cory Davis. *Plant Powered Protein: Nutrition Essentials and Dietary Guidelines for All Ages*. Healthy Living Publications, Tennessee, USA; 2023.

Henry Dimbleby. *Ravenous: How to get ourselves and the planet into shape.* Profile Books; 2024.

Dr Alan Desmond. *The Plant-Based Diet Revolution: 28 days to a happier gut and a healthier you.* Yellow Kite; 2024.

Giulia Enders. *Gut: the inside story of our body's most under-rated organ.* Scribe Publications, London; 2017.

Dr Booke Goldner. *Good Autoimmune Disease: How to Prevent and Reverse Chronic Illness and Inflammatory Symptoms using Supermarket Foods.* Express Results, Texas; 2019.

Professor George Jelinek. *Overcoming Multiple Sclerosis: The evidence-based 7 step recovery program, Second Edition.* Allen & Unwin; 2016.

Dr James Kinross. *Dark Matter: The New Science of the Microbiome.* Penguin Life; 2024.

Dr Shireen and Dr Zahra Kassam, *Eating Plant-Based: Scientific Answers to your Nutrition Questions.* Hammersmith Health Books, London; 2022.

Karen Lee. *Eat Well Live Well with The Sensitive Foodie: An accessible, practical guide to eating a whole-food plant-based diet with over 100 recipes.* Sensitive Foodie Books, UK; 2019.

Dr Valter Longo. *The Longevity Diet: Discover the New Science to Slow Ageing, Fight Disease and Manage Your Weight.* Penguin Random House; 2018.

George Monbiot. *Regenesis.* Penguin Random House; 2022.

Dr Gemma Newman. *The Plant Powered Doctor: A simple prescription for a healthier you.* Ebury Press; 2021

Mark Schatzker. *The Dorito Effect: The Surprising New Truth About Food and Flavour.* Simon & Schuster; 2016.

Gin Stephens. *Fast. Feast. Repeat: The Comprehensive Guide to Delay, Don't Deny Intermittent Fasting.* St Martins Publishing Group, New York; 2020.

Dr Chris van Tulleken. *Ultra-Processed People: Why Do We All Eat Stuff That Isn't Food…and Why Can't We Stop?.* Penguin Random House; 2023.

Bee Wilson. *The Way We Eat Now: Strategies for Eating in a World of Change.* 4th Estate; 2020

'How-to' food-related books

Bharat B Aggarwal. *Healing Spices: How to Use 50 Everyday and Exotic Spices to Boost Health and Beat Disease.* Sterling; 2011

Samantha Bax. *Gluten-Free Sourdough Bread Recipes for Beginners.* Prose Books; 2024.

Doug Evans. *The Sprout Book: Tap into the Power of the Planet's Most Nutritious Food.* Essential Publishing; 2020.

Rachel de Thample. *Fermentation: River Cottage Handbook No.18.* Bloomsbury Publishing; 2020.

Helpful websites and organisations

Autoimmune Association – www.autoimmune.org.
US-based non-profit supporting awareness and advocacy for people with autoimmune disease. Lots of free resources and online community for support.

Overcoming MS – www.overcomingms.org.
Full lifestyle-medicine program for managing multiple sclerosis. Website includes resources and research as well as a free community for people around the world, the Live Well Hub.

Plant-Based Health Professionals UK
www.plantbasedhealthprofessionals.com.
Free resources and factsheets about plant-based diets and health conditions. YouTube channel has lots of talks and other resources.

Plants For Health – www.plants-for-health.com.
Information based on the Plants for Joints research study in the Netherlands. Some resources in Dutch only.

Plants For Joints – https://www.amsterdamumc.org/en

Dr Micah Yu: My Autoimmune MD
www.myautoimmunemd.com. Website for US-based doctor with some free resources, including YouTube videos and articles.

Other resources

Finding a plant-based health professional: Where to find a plant-based doctor, dietitian or nutritionist? For the UK, Plant-Based Health Professionals have a list of practising health professionals promoting plant-based nutrition. Find it at www.plantbasedhealthprofessionals.com/directory-of-uk-plant-based-health-professionals

Flaxseed oil: Looking for high-quality omega 3 flaxseed oil? For readers in the UK, I recommend the Flax Farm in Sussex (this is the brand I use), it's the only one I have found that's palatable. Buying direct from the farm means you know it has been stored appropriately to maintain its freshness and minimise the risk of it going rancid. Delivery throughout the UK. www.flaxfarm.co.uk/

Whole grains and pulses: Hodmedod's supply UK-grown whole grains, including ancient and gluten-free grains, beans and legumes. Many are organic and include a wide variety of pulses not usually found in the supermarket. They also have a great supply of pea flours. www.hodmedods.co.uk

Whole foods online: There are a number of online stores selling dried whole foods, herbs and spices. My favourite is Buy Wholefoods Online for their wide choice of products and packet sizes. You can find them at www.buywholefoodsonline.co.uk

Plant-based community kitchens: There are a number popping up around the UK, but with no central database to consult so this list is not definitive:

London	Made in Hackney www.madeinhackney.org
Godalming	Joyful Greens www.joyfullgreen.com
Exeter	Love Food CIC www.lovefoodcic.co.uk
Cambridge	Cambridge Community Kitchen www.cckitchen.uk
Nottingham	Sumac www.sumac.org.uk
Glasgow	Kin Kitchen www.kinkitchenglasgow.org.uk
Greenock	Belville Community Garden www.belvillecommunitygarden.org.uk

References

Introduction

1. Jelinek G. *Overcoming Multiple Sclerosis. The evidence-based 7 step recovery program.* Allen & Unwin, Atlantic Books, London; 2016.
2. Institute for Health Metrics and Evaluation. *Global Burden of Disease 2021: Findings from the GBD 2021 Study.* Seattle, WA: IHME; 2024. https://www.healthdata.org/research-analysis/library/global-burden-disease-2021-findings-gbd-2021-study. (Accessed 27 May 2025.)
3. Conrad N, et al. Incidence, prevalence, and co-occurrence of autoimmune disorders over time and by age, sex and socioeconomic status: a population-based cohort study of 22 million individuals in the UK. *The Lancet* 2023; 401 (10391): 1879-1890.

Chapter 1: What exactly is autoimmune disease and why do I have it?

1. Xiang Y, et al. The role of inflammation in autoimmune disease: a therapeutic target. *Frontiers in Immunology* 2023; 14: 1267091. doi:10.3389/fimmu.2023.1267091
2. The Autoimmune Association. https://autoimmune.org/resource-center/about-autoimmunity/ (Accessed 27 May 2025)
3. Conrad N, et al. Incidence, prevalence, and co-occurrence of autoimmune disorders over time and by age, sex and socioeconomic status: a population-based cohort study of 22 million individuals in the UK. *The Lancet* 2023; 401 (10391): 1879-1890.
4. Thomas SL, et al. Burden of mortality associated with autoimmune diseases

among females in the United Kingdom. *Am J Public Health* 2010; 100(11): 2279-2287. doi:10.2105/AJPH.2009.180273.

5. Welsh S, et al. Autoimmune diseases: a leading cause of death among young and middle-aged women in the United States. *American Journal of Public Health* 2000; 90: 1463-1466. doi:10.2105/AJPH.90.9.1463
6. Furman D, et al. Chronic inflammation in the etiology of disease across the life span. *Nature Medicine* 2019; 25: 1822–1832. doi:10.1038/s41591-019-0675-0
7. Sloan M, et al. Prevalence and identification of neuropsychiatric symptoms in systemic autoimmune rheumatic diseases: an international mixed methods study. *Rheumatology* 2023; 63(5): 1259-1272. doi:10.1093/rhe/kead369
8. Rojas M, et al. Molecular mimicry and autoimmunity. *Journal of Autoimmunity* 2018; 95: 100-123. doi:10.1016/j.jaut.2018.10.012.
9. Pacheco Y, et al. Bystander activation and autoimmunity. *Journal of Autoimmunity* 2019; 103: 102301. doi:10.1016/j.jaut.2019.06.012.
10. Chiavolini D. Comorbidities in autoimmune disease and multiple autoimmune syndrome. Global Autoimmune Institute; 2013. https://www.autoimmuneinstitute.org/articles/comorbidities-in-autoimmune-disease-multiple-autoimmune-syndrome/ (Accessed 2 September 2025)

Chapter 2: Why gut health is so important

1. Wiertsema SP, et al. The Interplay between the Gut Microbiome and the Immune System in the Context of Infectious Diseases throughout Life and the Role of Nutrition in Optimizing Treatment Strategies. *Nutrients* 2021; 13(3): 886. doi:10.3390/nu13030886.
2. Sender R, et al. Revised estimates for the number of human and bacteria cells in the body. *PLOS Biology* 2016; 14 (8): e1002533. doi:10.1371/journal.pbio.1002533
3. Spector T. *The Diet Myth. The real science behind what we eat.* Weidenfeld & Nicholson, London; 2015.
4. Thursby E, Juge N. Introduction to the human gut microbiota. *Biochemical Journal* 2017; 474(11): 1823-1836. doi:10.1042/BCJ20160510.
5. Schlomann BH, Parthasarathy R. Timescales of gut microbiome dynamics. *Current Opinion in Microbiology* 2019; 50: 56-63. doi:10.1016/j.mib.2019.09.011.
6. Kelsey F, et al. Breastmilk Feeding Practices Are Associated with the Co-Occurrence of Bacteria in Mothers' Milk and the Infant Gut: the CHILD Cohort Study. *Cell Host and Microbe* 2020; 28(2): 285-297. doi:10.1016/j.chom.2020.06.009
7. Rinninella E, et al. The role of diet in shaping human gut microbiota. *Best Practice & Research Clinical Gastroenterology* 2023; 62-63: 101828.

References

doi:10.1016/j.bpg.2023.101828.

8. Wang H, et al. Gut microbiome host interactions in driving environmental pollutant trichloroethene-mediated autoimmunity. *Toxicology and Applied Pharmacology* 2021; 424: 115597. doi:10.1016.taap.2021.115597

9. Sutherland N, Coe S, Balogun B. The use of antibiotics on healthy farm animals and antimicrobial resistance. House of Commons Library, UK Parliament; 2023. https://researchbriefings.files.parliament.uk/documents/CDP-2023-0012/CDP-2023-0012.pdf (Accessed 28 May 2025)

10. Beurel E. Stress in the microbiome-immune crosstalk. *Gut Microbes* 2024; 16(1): 2327409. doi: 10.1080/19490976.2024.2327409.

11. Shaheen W, Quraishi M, Iqbal T. Gut microbiome and autoimmune disorders. *Clinical and Experimental Immunology* 2022; 209: 161-174. doi:10.1093/cei/uxac057.

12. National Institutes of Health (NIH). Human Microbiome Project. Reviewed 29 January 2025. https://commonfund.nih.gov/hmp (Accessed 28 May 2025)

13. McDonald D, Hyde E, Debelius JW, Morton JT, et al. American Gut: an Open Platform for Citizen Science. *Microbiome Research* 2018; 3(3): e00031-18. doi:10.1128/msystems.00031-18

14. Human Gut Microbiome Altas. www.microbiomeatlas.org. (Accessed 28 May 2025)

15. Enders G. *Gut: the inside story of our body's most under-rated organ*. Scribe publications, London; 2017.

16. Grondin J, et al. Mucins in intestinal mucosal defence and inflammation: learning from clinical and experimental studies. *Frontiers in Immunology* 2020; 11: 2054. doi:10.3389/fimmu.2020.02054

17. Lo Conte M, et al. Alterations of the intestinal mucus layer correlate with dysbiosis and immune dysregulation in human Type 1 Diabetes. *Lancet eBioMedicine* 2023; 91: 104567. doi:10.1016.j.ebiom.2023.104567.

18. Newman T, Leeming E. Why are short-chain fatty acids important? *Zoe* Updated 17 April 2024. https://zoe.com/learn/what-are-short-chain-fatty-acids (Accessed 4 September 2025)

19. Silva Y, Bernardi A, Frozza R. The role of short-chain fatty acids from gut microbiota in gut-brain communication. *Frontiers in Endocrinology* 2020; 11: 25. doi:10.3389/fendo.2020.00025

20. Candelli M, Franza L, Pignataro G, Ojetti V, et al. Interaction between lipopolysaccharide and gut microbiota in inflammatory bowel disease. *International Journal of Molecular Sciences* 2021; 22 (12): 6242. doi:10.3390/ijms22126242

21. Page M, Kell D, Pretorius E. The role of lipopolysaccharide-induced cell signalling in chronic inflammation. *Chronic Stress* 2022; 6: 1-18. doi:10.1177/24705470221076390
22. Christensen C, et al. Diet, food, and nutritional exposures and Inflammatory Bowel Disease or progression of disease: an umbrella review. *Advances in Nutrition* 2024; 15 (5): 100219. doi.org1016/j.advnut.2024.100219
23. Uyory C. Role of dietary fibre and short-chain fatty acids in preventing neurodegenerative diseases through the gut-brain axis. *Journal of Functional Foods* 2025; 129: 106870. doi:10.1016/j.jff.2025.106870.
24. Bulsiewicz W. *Fibre Fuelled: the plant-based gut health plan to lose weight, restore health and optimise your microbiome.* Vermillion, Ebury Publishing, London; 2020.
25. Marietta E, et al. Intestinal dysbiosis in, and enteral bacterial therapies for, systemic autoimmune diseases. *Frontiers in Immunology* 2020; 11: 573079. doi:10.2289/fimmu.2020.573079

Chapter 3: Inflammatory foods

1. Wang Z, Yuan C, Zhang Y, Abdelaty NS, et al. Food inflammation index reveals the key inflammatory components in foods and heterogeneity within food groups: how do we choose food? *Journal of Advanced Research* 2024; 74: 87-98. doi:10.1016/j.jare.2024.10.010
2. Tsigalou C, et al. Mediterranean Diet as a Tool to Combat Inflammation and Chronic Diseases. An Overview. *Biomedicines* 2020; 8(7): 201. doi:10.3390/biomedicines8070201.
3. Manzel A, et al. Role of 'Western Diet' in inflammatory autoimmune diseases. *Current Allergy and Asthma Reports* 2014; 14(1): 404. doi:10.1007/s11882-013-0404-6.
4. Garcia C, et al. The role of lipids in the regulation of immune responses. *Nutrients* 2023; 15: 3899. doi:10.3390/nu15183899.
5. Yihui S, et al. Metabolic activity induces membrane phase separation in endoplasmic reticulum. *Proceedings of the National Academy of Sciences (PNAS)* 2017; 114(51): 13394-13399. doi: 10.1073/pnas.1712555114
6. González F, et al. Saturated fat ingestion promotes lipopolysaccharide-mediated inflammation and insulin resistance in Polycystic Ovary Syndrome. *Journal of Clinical Endocrinology Metabolism* 2019; 104(3): 934-946. doi:10.1210/jc.2018-01143.
7. Ghezzal S, et al. Palmitic acid damages gut epithelium integrity and initiates inflammatory cytokine production. *Biochimica et Biophysica Acta*

References

(BBA) - Molecular and Cell Biology of Lipids 2020; 1865(2): 158530. doi: 10.1016/j.bbalip.2019.158530.

8. Pagliai G, et al. Nutrients, foods and dietary patterns in the management of autoimmune rheumatic diseases. *Clinical Nutrition Open Science* 2022; 44: 49-65. doi:10.1016/j.nutros.202206.002.
9. Simopoulos A. An increase in the Omega-6/Omega-3 fatty acid ratio increases the risk for obesity. *Nutrients* 2016; 8(3): 128. doi:10.3390/nu8030128
10. Erasmus U. *Fats that heal, fats that kill*. Alive books; 1993.
11. Chen Z. The chemistry behind fried foods: how frying affects flavour, texture and health. *Journal of Food: Microbiology, Safety and Hygiene* 2023; 8(2): 1000205. doi:10.35248/2476-2059.23.8.205
12. De Almeida AJPO, De Oliveira JCPL, da Silva Pontes LV, de Souza JF, et al. ROS: basic concepts, sources, cellular signalling, and its implications in aging pathways. *Oxidative Medicine and Cell Longevity* 2022; 2022: 1225578. doi:10.1155/2022/1225578.
13. Ma X, et al. Excessive intake of sugar: an accomplice of inflammation. *Frontiers in Immunology* 2022; 13: 988481. doi:10.3389/fimmu.2022.988481.
14. Henney AE, et al. Ultra-processed food intake is associated with non-alcoholic fatty liver disease in adults: a systematic review and meta-analysis. *Nutrients* 2023; 15(10): 2266. doi: 10.3390/nu15102266.
15. Plamada D, Vodnar CD. Polyphenols – gut microbiota interrelationship: a transition to a new generation of prebiotics. *Nutrients* 2021; 14(1): 137. doi:10.3390/nu14010137.
16. Kleinewietfeld M, et al. Sodium chloride drives autoimmune disease by the induction of pathogenic TH17 cells. *Nature* 2013; 496(7446): 518-522. doi:10.1038/nature11868.
17. Jobin K, et al. Sodium and its manifold impact on our immune system. *Trends in Immunology* 2021; 42(6): 469-479. doi:10.1016/j.it.2021.04.002
18. Borba V, et al. Bovine milk proteins as a trigger for autoimmune diseases: myth or reality? *International Journal of Celiac Disease* 2020; 8(1): 10-21. doi:1012691/ijed-8-1-3
19. BBC News. Is dairy healthy? Canada's new food guidelines says not necessarily. BBC; 2019. https://www.bbc.co.uk/news/world-us-canada-46964549#. (Accessed 26/5/1025)
20. World Population Review. Lactose intolerance by country 2025. *World Population Review* 2025. https://worldpopulationreview.com/country-rankings/lactose-intolerance-by-country (Accessed 26 May 2025)
21. Cusick M, Libbey J, Fujinami R. Molecular mimicry as a mechanism of

autoimmune disease. *Clinic Reviews in Allergy and Immunology* 2012; 42: 102-111. doi:10.1007/s12016-011-8294-7
22. Gottlieb S. Early exposure to cow's milk raises risk of diabetes in high risk children. *British Medical Journal* 2000; 321(7268): 1040.
23. Wang Y, et al. The effects of red meat intake on inflammation biomarkers in humans: a systematic r review and meta-analysis of randomised controlled trials. *Current Developmets in Nutrition* 2022; 6(S1): 994. doi: 10.1093/cdn/nzac068.023.
24. Zhang Y, et al. Arachidonic acid metabolism in health and disease. *MedComm* 2023; 4(5): e363. doi: 10.1002/mco2.363
25. Samraj A, et al. A red meat-derived glycan promotes inflammation and cancer progression. *PNAS* 2014; 112(2): 542-547. doi:10.1073/pnas.1417508112

Chapter 4: What is a whole-food plant-based diet and why does it help?

1. Remde A, et al. Plant-predominant eating patterns – how effective are they for treating obesity and related cardiometabolic health outcomes? – a systematic review. *Nutrition Reviews* 2022; 80(5): 1094–1104. doi:10.1093/nutrit/nuab060.
2. Slywitch E, et al. Iron deficiency in vegetarian and omnivorous individuals: analysis of 1340 individuals. *Nutrients* 2021; 13(9): 2964. doi:10.3390/nu13092964.
3. British Dietetic Association. Vegetarian, vegan and plant-based diets. BDA. www.bda.uk.com/resource/vegetarian-vegan-plant-based-diet.html (Accessed 27 May 2025)
4. Ritchie H, Rosado P, Roser M. Hunger and undernourishment. *Our World in Data* 2023. https://ourworldindata.org/hunger-and-undernourishment (Accessed 28 May 2025).
5. Rauber F, et al. Ultra-processed foods and excessive free sugar intake in the UK: a nationally representative cross-sectional study. *BMJ Open* 2019; 9(10): e027546. doi: 10.1136/bmjopen-2018-027546
6. Gibney MJ. Ultra-processed foods: definitions and policy issues. *Current Developments in Nutrition* 2018; 3(2): nzy077. doi:10.1093/cdn/nzy077.
7. Monteiro C, et al. *Ultra-processed foods, diet quality, and health using the NOVA classification system.* Rome: Food and Agriculture Organisation of the United Nations; 2019. https://openknowledge.fao.org/server/api/core/bitstreams/5277b379-0acb-4d97-a6a3-602774104629/content (Accessed 4 September 2025)

References

8. Naimi S, et al. Direct impact of commonly used dietary emulsifiers on human gut microbiota. *Microbiome* 2021; 9: 66. doi:10.1186/s40168-020-00996-6
9. Van Tulleken C. *Ultra-Processed People: why do we all eat stuff that isn't food…and why can't we stop?*. London, UK: Penguin; 2024.
10. Nutrition Science Team. *Government dietary recommendations*. Public Health England; 2016. https://assets.publishing.service.gov.uk/media/5a749fece5274a44083b82d8/government_dietary_recommendations.pdf. Accessed 28 May 2025
11. Cooper H, et al. UK still failing to meet basic dietary guidelines. The Food Foundation. https://foodfoundation.org.uk/news/uk-still-failing-meet-basic-dietary-guidelines (Accessed 31 August 2025)
12. Chiba M, Ishii H, Komatsu M. Recommendation of plant-based diets for inflammatory bowel disease. *Translational Pediatrics* 2018; 8(1): 23-27. doi:10.21037/tp.2018.12.02
13. Berer K, et al. Dietary non-fermentable fibre prevents autoimmune neurological disease by changing gut metabolic and immune status. *Nature – Scientific Reports* 2018; 8: 10431. doi:10.1038/s41598-018-28839-3
14. Zegarra-Ruiz D, et al. A diet-sensitive commensal Lactobacillus strain mediates TLR7-dependent systemic autoimmunity. *Cell Host and Microbe* 2019; 1: 113-127. doi:10.1016/j.chom.2018.11.009.
15. Gallicchio L, et al. Carotenoids and the risk of developing lung cancer: a systematic review. *American Journal of Clinical Nutrition* 2008; 88(2): 372-383. doi:10.1093/ajcn/88.2.372
16. Golpour F, et al. Short chain fatty acids, a possible treatment option for autoimmune diseases. *Biomedicine and Pharmacotherapy* 2023; 163:114763. doi:10.1016/j.biopha.2023.114763.
17. Kent K, et al. Food-based anthocyanin intake and cognitive outcomes in human intervention trials: a systematic review. *Journal of Human Nutrition and Dietetics* 2016; 30(3): 260-274. doi:10.1111//jhn.12431.
18. Khan H, et al. Polyphenols in the treatment of autoimmune diseases. *Autoimmune Review* 2019; 18(7): 647-657. doi:10.1016/j.autrev.2019.05.001.
19. Heidt C, et al. MCT-induced ketosis and fibre in Rheumatoid Arthritis (MIKARA) – study protocol and primary endpoint results of the double blind randomised controlled intervention study indication effects on disease activity in RA patients. *Nutrients* 2023; 15(17): 3719. doi:10.3390/nu1513719.
20. Zhang Q, Sun W, Wang Q, et al. A high MCT-based ketogenic diet supresses Th1 and Th17 responses to ameliorate experimental autoimmune encephalomyelitis in mice by inhibiting GSDMD and JAK2-STAT3/4 pathways.

Molecular Nutrition and Food Research 2023; 68(3): e2300602. doi:10.1002/mnfr.202300602

21. Baker E, et al. Metabolism and functional effects of plant-derived omega-3 fatty acids in humans. *Progress in Lipid Research* 2016; 64: 30-56. doi:10.1016/j.plipres.2016.07.002.

22. Cheng Y, Yang Y, Bai L. Cui J. Microplastics: an often-overlooked issue in the transition from chronic inflammation to cancer. *Journal of Translational Medicine* 2024; 22(1): 959. doi:10.1186/s12967-024-05731-5

Chapter 5: Starting your healing journey

1. Gregory A. One in three adults in UK and Ireland eat five or more daily portions of fruit and veg. *The Guardian* 1 January 2024. https://www.theguardian.com/lifeandstyle/2024/jan/01/adults-uk-ireland-five-daily-portions-fruit-and-veg (Accessed 15 August 2025)

2. Aune D, et al. Fruit and vegetable intake and the risk of cardiovascular disease, total cancer and all-cause mortality – a systematic review and dose-response meta-analysis of prospective studies. *International Journal of Epidemiology* 2017; 46(3): 1029-1056. doi:10.1093/ije/dyw319

3. Schnorr S, et al. Gut microbiome of the Hazda hunter-gatherers. *Nature Communications* 2014; 5: 3654. doi:10.1038/ncomms4654.

4. Varela A, et. Patient empowerment: a critical evaluation and prescription for a foundational definition. *Frontiers in Psychology* 2025; 15: 1064-1078, doi:10.3389/fpsyg.2024.1473345

Chapter 6: But what about…? Myth busting

1. Pardali E, et al. Autoimmune protocol diet: a personalised elimination diet for patients with autoimmune diseases. *Metabolism Open* 2024; 25: 100342. doi:101016.j.metop.2024.100342.

2. Chandrasekaran A, Groven S, Lewis JD, Levy SS, et al. An Autoimmune Protocol diet improves patient-reported quality of life in Inflammatory Bowel Disease. *Crohns Colitis* 2019; 360, 1(3): otz019. doi:10.1093/crocol/otz019.

3. Abbot R, Sadowski A, Alt A. Efficacy of the Autoimmune Protocol diet as part of a multi-disciplinary, supported lifestyle intervention for Hashimoto's thyroiditis. *Cureus* 2019; 11(4): e4556. doi:10.7759/cureus.4556.

4. Devlin, H. Hunter-gatherers were mostly gatherers, says archaeologist. *The Guardian*; 24 January 2024. https://www.theguardian.com/science/2024/

References

jan/24/hunter-gatherers-were-mostly-gatherers-says-archaeologist (Accessed 4 September 2025)

5. Revedin A, et al Thirty thousand-year-old evidence of plant food processing. *PNAS* 2010; 107(44): 18815-18819. doi: 10.1073/pnas.1006993107.
6. The Food Foundation. *The Broken Plate 2025.* https://foodfoundation.org.uk/publication/broken-plate-2025. 29 January 2025. (Accessed 16 August 2025)
7. Buettner D, Skemp S. Blue Zones: Lessons from the world's longest lived. *American Journal of Lifestyle Medicine* 2016; 10(5): 318-321. doi:10.1177/1559827616637066
8. World Health Organization. Cancer: carcinogenicity of the consumption of red meat and processed meat. WHO; 26 October 2015. https://www.who.int/news-room/questions-and-answers/item/cancer-carcinogenicity-of-the-consumption-of-red-meat-and-processed-meat (Accessed 16 August 2025)
9. Rodhouse J, et al. Red kidney bean poisoning in the UK: an analysis of 50 suspected incidents between 1979 and 1989. *Epidemiology and Infection* 1990; 105(3): 485-491.
10. UK Health Security Agency. Non-typhoidal Salmonella data 2013 to 2022. Gove.UK; updated 26 June 2025. https://www.gov.uk/government/publications/salmonella-national-laboratory-and-outbreak-data/non-typhoidal-salmonella-data-2013-to-2022#foodborne-outbreak-data-in-2022 (Accessed 16 August 2025)
11. Nciri N, et al. Toxicity assessment of common beans (Phaseolus vulgaris L.) widely consumed by Tunisian population. *Journal of Medicinal Food* 2015; 18(():1049-1064. doi:10.1089/jmf.2014.0120.
12. Nciri N, Cho N, Bergaoui N, Ammar AB, et al. Effect of white kidney bean (Phaseolus vulgaris L. var. Beldia) on small intestine morphology and function in Wistar rats. *Journal of Medicinal Food* 2015; 18(12): 1387-1399. doi:10.1089/jmf.2014.0193.
13. NHS Website. Causes: Kidney stones. NHS, UK; updated 30 November 2022. https://www.nhs.uk/conditions/kidney-stones/causes/. (Accessed 28 May 2025.)
14. Lopez-Moreno M, Garces-Rimon M, Miguel M. Antinutrients: Lectins, goitrogens, phytates and oxalates, friends or foe?. *Journal of Functional Foods* 2022; 89:104938. doi:10.1016/j.jff.2022.104938.
15. Kayashima T, Katayama T. Oxalic acid is available as a natural antioxidant in some systems. *Biochimica et Biophysica Acta (BBA) – General Subjects* 2002; 1573(1): 1-3. doi:10.1016/S0304-4165(02)00338-0.
16. Liu M, et al. Microbial genetic and transcriptional contributions to oxalate degradation by the gut microbiota in health and disease. *Elife* 2021; 26(10):

e63642. doi:10.7554/eLife.63642.
17. Guerlain J, et al. Localization and characterization of thyroid microcalcifications: a histopathological study. *PLoS One* 2019; 24(10): e0224138. doi:10.1371//journal.pone.0224138.
18. Kapała A, Szlendak M, Motacka E. The anti-cancer activity of lycopene: a systematic review of human and animal Studies. *Nutrients* 2022;14(23): 5152. doi:10.3390/nu14235152
19. Przybylska S, Tokarczy G. Lycopene in the prevention of cardiovascular diseases. *International Journal of Molecular Science* 2022; 23(4): 1957. doi:10.3390/ijms23041957.
20. Xiang Y, et al. Beneficial effects of dietary capsaicin in gastrointestinal health and disease. *Experimental Cell Research* 2022; 417(2): 113227. doi:10.1016/j.excr.2022.113227.
21. Iablokov V, et al. Naturally occurring glycoalkaloids in potatoes aggravate intestinal inflammation in tow mouse models of inflammatory bowel disease. *Digestive Diseases and Sciences* 2010; 55(11): 3078-3085. doi:10.1007/s10620-010-1158-9.
22. Patel B, et al. Potato glycoalkaloids adversely affect intestinal permeability and aggravate inflammatory bowel disease. *Inflammatory Bowel Diseases* 2002; 8(5): 340-346. doi:10.1097/00054725-200209000-00005.
23. Chipman J, et al. Risk assessment of glycoalkaloids in feed and food, in particular in potatoes and potato-derived products. *EFSA Journal* 2020; 18(8): e06222. doi:10.2903/j.efsa.2020.6222.
24. Petroski W, Minich D. Is there such a thing as 'anti-nutrients'? A narrative review of perceived problematic plant compounds. *Nutrients* 2020; 12: 2929. doi:10.3390/nu12102929.
25. Celiac Disease Foundation. Autoimmune disorders. https://celiac.org/about-celiac-disease/related-conditions/autoimmune-disorders/ (Accessed 17 August 2025)
26. Philip A, White N. Gluten, inflammation and neurodegeneration. *American Journal of Lifestyle Medicine* 2022; 16(1): 32-35. doi.10.1177/1559827611049345.
27. Lerner, A, et al. Gluten-free diet can ameliorate the symptoms of non-celiac autoimmune diseases. *Nutrition Reviews* 2022; 80(3): 525-543. doi:10.1093/nutrit/nuab039.
28. Novick J. The myth of complementary protein. *Forks over Knives*. Updated 5 August 2024. https://www.forksoverknives.com/wellness/the-myth-of-complementary-protein/ (Accessed 17 August 2025)
29. British Dietetic Association. Vegetarian, vegan and plant-based diets. BDA.

https://www.bda.uk.com/resource/vegetarian-vegan-plant-based-diet.html (Accessed 27 May 2025)

Chapter 7: What am I actually going to eat?

1. EWG's Shoppers Guide. The 2025 Dirty Dozen. https://www.ewg.org/foodnews/dirty-dozen.php (Accessed 29 May 2025)
2. PAN UK. *Dirty Dozen 2023*. https://www.pan-uk.org/site/wp-content/uploads/Dirty-Dozen-2024.pdf (Accessed 30 May 2025.)
3. Govers C, et al. Review of the health effects of berries and their phytochemicals on the digestive and immune systems. *Nutrition Reviews* 2018; 76(1): 29-46. doi:10/1093/nutrit/nux039.
4. Oliveira AL, et al. Resveratrol role in autoimmune disease – a mini-review. *Nutrients* 2017; 9: 1306. doi:10.3390/nu912306.
5. Jiang Y, Wu S-H, Shu X-O, Xiang Y-B, et al. Cruciferous vegetable intake is inversely correlated with circulating levels of proinflammatory markers in women. *Journal of the Academy of Nutrition and Dietetics* 2014; 114(5): 700-8.e2. doi:10.1016/j.jand.2013.12.019.
6. Petroski W, Minich D. Is there such a thing as 'anti-nutrients'? A narrative review of perceived problematic plant compounds. *Nutrients* 2020; 12:2929.
7. Martins T, et al. Enhancing health benefits through chlorophylls and chlorophyll-rich agro-food: a comprehensive review. *Molecules* 2020; 28(14): 5344. doi:10.3390/molecules28145344.
8. University of Arkansas. Cook your carrots for more antioxidants. *Science Daily* 7 September 2000. www.sciencedaily.com/releases/2000/09/000904124728.htm . (Accessed 30 May 2025.)
9. Lull C, Wichers H, Savelkoul H. Anti-inflammatory and immunomodulating properties of fungal metabolites. *Mediators of Inflammation* 2005; 2: 63-80. doi:10.1155/MI.2005.63.
10. Schwartz B, Hadar Y. Possible mechanisms of action of mushroom-derived glucans on inflammatory bowel disease and associated cancer. *Annals of Translational Medicine* 2014; 2(2): 19. doi:10.3978/j.issn.2305-5839.2014.01.03.
11. Meng M, et al. Potential anti-rheumatoid arthritis activities and mechanisms of *Ganoderma lucidum polysaccharides. Molecules* 2023; 28(6): 2483. doi:10.3390/molecules28062483
12. Zhao S, et al. Immunomodulatory Effects of Edible and Medicinal Mushrooms and Their Bioactive Immunoregulatory Products. *Journal of Fungi* 2020; 6(4): 269. doi: 10.3390/jof6040269.

13. Chang CJ, et al. *Ganoderma lucidum reduces obesity in mice by modulating the composition of the gut microbiota*. Nature Communications 2025; 6: 7489. doi:10.1038/ncomms8489
14. Zargarzadeh N, et al. Legume consumption and risk of all-cause and cause-specific mortality: a systematic review and dose-response meta-analysis of prospective studies. *Advances in Nutrition* 2023; 14(1): 64-76. doi:10.1016/j.advnut.2022.10.009.
15. Bambridge-Sutton A. Soy animal feed's trail of deforestation: what are the solutions? *Food Navigator Europe* 14 June 2023. https://www.foodnavigator.com/Article/2023/06/14/soy-animal-feed-s-trail-of-deforestation-what-are-the-solutions/ (Accessed 30 May 2025.)
16. Khan D, Ansar Ahmed S. The Immune System Is a Natural Target for Estrogen Action: Opposing Effects of Estrogen in Two Prototypical Autoimmune Diseases. *Frontiers of Immunology* 2016; 6: 635. doi: 10.3389/fimmu.2015.00635
17. Khan D, Ansar Ahmed S. The immune system is a natural target for estrogen action: opposing effect of estrogen in two prototypical autoimmune diseases. *Frontiers in Immunology* 2016; 6: 635. doi:10.3389/fimmu.2015.00635.
18. Chakraborty D, Gupta K, Biswas S. A mechanistic insight of phytoestrogens used for Rheumatoid arthritis: an evidence-based review. *Biomedicine and Pharmacotherapy* 2020; 233: 111039. doi:10.1016/j.biopha.202.111039.
19. Balakrishna R, et al. Consumption of nuts and seeds and health outcomes including cardiovascular disease, diabetes and metabolic disease, cancer and mortality: an umbrella review. *Advances in Nutrition* 13(6): 2136-2148. doi:10.1093/advances/nmac077.
20. De Vito R, et al. Olive oil and nuts in Rheumatoid Arthritis activity. *Nutrients* 2023; 15(4): 963. doi:10.3390/nu150400963.
21. Barbhaiya M, et al. Association of dietary quality with risk of incident systemic lupus erythematosus in the Nurses' Health Study and Nurses' Health Study II. *Arthritis Care and Research* 2020; 73(9): 1250-1258. doi:10.1002/acr.24443.
22. Sharifi M, et al. Association between multiple sclerosis and dietary patterns based on the traditional concept of food nature: a case-control study in Iran. *BMC Neurology* 2021; 21: 453. doi:10.1186/s12883-021-02483-3.
23. Negi R, et al. Efficacy of Ginger in the Treatment of Primary Dysmenorrhea: A Systematic Review and Meta-analysis. *Cureus* 2021; 13(3): e13743. doi:10.7759/cureus.13743.
24. Sun J, et al. A comprehensive review on the effects of green tea and its components on the immune function. *Food Science and Human Wellness* 2022; 11(5): 1143-1155. doi:10.1016/j.fshw.2022.04.008.

25. Alok P, et al. Are fermented foods effective against Inflammatory Diseases? *International Journal of Environmental Research and Public Health* 2023; 20(3): 2481. doi:10.3390/ijerph20032481.
26. Yong C, et al. Effect of Lactobacillus Fermentation on the anti-inflammatory potential of turmeric. *Journal of Microbiology and Biotechnology* 2019; 29(10): 1561-1569. doi:10.4104/jmb.1906.06032.
27. Matas A, et al. Urinary tract infection and autoimmune disease. *Handbook of Systemic Autoimmune Diseases* 2020; 16:49-57. doi:10.1016/B978-0-444-64217-2.000003-8.
28. Caslin B, et al. Alcohol as friend or foe in autoimmune diseases: a role for gut microbiome? *Gut Microbes* 2021; 13(1): 1916278. doi:10.1080/19490976.2021.1916278.

Chapter 8: Final things to consider

1. Bishehsari F, et al. Circadian rhythms in gastrointestinal health and diseases. *Gastroenterology* 2016; 151: e1-e5. doi:10.1053/j.gastro.2016.07.036.
2. Stenger S, et al. Potential effects of shift work on skin autoimmune diseases. *Frontiers in Immunology* 2023; 13: 1000951. doi:10.3389/fimmu.2022.1000951.
3. Cleveland Clinic. Autophagy. https://my.clevelandclinic.org/health/articles/24058-autophagy Last updated 23 August 2022. (Accessed 30 May 2025.)

Index

acrylamide 56, 156
adaptive (learned) immune system 18–19, 41, 64, 137, 147
additives 78
adipose tissue 59
agriculture *see* farming/agriculture
air fryer 57, 156
alcohol 151
algae and algae oil 65, 89–90, 96, 137–138
Alliaceae and Allium 125
almond
   and apricot chia breakfast pot 179–180
   broccoli and almond soup 190–191
   and cardamom balls 276–277
   'ricotta' 309, 310
aloo tikki balls 231–232
alpha-lipoic acid (ALA) 88, 89
amaranth and millet pancakes 220–221
Amazon, deforestation 67
American Gut Project 99
amino acids 73, 120, 121
   essential 119, 120
ancient/early/prehistoric/ancestors 76, 99, 108, 108–109, 127, 137, 144
animal agriculture
   antibiotics 36*fn*, 63
   subsidies 76
antacids 37
anthocyanins 86, 97, 114, 127, 200
antibiotics (and antibacterial drugs) 35, 36, 44
   animal agriculture 63, 66
   resistance 36, 63
antibodies 14, 18, 19
   autoimmune (autoantibodies) 19, 26
anti-nutrients 108, 109–110, 111, 116

antioxidants 84
   coloured food 136
apple(s) 70–71
   and apricot and oat bars 262–264
   and blackberry traybake 286–287
   and salted caramel slice 292–294
apricot
   and almond chia breakfast pot 179–180
   and apple and oat bars 262–264
   tempeh and hazelnut and apricot bake 247–248
arachidonic acid (AA) 66–67
arthritis
   psoriatic 10, 21, 115
   rheumatoid (RA) 14, 15, 21, 60, 64, 66, 67, 83, 87, 129, 137, 139, 142, 144
artichokes, Jerusalem 103
artificial sweeteners (sugar substitutes) 82, 319
ashwagandha 146
asparagus 138
   and broccoli pasta with white bean sauce 238–239
   and pea and rocket salad 213–214
aubergine (eggplant) 114
   for moussaka 248, 249, 250
autoantibodies (autoimmune antibodies) 19, 26
Autoimmune Association 323
autoimmune disease 13–27
   causes and risk factors 5, 13, 22–26, 38, 59
   definition 13–15
   diagnosis of and difficulties in 16
   disease-modifying therapies 162–163

nightshades and 114
polyphenols and 86
seven steps to healing 91–106, 154, 165
signs and symptoms 15–16
types 15–16
Autoimmune Protocol 107–108
autophagy 158–159, 160
avocado 55, 94, 161, 162

B cells 19, 41
babies and infants
    birth and feeding and the microbiome 34–35
    diarrhoea 36
'bacon', tempeh 185
bacteria 17–18, 19, 65, 77, 86–87, 149
    bad/pathogenic 37, 38, 41, 43, 44, 48, 63, 85, 86, 103, 104, 118, 124, 135, 154
    friendly/beneficial 30, 35, 36, 38, 43, 61
    infection by 23
    meat and 65
Bakewell flapjacks, cherry 268–269
Bakewell raspberry tart 284–286
baking (in oven) 156
banana 130, 161, 162
    banana breakfast bars 186–187
beans 110–111, 138–142
    black bean soup 200–201
    greens and mushrooms and 184–185
    Italian bean soup 198–199
    kidney, red 110–111
    portions per day of 166
    smoky 223
    sprouting see soaking and sprouting
    two-bean salad 204–205
    white see white bean
bechamel sauce for moussaka 249, 250
beetroot 134
    and watercress salad 212
berbere 231
berries 127–128
beta-carotene 85, 114, 133, 134

beta-glucans (β-glucans) 318
bhajis, tempeh onion 217–219
birth and the microbiome 34–35
bisphenol A (BPA) 36
black beans
    black bean chocolate brownies 264–266
    black bean soup 200–201
Black Forest fruit smoothie 176–177
black grapes 129
black pepper 146
blackberry and apple traybake 286–287
bloating 79–80, 81, 104, 105
blood vessels, leaky 18, 46
blue foods 98
Blue Zones 109
blueberry lemon tarts (raw) 282–283
boswellia 146
bottle-feeding and infant microbiome 35
bowel see intestine
BPA (bisphenol A) 36
brain–gut interactions 37–38, 47
bread-making 116, 117
breads and spreads 304–315
breakfast 176–187
    three-day sample menu 175
breast-feeding and infant microbiome 35
broad bean, mangetout and new potato salad with crispy smoked tofu 202–204
broccoli
    and almond soup 190–191
    asparagus and broccoli pasta with white bean sauce 238–239
    and kale tart 254–256
    quick, and smoked tofu rice 239–241
brown foods 97, 98
brownies, black bean chocolate 264–266
bubble and squeak, baked 224
buckwheat bread 313–314
bulbs and stems 135
butter, alternatives 271, 284
butter beans 139
butternut squash rings with smoky chickpeas 258–259

Index

butyrophilin 63, 64
bystander activation 21–22, 63–64

cabbage slices (roasted), aromatic millet and tahini dressing 260–261
Caesarean section and infant microbiome 34
calcium 112, 145, 161
calcium oxalate compounds 112
calorie intake 52
    ensuring sufficiency 174
    low *see* low-calorie intake
cancer risk and soya 142
capsaicin 114
caramel (salted) and apple slice 292–294
carbohydrate 58, 60, 73
    complex 58, 78
    differentiating 'good' from 'bad' carbs 79–81
    see also fibre
cardamom
    almond and cardamom balls 276–277
    plum and cardamom balls 273–274
β-carotene (beta-carotene) 85, 114, 133, 134
carotenoids 320
carrot 134
    flapjacks 226–227
    and maple muffins 274–276
    rainbow 134
        and thyme salad 209–210
    sweet carrot scones 271–272
casein 26, 64
cashew 'cheese' sauce 235
cashew cream 283, 301
catechins 147
cauliflower
    baked mini Romanesco cauliflower 234–235
    creamy cauliflower curry 229–231
    crunchy cauliflower bites 216–217
celeriac soup with chickpea croutons 191–193
cell membranes 52, 53, 63, 63

cellulose 318
chard
    chickpeas and 219–220
    Swiss 132
cheese (alternatives to dairy cheese) 61–62, 154
    melty vegan 'cheese' 308–309
    'ricotta' 309–310
'cheesecake', baked 288–291
cherry Bakewell flapjacks 268–269
chia (seeds) 90, 94, 95, 145
    almond and apricot chia breakfast pot 179–180
    chocolate and chia pudding 281
chickpeas
    celeriac soup with chickpea croutons 191–193
    chard and 219–220
    sesame-baked butternut squash rings with smoky chickpeas 258–259
    smashed 215–216
    turmeric hummus 304–305
    vegetable curry with chickpea dumplings 243–245
children
    'hygiene hypothesis' 35–36
    trauma 24
    see also babies and infants
chillies/chilli peppers 114
chlorella 89, 95, 96
chlorophyll 132
chocolate
    black bean brownies 264–266
    sauce 301–302
citrus fruits 129–130
coeliac disease 14, 29, 110, 113, 118, 143, 144
colon (and large intestine) 30, 39, 43, 78
colours of food *see* rainbow colours
community 163
    kitchens 69, 164, 324
constipation 31, 104
cookies, spiced 269–271
cooking and heating 56–57, 155–157

coriander, spinach and squash soup 194–195
corticosteroids (referred to as 'steroids') 162–163
Covid 19 pandemic 23, 148
cow's milk *see* dairy
Crohn's disease 10, 29, 44, 93, 120, 140, 183
cruciferous vegetables 104–105, 130–132, 162
cumin 146
    and turmeric traybake 256–257
curry
    creamy cauliflower 229–231
    vegetable, with chickpea dumplings 243–245

dairy (incl. cow's milk) 61–64
    avoidance/replacement 63–64, 154
    intolerance and sensitivities 11, 61, 63, 81, 104, 124, 139, 144
    see also cheese
dates
    in apple and apricot oat bars 263
    in apple and salted caramel slice 292, 293
    in cumin and turmeric traybake 257
    sticky date and ginger cake 267–268
deforestation (Amazon) 67
desserts 278–294
DHA 88, 89, 95, 96
diabetes type 1 2, 42, 64, 83, 117, 129
    time-restricted eating and 159fn)
diarrhoea 82–83
    infants 36
diet 26
    elimination 108, 124
    keto 50, 159
    Mediterranean 50, 109, 113, 136, 144–145
    microbiome and 35
    paleo 107, 108
    supplements *see* supplements
    Western 6, 31, 35, 54, 55, 57–58, 59, 74, 88, 130, 167
    whole-food plant-based *see* whole-food plant-based diet
    see also food; nutrients; nutritional advice
Dietary Inflammatory Index (Food Inflammatory Index; FII) 49–50
dimethyl fumarate (Tecfidera) 162
dinner and main meals 243–261
    friends and guests 102, 164, 278, 292, 304, 306
    recipes 243–261
    three-day sample menu 175
disaccharides, fermentable 81
disease-modifying therapies 162–163
docosahexaenoic acid (DHA) 88, 89, 95, 96
dopamine 38, 58, 75
dressings 295–303
    salads 205, 208, 212, 213, 214, 298
    tahini *see* tahini dressing
    see also sauces
drinks 150–151
drugs *see* medications
dysbiosis 33, 38–48, 81, 138, 139

Eat Well Live Well course 155
Eat Well Live Well with The Sensitive Foodie 165
eggplant *see* aubergine
eicosapentaenoic acid (EPA) 88, 89, 95, 96
8:16 diet plan 159, 161
elderflower dressing 300
elimination diet 108, 124
empowerment 105–106
emulsifiers 77–78
endotoxin (lipopolysaccharide; LPS) 44, 45
energy source 43
    fats as 43, 52
    sugar (glucose as) 57
environment
    microbiome and 35–36, 99
    toxins 23–24, 36
EPA 88, 89, 95, 96
epigenetic modulation 86

Index

Epstein Barr virus (EBV) 23
essential amino acids 119, 120
essential fatty acids 55–57, 88–89, 94
Ethiopian split pea stew 231–232
evidence-based nutritional advice 8

farming/agriculture 108
    animal *see* animal agriculture
    fish 89
    soya bean 141
farting (wind; flatulence) 43*fn*, 103, 105, 135, 139, 141
fasting 159, 159–161
fat (and fatty acids) 52–57, 73, 74, 87–90
    cooking and heating 56–57, 155–157
    as energy source 43, 52
    essential 55–57, 88–89, 94
    healthy 55, 57, 87–90, 94–96
    high-fat foods 50, 57, 159
    ice cream 58
    saturated 52–54
    short-chain fatty acids (SCFAs) 43, 46–48, 59, 79, 86–87, 148, 149
    unsaturated *see* unsaturated fat/fatty acids
    see also oil
fatty liver disease 59, 126
fava beans 139
female (being a) as autoimmune disease risk factor 25
fermentable fibre (prebiotics) 81, 103, 104, 135
fermentable oligosaccharides, disaccharides, monosaccharides and polyols 81
fermented foods 148–150
    turmeric 149
fibre 73, 78–83, 102–105, 318–319
    added-back 319
    complex 43, 70, 83, 108
    fermentable (prebiotics) 80, 81, 103, 104, 135
    high-fibre foods/diet 126, 139, 162
    increasing your intake 102–105
    insoluble 43, 47, 80, 129, 318

    recommended intake 79
    roles in gut 30, 43, 79
    soluble 73, 80, 104, 318
fish farming 89
fish oil 89, 96
5:2 diet plan 159, 160
flapjacks
    carrot 226–227
    cherry Bakewell 268–269
flatbread, sweet potato 311–312
flatulence (wind; farting) 43fn, 103, 105, 135, 139, 141
flavonoids 127, 129, 131, 133
flaxseed(s) 95, 145
    oil 55, 90, 96, 145, 323–324
FODMAPs 81–83, 124, 139
food(s) 49–67
    additives 78
    book's focus on 5, 70, 146, 164
    choosing 125–151
    fermented *see* fermented foods
    groups and types 69, 125
    inflammatory 49–67
    processed and refined *see* processed and refined food
    rainbow colours *see* rainbow colours
    supplements *see* supplements
    varieties and diversity 99–100
    see also diet; nutrients; nutritional advice; whole-food plant-based diet
food allergies/intolerances/sensitivities 11, 81, 91, 124, 144
    dairy (milk and lactose) 11, 61, 63, 81, 104, 124, 139, 144
Food Inflammatory Index 49–50
formula-feeding and infant microbiome 35
14:10 (10:14) diet plan 159, 160
frangipane for raspberry Bakewell tart 284, 285
free radicals 56, 84
friends 164
    and guests and dinner or main meals 102, 164, 278, 292, 304, 306

frozen items
    soups 188–201
    vegetables 174, 177, 233, 256
fructose 58, 82, 126
fruit 126–130
    increasing your intake 92–94, 104, 130
    mistaken as vegetables 136
    portions per day of 166
frying food 56–57, 155–157
fungi 137–138
    see also mushrooms

galactooligosaccharides 82
garlic, white bean, thyme and roasted garlic dip 305–306
gastritis, autoimmune 23
gastrointestinal tract see gut
genetics 22–23
    see also epigenetic modulation
ginger 146–147
    ginger and pear muffins 266–267
    ginger and pear rice pudding 291–292
    ginger and sticky date cake 267–268
    ginger tea 105
    ginger turmeric tahini dressing 298–299
Ginkgo biloba 146
GLP-1 (glucagon-like peptide-1) 47, 102
glucagon-like peptide-1 (GLP-1) 47, 102
β-glucans (beta-glucans) 318
glucose (dietary sugar) see sugar
glucosinolates 131, 320
gluten (and its avoidance) 117–119, 142–143
gluten-free foods
    grains 143
    pancakes 180–181
    whole grains 104
glycoalkaloids 114, 115
glycoproteins 41, 111
goblet cells 42, 44
goitrogens 132
golden soup 195–196
grains 142–144

gluten-free whole grains 104
    portions per day of 166
    sourcing 324
granolas 178, 287
grapefruit 130, 162
grapes 129
Graves' disease 67, 83, 113, 117
green(s) (and green foods) 97, 98
    beans and greens and mushrooms 184–185
    leafy see leafy greens
green kitcheri 237–238
green peas
    dip 307–308
    split green pea soup 193–194
green smoothies 94, 95
    recipe 177–178
green tea 147
growth hormones 63
    in meat 66
Guillan-Barre syndrome 23
gums 318, 319
gut (gastrointestinal tract; GIT) 17, 29–48
    barrier function 17, 24, 30, 41
    brain interactions with 37–38, 47
    dysbiosis 33, 38–48, 81, 138, 139
        gut lining and 44–46
    fibre and its roles in 30, 43, 79
    giving gut a rest 157–161
    health 29–48, 99, 108
        fats and 54–57
        fruit and vegetables and 93
        polyphenols and 86, 99
    health fungi and 138
    immune system and 29, 31, 35, 41, 42, 44, 45, 46, 47, 54
    leaky 11, 24–25, 66, 81, 91, 110, 112, 124, 144
    lectins and lining of 111
    microbiome see microbiome
    sections and their role 30–31
    wall structure 39–42

haem-iron 66
haemolytic anaemia, autoimmune 66

Index

haricot beans 139
Hashimoto's disease 83, 108
Hazda tribe 99–100, 102
health/medical professionals 164
    plant-based 323
heating and cooking 56–57, 155–157
Helicobacter pylori 23
hemicellulose 318
hemp seeds and oil 90, 94, 95, 145
herbs 145–147
    portions per day of 166
high-fat foods 50, 57, 159
high-fibre foods/diet 126, 139, 162
histamine and nightshades 115, 136
homeostasis 51
humans
    ancient/early ancestors 76, 99, 108, 108–109, 127, 137, 144
    choosing your tribe 163–165
    programmed for survival 51
hummus, turmeric 304–305
hunter-gatherers 99, 107–108, 108
hygiene hypothesis 35–36

ice cream 58
immune system 14–15, 117–120
    adaptive 18–19, 41, 64, 137, 147
    drugs depressing 37
    gut and 29, 31, 35, 41, 42, 44, 45, 46, 47, 54
    innate (natural) 17–18, 19, 41, 54, 63, 137, 147
    self/non-self (us/them) in 20, 46, 64, 67
    see also autoimmune disease
infants *see* babies and infants
infections 23
    see also bacteria; viruses
inflammation
    acute/short episodes 17, 44–45, 103
    chronic 24, 25, 26, 55, 66–67, 87, 146
    gluten and 118
inflammatory bowel disease (IBD) 67, 100, 113, 114, 129, 131, 137
    fibre and 82–83, 103

LPS and 44–45
    see also Crohn's disease; ulcerative colitis
innate immune system 17–18, 19, 41, 54, 63, 137, 147
insoluble fibre 43, 47, 80, 129, 318
intermittent fasting 159, 159–161
internet *see* online
intestine (bowel)
    epithelium 42, 44, 45, 46
    large (and colon) 30, 39, 43, 78
    small 30, 39, 40, 41, 81, 104, 119, 122, 135
inulin 103, 318
iodine 122, 123, 138
iron 66
isoflavones 144, 145
Italian bean soup 198–199

jam for raspberry Bakewell tart 285
Jambalaya, quick 233–234
Jerusalem artichokes 103

kale 131
    broccoli and kale tart 254–256
    mushrooms and squash and kale root vegetable pie 241–242
    pear and red kale salad 210–211
    and sweet potato salad 205–206
Kate's story 10, 25, 57, 77, 92, 106, 115, 129, 149, 153
keto diet 50, 159
kidney beans, red 110–111
kimchi 146, 149
kitcheri, green 237–238
knowledge and power 105–106
kombucha 148–149
krill oil 89

lacteals 40, 41
lactose 82
large intestine/bowel (incl. colon) 30, 39, 43, 78
leafy greens 132–133, 162
    sauce 299–300

leaky blood vessels 18, 46
leaky gut 11, 24–25, 66, 81, 91, 110, 112, 124, 144
lectins 110–112
legumes 138–142
    soaking and sprouting *see* soaking and sprouting
lemon
    herb and lemon dressing 298
    raw blueberry lemon tarts 282–283
lentils (incl. red lentils) 138–142
    bread 314–315
    dip 306–307
    salad 208–209
    sauce for moussaka 249, 250
    and sweet potato soup 199–200
lifestyle behaviour 4, 5, 6, 25–26, 164–165
    changes in 5, 6, 26, 105, 108
    genes and 23
light meals *see* lunch and light meals
lignans 55
lignin 318
lima beans 139
limonoids 320
α-lipoic acid (alpha-lipoic acid) 88, 89
lipopolysaccharides (LPS; endotoxin) 44, 45
liquorice 162
liver disease, fatty 59, 126
low-calorie intake 159, 160
    very 159
lunch and light meals 215–227
    three-day sample menu 175
lupus (SLE) 14, 15, 21, 22, 23, 26, 60, 67, 83, 129, 137, 142, 144
lycopene 114, 116, 320
lymphocytes 19
    B cells/lymphocytes 19, 41
    T cells/lymphocytes 19, 22, 41, 54, 61, 63, 64

macronutrients 73, 74
Maillard reaction 56
main meals *see* dinner and main meals
malnutrition 74
mangetout, broadbean and new potato salad with crispy smoked tofu 202–204
maple and carrot muffins 274–276
mastitis 63
meat 64–67
medical professionals *see* health/medical professionals
medications (drugs; pharmaceuticals) 161–163
    in autoimmune disease treatment 161–163
    side-/adverse effects 23, 36–37, 91, 161
Mediterranean diet 50, 109, 113, 136, 144–145
medium-chain triglycerides (MCTs) 87–88
membranes, cell 52, 53, 63, 63
microbiome (gut) 29, 32–38
    dysbiosis and 33, 38–48, 81, 138, 139
    environment and 35–36, 99
    fibre consumption (increases) and 102, 103
    food varieties and 99
    polyphenols and 86–87
    see also bacteria; viruses
micronutrients 71, 73
microplastics 24, 36, 89
microvilli 40, 41
milk
    breast 35
    dairy *see* dairy
millet
    and amaranth pancakes 220–221
    herby millet tabbouleh 211–212
    roasted cabbage slices with aromatic millet and tahini dressing 260–261
minerals 73, 74
    in nuts and seeds 145
    oxalic acid binding to 112
    phytates binding to 116
minimally-processed food 100–102, 142

Index

food groups and 69
mint tea 105
miso 148, 149
molecular mimicry 20, 21, 46, 63, 64, 67, 111
monosaccharides, fermentable 81
monounsaturated fatty acids 53, 87
'Moroccan soup' 189–190
moussaka 248–250
mucilage 318
mucin 41, 42, 44, 86
muffins
    carrot and maple 274–276
    pear and ginger 266–267
multiple sclerosis (MS) 2, 4, 14, 15, 21, 22, 23, 26, 60, 63, 67, 83, 86, 87–88, 117, 142, 144, 162
    author's 2, 3, 4, 5, 6, 7, 62, 155
    Overcoming MS 3, 4, 164, 323
mung bean (sprouted) salad 206–207
mushrooms 137, 138
    greens and beans and 184–185
    pate 310–311
    Shiitake, and tofu noodle bowl 252–253
    squash and mushroom and kale root vegetable pie 241–242
My Autoimmune MD 323
myelin 2, 21, 64, 88
myrosinase 131

natto 148
natural (innate) immune system 17–18, 19
natural killer (NK) cells 17
nectarines, baked crunchy 287–288
Neu5GC 67
neurotransmitters 38
nicotine 114
nightshades 113–115, 130, 136
nightshift workers 158
NK (natural killer) cells 17
non-steroidal anti-inflammatory drugs (NSAIDs) 36–37
nori 89, 95, 138

NOVA classification of food processing levels 76, 77
NSAIDs 36–37
nurse, author as 1, 3
nut(s) 90, 94–95, 144–145
    bulk-buy 174
    portions per day of 166
nutrients 84–85
    groups 72–74
    healing 84–85
nutritional advice, seven-step decision-making tool 7, 8–9

oats 104, 144
    apple and apricot oat bars 262–264
obesity 26, 59
oestrogens 141–142
    in milk 63
    see also phytoestrogens
oil (dietary) 55–56, 95
    cooking and heating 56–57, 155–157
    omega-3 and -6 fatty acid-containing 55, 89–90, 96
oligofructose 318
oligosaccharides 82, 139, 140
    fermentable 81
omega-3 fatty acids 4, 55, 88
    supplementation 89, 89–90, 96
omega-6 fatty acids 55, 56, 88, 96
omelette 181–182
online (internet)
    groups 107, 163
    helpful websites 323
orange foods 98
osweeteners, artificial (sugar substitutes) 82, 319
Overcoming MS 3, 4, 164, 323
over-nutrition 74
oxalates and oxalic acid 112–113
oxidative stress 84, 86, 118
oxygen, reactive species of (ROS) 56, 84

paleo diet 107, 108
palmitic acid 54
pan frying 57

pancakes
    amaranth and millet 220–221
    gluten-free 180–181
Paneth cells 42
pasta, asparagus and broccoli pasta with white bean sauce 238–239
pastry for raspberry Bakewell tart 284, 285
pear
    and ginger *see* ginger
    and red kale salad 210–211
peas
    asparagus, pea and rocket salad 213–214
    split *see* split peas
    split green pea soup 193–194
pectin 127, 129, 318
PHA (phytohaemagglutinin) 110–111
pharmaceuticals *see* drugs
phytates 116
phytoestrogens 141, 142, 145
phytohaemagglutinin (PHA) 110–111
phytonutrients 73, 84–85
    leafy greens 133
pineapple 129–130
planning meals 174
plant-based diet *see* food; whole-food plant-based diet
plant-based health professionals 323
Plants for Health (website) 323
platelet production 59
plum and cardamom cake 273–274
polyols 82
    fermentable 81
polyphenols 60, 85–87, 93, 99, 113, 127, 320
polyunsaturated fatty acids 53, 55, 66, 87
pomegranate seeds 261
potato
    glycoalkaloids 114–115
    mangetout and broad bean and crispy smoked tofu with new potato salad 202–204
prebiotics 81, 103, 104, 135
prehistoric/ancient/early/ancestors 76, 99, 108, 108–109, 127, 137, 144

probiotics 34, 35, 148, 149
processed and refined food 74–78
    levels of food processing 75–78, 101
    sugar 35, 58, 59, 104
    see also minimally-processed food; ultra-processed food
protein 73, 73–74, 119–122
    incomplete 120
proton pump inhibitors 37, 122
proving (in bread-making) 117fn
pseudo-grains 101, 143
psoriatic arthritis 10, 21, 115
psyllium 319
pulses
    bulk-buy 174
    portions per day of 166
    sourcing 324
purple foods 97, 98
pus in cow's milk 63

quinoa
    crust, for broccoli and kale tart 254, 255
    and vegetable patties 221–223

radishes 133–134
rainbow colours of food 96–97, 98, 136, 151
    carrot *see* carrot
raspberry
    Bakewell tart 284–286
    mousse 280
    sauce 302–303
reactive species of oxygen (ROS) 56, 84
recipes 169–315
    baking 262–278
    breakfast 176–187
    desserts 278–294
    dinner/main meals *see* dinner and main meals
    easy 228–244
    introduction to 173–175
    lunch/light meals *see* lunch and light meals
    notes on 172

Index

salads 202–214
sauces and dressings 295–303
soups 188–201
spreads and breads 304–315
three-day sample menu 175
red foods 97, 98
    kidney beans 110–111
    lentils *see* lentils
    red grapes 129
    red kale and pear salad 210–211
refined food *see* processed and refined food
religion and fasting 159
resistant starch 43, 73, 79, 318
resveratrol 129
rheumatoid arthritis (RA) 14, 15, 21, 60, 64, 66, 67, 83, 87, 129, 137, 139, 142, 144
rhubarb and strawberry crumble 278–279
rice 144
    ginger and pear rice pudding 291–292
    quick broccoli and smoked tofu rice 239–241
rice cooker 157
'ricotta' 309–310
rocket salad, asparagus and pea and 213–214
Romanesco cauliflower, baked mini 234–235
roots (root vegetables) 134
    mushroom and squash and kale root vegetable pie 241–242
    stew, with herby dumplings 250–252
Rosa's story 7, 16, 25, 27, 65, 75, 154, 163, 167
rosemary 147
    and spinach soup 197–198

St John's wort 146
salads 202–214
    dressings 205, 208, 212, 213, 214, 298, 300

salmonella poisoning 111
salt 60–61
sarcoidosis 7, 16, 27, 113, 163
saturated fat/fatty acids 53–54, 54, 57, 59, 87
    meat 65
sauces 295–303
    for moussaka 249, 250
    white bean *see* white bean
    see also dressings
sauerkraut 148, 149
scones, sweet carrot 271–272
scrambled tofu 182–184
sea vegetables/edible seaweed 95, 96, 123, 137, 138
seeds 90, 94–95, 144–145
    bulk-buy 174
    portions per day of 166
serotonin 38
sesame-baked butternut squash rings with smoky chickpeas 258–259
Shiitake mushrooms and smoke tofu noodle bowl 252–253
short-chain fatty acids (SCFAs) 43, 46–48, 59, 79, 86–87, 148, 149
16:8 (8:16) diet plan 159, 161
Sjögren's syndrome 86, 117
sleep 158
small intestine/bowel 30, 39, 40, 41, 81, 104, 119, 122, 135
smoking 25
smoothies 94, 95, 176–178
snacks 94, 126, 157, 158
soaking and sprouting (beans/legumes) 140
    mung bean sprouted salad 206–207
social media 107, 163
sodium chloride (salt) 60–61
Solanaceae 113
solanine 114
soluble fibre 73, 80, 104, 318
sorbitol 82, 319
soups 188–201
soya bean 101, 141–142, 148, 149
Spanish omelette/tortilla 181–182

spices 145–147
   portions per day of 166
spinach 132, 133
   frozen 177
   'ricotta' and 309–310
   soups with 194–195, 197–198
spirulina 89, 95, 136
split peas
   Ethiopian split pea stew 231–232
   green pea soup 193–194
spreads and breads 304–315
sprouting *see* soaking and sprouting
squash
   mushroom and squash and kale root vegetable pie 241–242
   sesame-baked butternut squash rings with smoky chickpeas 258–259
   spinach and squash and coriander soup 194–195
starch, resistant 43, 73, 79, 318
steaming 157
stems and bulbs 135
steroids 162–163
sterols 320
stock, cooking in 155–156
strawberry and rhubarb crumble 278–279
stress (psychological; emotional) 24, 37–38, 51
stress hormones in meat 66
sucrose 58
sugar 57–60
   added, problem of 59–60
   in fruit 126
   refined 35, 59, 104
   substitutes (artificial sweeteners) 82, 319
sulphoraphane 130–131
supplements 122–123
   omega-3 fatty acids 89, 89–90, 96
   vitamin D 26, 72, 123
survival, animals incl. humans programmed for 51
sushi 90, 138

sustainability of nutritional advice 8
sweet and sour sauce 296
sweet potato
   flatbread 311–312
   and kale salad 205–206
   and red lentil soup 199–200
   stuffed 235–237
sweeteners, artificial (sugar substitutes) 82, 319
Swiss chard 132
systemic lupus erythematosus (SLE; lupus) 14, 15, 21, 22, 23, 26, 60, 67, 83, 129, 137, 142, 144

T cells/lymphocytes 19, 22, 41, 54, 61, 63, 64
tabbouleh, herby millet 211–212
tahini dressing
   roasted cabbage slices with aromatic millet and 260–261
   turmeric and ginger and 298–299
tamarind stir-fry 297
tastebuds 61, 78
tea
   ginger 105
   green 147
   mint 105
Tecfidera 162
tempeh 142, 148
   tempeh and hazelnut and apricot bake 247–248
   tempeh and vegetable skewers 228–229
   tempeh 'bacon' 185
   tempeh onion bhajis 217–219
temperature
   conversions 172
   refined oils 55
   see also cooking and heating
10:14 (14:10) diet plan 159, 160
thiocyanates 320
thyme 147
   and carrot salad 209–210
   and white bean and roasted garlic (dip) 305–306

Index

thyroid disease (autoimmune) 117, 123, 132
thyroxine 145, 161
time-restricted eating 158, 159–161
TNF (tumour necrosis factor) 54, 59, 63
tofu
    mousse 280
    quick broccoli and smoked tofu rice 239–241
    'ricotta' 309, 310
    scrambled 182–184
    Shiitake mushrooms and smoked tofu noodle bowl 252–253
    warm broad bean and mangetout and new potato salad with crispy smoked tofu 202–204
tomatoes 85, 97, 114, 115, 136
tortilla (Spanish) 181–182
toxins
    environmental 23–24, 36
    in gut 30–31
transglutaminase 118
trauma (emotional) in childhood 24
traybake
    blackberry and apple 286–287
    cumin and turmeric 256–257
Tricia's story 10, 25, 83, 100, 102, 120, 131, 140, 167
triglycerides 52, 53
    medium-chain (MCTs) 87–88
tropical fruit 126–127
tubers 133–134
tumour necrosis factor (TNF) 54, 59, 63
turmeric 85, 146
    and cumin traybake 256–257
    fermented 149
    and ginger tahini dressing 298–299
    hummus 304–305
12:12 diet plan 159, 160

ulcerative colitis 44, 86, 93
ultra-processed food (UPF) 74, 75–76, 77
    avoiding/removing in one's diet 77, 104
undernourishment 74

unsaturated fat/fatty acids 53, 54, 55, 87
    monounsaturated fat 53, 87
    polyunsaturated fat 53, 55, 66, 87

vaginal delivery and infant microbiome 34
vanilla baked cheesecake 289
vegan diet and protein 121
vegan melty 'cheese' 308–309
vegan Spanish omelette/tortilla 181–182
vegetables 92–94, 130–138
    cruciferous 104–105, 130–132, 162
    curried, with chickpea dumplings 243–245
    frozen 174, 177, 233, 256
    fruits mistaken for 136
    green leafy *see* leafy greens
    increasing your intake 92–94, 174
    portions per day of 166
    quinoa and vegetable patties 221–223
    root *see* roots
    squash and mushroom and kale root vegetable pie 241–242
    tempeh and vegetable skewers 228–229
veggie scramble, morning 182–184
villi 41
viruses 17, 18, 23
    infection by 23
    meat and 65–66
vitamin(s) 73
    leafy greens 132
vitamin A 134, 226, 320
vitamin B12 72, 122
vitamin D 25–26, 122, 123, 137
    supplementation 26, 72, 123
vitamin K 133, 162

walnuts 90, 94
    and white bean bake 245–246
water
    cooking in 155–156
    drinking 104, 150–151
    water fasts 160

watercress and beetroot salad 212
websites, helpful 323
Western diet 6, 31, 35, 54, 55, 57–58, 59, 74, 88, 130, 167
white bean
   sauce 295–296
      asparagus and broccoli pasta with 238–239
   and thyme and roasted garlic dip 305–306
   and walnut bake 245–246
white foods (in general) 97, 98
whole-food plant-based diet 69–90
   groups of food in 25, 69
   myth-busting 107–124
   portions of whole plant foods per day 166
   recipes *see* recipes
   why we need whole foods 70–72
wind (flatulence; farting) 43fn, 103, 105, 135, 139, 141
woman (being a) as autoimmune disease risk factor 25

yellow foods (in general) 97, 98
yellow split peas 231, 232
yoghurt pot, crunchy fruit 178–179